NORMAL AND PATHOLOGIC DEVELOPMENT OF THE HUMAN BRAIN AND SPINAL CORD

The Authors

Maria Dąmbska, M.D., Ph.D.

Department of Developmental Neuropathology, Medical Research Centre P.A.S., Warsaw, Poland

and

Krystyna E. Wiśniewski, M.D., Ph.D.

Department of Pathological Neurobiology,
Associate Director of Clinical Services at the George Jervis Diagnostic and Research Clinic, NYS Institute for Basic Research in Developmental Disabilities, Staten Island, New York; and Professor of Pediatric Neurology at State University of New York – Health Science Center at Brooklyn

NORMAL AND PATHOLOGIC DEVELOPMENT OF THE HUMAN BRAIN AND SPINAL CORD

Maria Dąmbska

and

Krystyna E. Wiśniewski

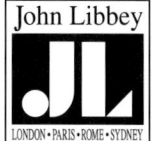

British Library Cataloguing in Publication Data

Normal and pathologic development of the human brain and spinal cord
1. Brain 2. Spinal cord
I. Dąmbska, Maria II. Wiśniewski, K.E. (Krystyna E.
611.8'1

ISBN: 0 86196 591 4 (paperback)

Published by

John Libbey & Company Ltd, 13 Smiths Yard, Summerley Street,
London SW18 4HR, England
Telephone: +44 (0)181–947 2777; Fax: +44 (0)181–947 2664
e-mail: johnlibbey@aol.com

John Libbey & Company Pty Ltd, 15–17 Young Street, Sydney, NSW 2000, Australia
John Libbey Eurotext Ltd, 127 avenue de la République, 92120 Montrouge, France
John Libbey at C.I.C. Edizioni s.r.l., via Lazzaro Spallanzani 11, 00161 Rome, Italy

© 1999 John Libbey & Company Limited. All rights reserved.

Unauthorised duplication contravenes applicable laws.
Printed in Malaysia by Kum-Vivar Printing Sdn Bhd, 48000 Rawang, Selangor.

Table of Contents

Acknowledgment ix
Preface xi
Forward xiii
Introduction xv

Part One: Normal development of the central nervous system (CNS)

Chapter 1: Elements constituting the nerve tissue and their differentiation and maturation 3
    Neurons 3
    Neuroglia 10
        Astroglia 11
        Oligodendroglia and formation of myelin sheaths 13
    Ependymal cells 17

Chapter 2: Mesodermal elements in the CNS 20
    Microglia 20
    Vessels 22

Chapter 3: Consecutive morphogenesis and maturation of CNS structures 23
    Initial stages of CNS development 23
    Spinal cord 28
    Brain stem 29
    Cerebellum 32
    Prosencephalon (forebrain) 35
        Diencephalic structures 36
            Hypothalamus 37

Subthalamus	37
Ventral thalamus	37
Epithalamus	38
Dorsal thalamus	28
Telencephalic structures	39
Pallium	39
Paleocortex (olfactory cortex)	40
Archicortex (hippocampal complex)	43
Neocortex (isocortex)	47
Insular cortex	56
Other telencephalic derivatives	57
Myelination of the CNS structures	60
Vascularization of the CNS	64
Meninges – skull bones	68
The parameters for evaluation of CNS development	70

References: Part One — 71

Part Two: Abnormal brain and spinal cord development 2

Chapter 4: Etiologic factors of abnormal CNS development — 89
- Genetic factors — 89
- Exogenous factors — 90
- Correlations between time and type of developing brain damage — 91

Chapter 5: The phakomatoses – the ecto-mesodermal syndromes — 93
- Tuberous sclerosis (Bourneville disease) — 94
- Neurofibromatosis — 95
  - Neurofibromatosis Type 1 – von Recklinghausen disease (the peripheral form) — 96
  - Neurofibromatosis Type 2 – the central form — 96
- von Hippel–Lindau disease — 97
- Sturge–Weber disease — 97
- The Jadassohn linear nevus — 98
- Hemimegalencephaly — 98
- Neurocutaneous melanosis — 98
- Lhermitte–Duclos disease — 98

Chapter 6: Malformation of the CNS — 101
- Neural tube defects – the dysraphic syndromes — 101
  - Dysraphic cerebral changes — 103
  - Chiari (Arnold–Chiari) malformation — 106
  - Dysraphic and related anomalies of the spinal cord — 108

Other anomalies belonging to the same group	112
Midline malformations	113
Holoprosencephaly – arhinencephaly	113
Developmental anomalies of commissural system	115
Other anomalies of midline structures	117
Cortical malformations and dysplasia	118
Cortical, early-occurring dysplasia	118
Agyria and pachygyria (lissencephaly type I)	119
Subcortical heterotopia	122
Polymicrogyria	123
Disorganized cortical structure – (lissencephaly type II)	127
Other cortical anomalies	129
Laminar and focal cortical developmental anomalies	129
Particular or complex cortical anomalies	131
Cerebellum: Primitive and secondary developmental abnormalities	132
Cerebellar aplasia and hypoplasia, including Dandy–Walker malformation	132
Agenesis of the cerebellum	133
Aplasia of the cerebellar vermis	133
Dandy–Walker malformation	133
Joubert syndrome	135
Tectocerebellar dysraphia	135
Rhomboencephalosynapsis	135
Hypoplasia of the cerebellum	135
Malformations of cerebellar cortex	136
Micrencephaly and megalencephaly	139
Micrencephaly caused by genetic factors	140
Autosomal dominant inheritance	140
Autosomal recessive inheritance	140
Chromosomal abnormalities	140
Micrencephaly induced by environmental factors	140
Megalencephaly	141
Anomalies of the brain stem and spinal cord	142
Hydrocephalus	143
Non-communicating	144
Communicating	144
Changes related to vascular, skull bone and meningeal anomalies	146
Vascular anomalies	146
Skull bone anomalies	147
Meningeal anomalies	148

Chapter 7: Developmental disturbances due to chromosomal aberrations   149

Trisomy 13 (Patau syndrome)	149
Trisomy 18 (Edwards syndrome)	150

	Trisomy 21 (Down syndrome)	150
	Fragile X syndrome	152

Chapter 8: Late and secondary developmental anomalies   153
         Hydranencephaly   154
         Schizencephaly and porencephaly   154
         Variants of cystic encephalopathy   156

Chapter 9: Delay of CNS maturation   157

References: Part Two   159

Acknowledgments

We were helped by many people during the preparation of this book. We are grateful to Prof. Henryk M. Wiśniewski, M.D., Ph.D., Director of the New York State Institute for Basic Research (IBR) in Developmental Disabilities, Staten Island, New York, for his endorsement, encouragement and suggestions. For the preparation of pictures, we thank Ryszard Szopiński, who used not only our material, but also some slides from the collections of Bogna Schmidt-Sidor, MD, from the Department of Neuropathology of the Institute of Psychiatry and Neurology in Warsaw, Poland, and Piotr B. Kozłowski, MD, PhD, from the Department of Pathological Neurobiology, IBR. We also thank Maureen Stoddard Marlow for copy-editing the manuscript; Lawrence Black for bibliographical assistance; and Jo-Ann Woodbridge Buttafuoco, Janis Kay and Danuta Krysztofiak for their secretarial help in the preparation of this manuscript.

Figure illustrations 16–21, 23, 27, 29, 30–33, 45, 47 have been adapted and combined from:

Pansky, B. & Allen, D.J. (1980): *Review of Neuroscience*. Macmillan Publ. Co. Inc., NY; Sidman, R.L. & Rakic, P. (1982): Development of the human central nervous system. In: *Histology and Histopathology of the Neurons System*, vol. 1, eds. W. Haymaker & R.D. Adams, pp. 13–145. Springfield, Illinois: Thomas; Langman, J. (1963): *Medical Embriology*. Baltimore: William & Wilkins Company.

Preface

As we close a century in which we have learned more about the development of the nervous system than in all previous centuries combined, and as we close a decade in which almost the entire study of normal and abnormal developmental neuroanatomy has been focussed on the exciting new molecular genetic data on the programming of the neural tube, it is refreshing to remember that organizer genes and homeoboxes that explain morphogenesis become rather meaningless outside the context of classical neuroembryology. Professors Dąmbska and Wiśniewski have written a contemporary statement of what is known about morphological development of the normal and abnormal human nervous system and have put into perspective the continued importance of documenting the sequences of architectural changes that occur in the course of fetal development and how these processes may become defective.

Though genetic processes are mentioned, and the authors do not ignore the molecular basis of many changes, citing various growth factors, interleukins, intermediate filament proteins of cytoarchitecture and retinoic acid induction as examples, their principal emphasis is on gross and microscopic morphogenesis. Carefully selected references are representative of the most important publications in this field of the 20th century. The organization of the book, in two parts to cover first normal embryology and then cerebral dysgeneses, corresponds to the systematic way in which we are taught to think in the study of anatomy and pathology. This volume will serve as an excellent and appropriate summary text and introduction for students of human neuroembryology and developmental neuropathology of the early 21st century, and is an insightful review of these topics even for seasoned students, who also are involved in developmental molecular genetic research. I commend Professors Dąmbska and Wiśniewski for this intellectual gift so needed at this time.

Harvey B. Sarnat, MD, FRCPC

Professor of Neurology, Pediatrics and Pathology (Neuropathology), University of Washington School of Medicine, Seattle, USA

Foreword

This is a valuable contribution to the literature on developmental neuropathology. It is largely based on the extensive personal experience of two distinguished workers in the field, Prof. M. Dąmbska, a neurologist/developmental neuropathologist, and Prof. K.E. Wiśniewski, a pediatric neurologist/neuropathologist. The great merit of this work is that it deals with both the normal and abnormal development of the CNS in one volume. Both parts are written by the same authors and are therefore well integrated, the malformations being presented as aberrations of the normal development. The emphasis is morphologic, but adequate information is provided on etiology and pathogenesis, as far as known at present. The book will be a valuable asset to the library of any worker in the field, and the clear presentation of a complex subject is particularly valuable to persons in training. It gives me great pleasure to recommend this book for publication.

Henryk Urich, MD, FRCP, FRC Path

Professor Emeritus of Neuropathology, University of London, England

Introduction

This book is addressed to two groups of readers. First, we hope that it will be useful on a daily basis to neuropathologists, general pathologists and child neurologists as a short review of normal and disturbed brain development. The complexity of the central nervous system (CNS) structures overlaps with the differing times and rates of maturation of those structures. This results in variations in the times of the background of normal and pathologic processes occurring in the CNS over the long term, which extends over the course of several years, but is most evident until three years of age, when the changes demonstrating brain maturation are visible by means of light microscopy. We present these changes in this text. With the rapid progress in such modern branches of science as neurochemistry, genetics and molecular biology, we hope that our publication will be useful also for researchers working in those fields. Using young nervous tissue in their studies, they must understand and estimate correctly the formation of the CNS in normal and pathological conditions. Otherwise, they risk performing their studies on 'unknown' tissue. If our book proves useful for these readers, we will be totally satisfied.

Maria Dąmbska
and
Krystyna E. Wiśniewski

Part One

Normal development of the central nervous system (CNS)

Chapter 1

Elements Constituting Nerve Tissue, their Differentiation and Maturation

Neurons
Origin and characteristics of neuronal development

Neurons are highly differentiated and specialized among the elements of nerve tissue of neuroectodermal origin. The nerve cells originate from germinal ('matrix') cells lining the central canal of the neural tube and their derivatives (the lateral, third and fourth ventricles), as well as from some secondary germinal centers, such as the external germinal layer in the cerebellum and the neural crest; however, it is believed that neural tube and neural crest lineage are induced independently (Okamoto & Mitani, 1992). The same neuroepithelium gives rise to both neurons and glia. The majority of precursor cells are destined to develop as neurons, astrocytes or oligodendrocytes. Experiments on animals using retroviral vectors suggest that one exception is the N-O cells, which are able to generate both neurons and oligodendrocytes (Price et al., 1992).

The early morphological differentiation of matrix cells is difficult to observe, and the final destination of germinal cells is difficult to distinguish (Rakic, 1982). The consecutively appearing, positive reactions for some substances that are characteristic for given stages of development are diagnostically helpful. At early stages, the undifferentiated neuroepithelial cells are positive in reaction for vimentin, the intermediate filament protein (Sasaki et al., 1988). At a further developmental level, specific markers, e.g. neuron-specific enolase, allow differentiation between nerve and glial cells.

Morphological and immunohistochemical investigations have resulted in the conclusion that in the human brain, neuronal differentiation occurs much earlier than glial differentiation (Fujita, 1992; Ogawa, 1992) and that even neuronal and glial cell classes do not coexist at the early stage in the ventricular zone of the human fetal brain (Sasaki et al., 1988).

The first step of neuronal differentiation takes place in the ventricular zone of germinal centers (Fig. 1).

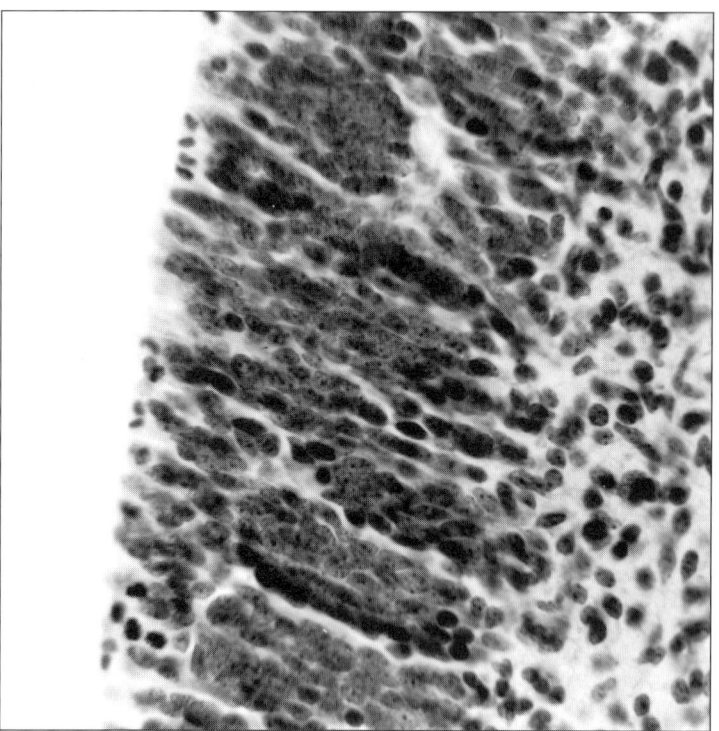

Fig. 1. Germinal layer in the ventricular zone. Cresyl violet, × 400.

The neuronal precursor cells multiply during the period before migrating until the end of their final division. Then, as postmitotic cells, they begin the migration process, with the aim of reaching their definite position. The stable population of neurons in primates, including humans, had been verified experimentally in monkeys with the use of auto-radiograms (Rakic, 1985). An exception is the primary olfactory neurons, whose precursors maintain some possibilities of neurogenesis during further life. This capability seemed to exist for support of olfactory function despite frequent damage to olfactory receptor cells (Farbman, 1990; Sarnat, 1992c). Most recent investigations suggest that some neural stem cells – the eventual neuronal precursors – exist in the adult mouse forebrain (Weiss et al., 1996). We have no data indicating whether this is a property of this species only.

The question arises as to what kind of instruction governs this early differentiation and further specialization of different types of neurons. Purves and Lichtman (1985) analyzed these complex mechanisms and found that most probably three types of instructions interact on developing neurons: (1) genetic, (2) arising from the cell cytoplasm, and (3) coming from the extracellular environment. Aboitiz (1988) formulated the hypothesis that nerve cell proliferation is regulated by genome. Then, as postulated by Fine and Rubin (1988), very early in development, the nerve cell becomes dependent for guidance and survival on external factors, mainly neuropeptides. Investigation of the developing cerebral cortex allows observation of how the cell fates are defined progressively during development (McConnell, 1992). At the same time, Fine and Rubin (1988) emphasized that the cell retains for a long time, and possibly for its lifetime, the entire set of genetic instructions. The term genetic instruction, although not precise, has to be used until the essence and the means of information transfer become finally clarified. On the basis of the understanding that has been gained of primitive animal species, it can be assumed that the consecutive steps of development are controlled by particular genes (Rorke, 1994).

Neuronal migration constitutes a particularly important and long-lasting process (Sidman & Rakic, 1973). The process of migration depends on phylogenetically conditioned development of particular brain structures. The data concerning the course of neuronal migration will be presented in the second part of this study as an essential component of morphogenesis in all parts of the CNS. Here, we would like to review the general rules of neuronal migration.

It has been established that neuronal precursors migrate in large numbers along radial glia, but others migrate without such guides. The long processes of radial glia extending between the matrix centers and target areas constitute the pathways for migrating young nerve cells. The neuroblasts move along the surface of glial cells, and their processes, appearing at the proper time, provide a given orientation (Kadhim et al., 1988). The migrating neuroblasts tightly adhere to the glial cells and processes, as a result of special membrane proteins on their surface (Lehmann et al., 1990; Cameron & Rakic, 1994).

The neuroblasts deprived of such preexisting guides may only use their ability to extend the axons with the growth cone located at their tips, particularly when the distance to the target is short, that is, the level of development at which the processes and immature cell axons and dendrites grow and experience cell movement. The movements of the growth cone controlled by the cell body determine the direction of axon growth. Growth cones are considered to be the site of interaction between neurons and their environment (Jacobson, 1991). It is believed that some neurons also migrate along fasciculi of axons (Garcia-Segura & Rakic, 1985; Klose & Bentley, 1989) or use other mechanisms not yet elaborated definitely (Kishi et al., 1990; Herrup & Silver, 1994). In general, the ability to make adhesive contacts and then to push the cell forward is believed to be a mechanism of migration. The mechanism itself cannot explain which or how many factors effect the proper orientation of neuroblasts to the areas of final destination. It was found that the factors influencing the migration and the formation of the final structure of neurons are intercellular interaction (in which nerve cell adhesion molecules [N-CAMs] play an important role), electrical signals and chemical trophic substances (Jacobson, 1991). Among them, nerve growth factor (NGF), recognized many years ago by Levi-Montalcini and Angeletti (1968), represents a large family of neurotrophins. The neurotrophic factors are localized as much in the nerve as the glial cells, or in both of them.

The morphologic features of nerve cells during development represent all stages of their early differentiation. The mitotic cell passes the phase of apolar neuroblast, then extends the primary neurite, and as a bipolar neuroblast, a postmitotic cell, is able to begin the migration. The term for such postmitotic cells should actually be 'immature neuron,' but long-lasting usage justifies retention of the term 'neuroblast' (Sarnat, 1992c). At that phase, the neuroblast has scanty cytoplasm, and its developmental process consists of increasing its entire content of cytoplasm and processes. Despite its small size, a young cell is already endowed with many organelles: mitochondria, Golgi membranes and neurofilaments can be detected in post-mitotic nerve cells. According to some classical descriptions, the silver-stained fibrils can be seen on light microscopy at this stage of development (Jacobson, 1991).

The bipolar neuroblast, a migrating cell, has to find appropriate targets. After reaching its place, the neuroblast is characterized by accelerated somal and nuclear growth and further development of organelles. On light microscopy, the first Nissl bodies are noted. Finally, the cell reaches the phase during which the dendritic tree arises, and multipolarity of the cell indicates it to be a maturing neuron. The maturing neurons are characterized by a small amount of cytoplasm around the nucleus. Changes in the nuclear to cell cytoplasm ratio are one of the parameters of neuronal development. The neurons complete their maturation by achieving their nuclear and somal size, although some further increase of volume is possible during further human life (Fig. 2).

Morphologically, adult neurons present a great diversity of types. Each neuron consists of the cell body, the so-called perikaryon, and two types of processes: one axon and numerous dendrites. The perikaryon includes the nucleus surrounded by cytoplasm, and its size varies from 5–8 µm to 100–200 µm in diameter. The amount of cytoplasm is responsible, in great part, for the size of cells, which is one criterion for division of neurons into three principal groups: (1) somatochromatic with abun-

Fig. 2. Motor neurons of the VII nerve. (a) at 7 months of gestation; (b) at 10 months of gestation. Cresyl violet, × 200.

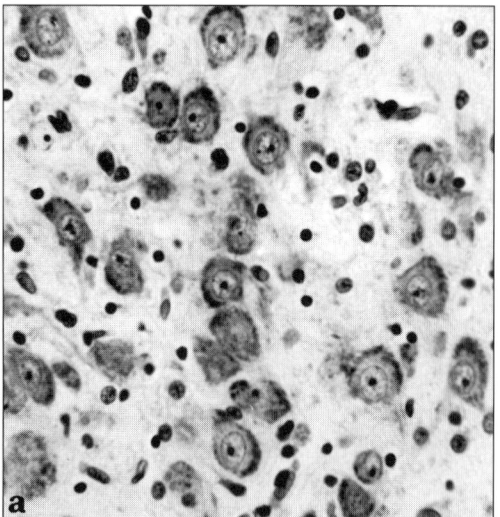
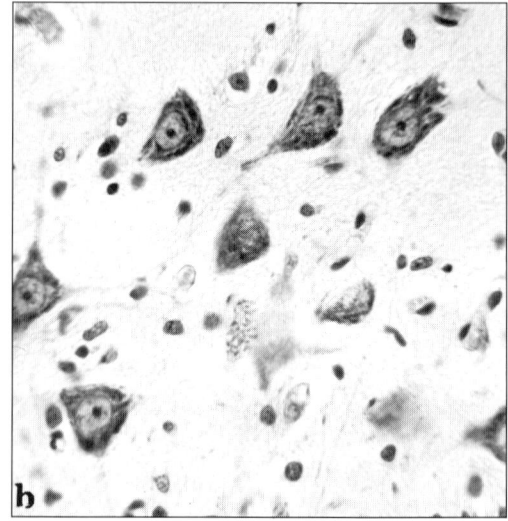

Fig. 3. A motor neuron with abundant cytoplasm. Cresyl violet, × 400.

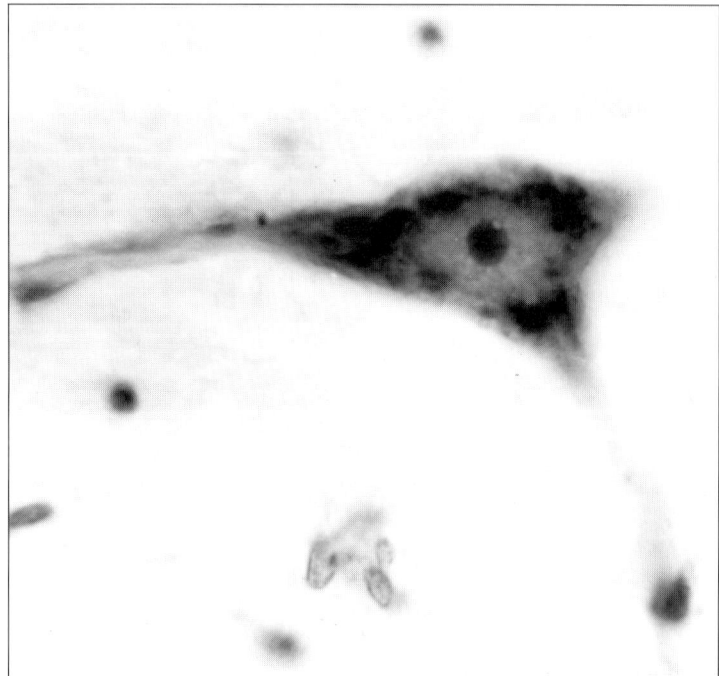

dant cytoplasm (Fig. 3), (2) cytochromatic, with a small nucleus and only scarce cytoplasm, and (3) karyochromatic, with a large nucleus surrounded by scarce cytoplasm.

The number of neurons, which are of various types in the entire brain, is estimated at several hundred thousands (Jacobson, 1991). A particular brain structure usually contains no more than five types of neurons.

Among them, the principal type – the big neurons – appear earlier than medium-sized and small neurons. During the migration process to each structure, the large neurons arriving could be 'dormant' for a long time, maturing at the proper moment. This sequence of migration and maturation is very well illustrated by Purkinje cells in the cerebellar cortex.

The cytoplasm of neurons includes organelles partially visible on light microscopy, in part only at the ultrastructural level (Fig.4).

Nearly all organelles are common to the majority of cells in the human body, but two organelles are particular to the nerve cells. The first one is the most characteristic element of neuronal cytoplasm called Nissl bodies or tigroid, which is visible on light microscopy as basophilic granular structures. At the ultrastructural level, the channels of rough endoplasmic reticulum with lining membranes studded with aggregations of ribosomes correspond to this structure. They are involved in synthesis of cellular proteins.

The other type of elements characteristic for nerve cells are neurofibrils, argentophilic structures that are visible on light microscopy. It is assumed that they correspond to the bundles of neurofilaments,

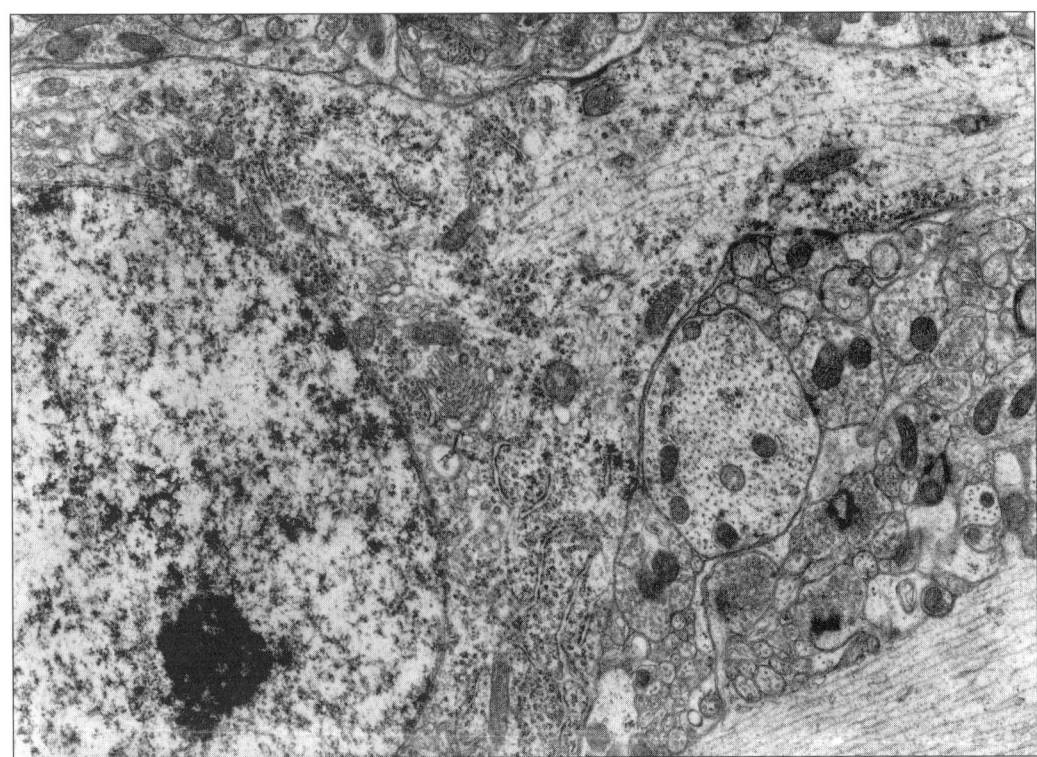

Fig. 4.
Ultrastructural picture of a neuron, × 18,000.

which have the character of intermediate filaments 6–10 nm in diameter, and are involved in intracellular transport and maintenance of cell shape. They are distributed in the dendrites, cell body and axon and are composed of specific neurofilament proteins (Jacobson, 1991; Sarnat, 1992).

The neurotubules, consisting of 5–7 μm-thick rings, with 20–25 nm outer diameter, form with neurofilaments components of the cytoskeleton. They are similar to tubules encountered in other cells and appear to be associated with movements of organelles through the cytoplasm.

The Golgi apparatus, a stack of curved, membrane-bound sacs specialized in concentration of synthesized material and production of polysaccharides and mucopolysaccharides, are abundant.

Mitochondria, surrounded by a double membrane, the inner one forming folds called cristae, are relatively small (2–6 μm × 0.2–0.5 μm in diameter), but numerous.

They are involved in the active metabolism necessary for neuronal survival and function, particularly with ATP production.

The lysosomes, appearing as small membrane-bound structures endowed with hydrolytic enzymes, are found in all nerve cells. As clear vesicles, they are called primary lysosomes. Others, containing phagocytic material, are called secondary lysosomes, and may ultimately become the residual bodies. The structures appearing in neurons as features of their particular activity or age are neurosecretory granules, melanin and lipofuscin.

The nuclei of nerve cells are clear because of their sparse chromatin content. They contain the genetic material located in chromosomes, which consists of a complex of DNA with proteins. The nuclei are enveloped by a bilayered nuclear membrane. The external layer is in many places connected to channels of rough endoplasmic reticulum. A characteristic feature of the neuronal nucleus is a very prominent dark

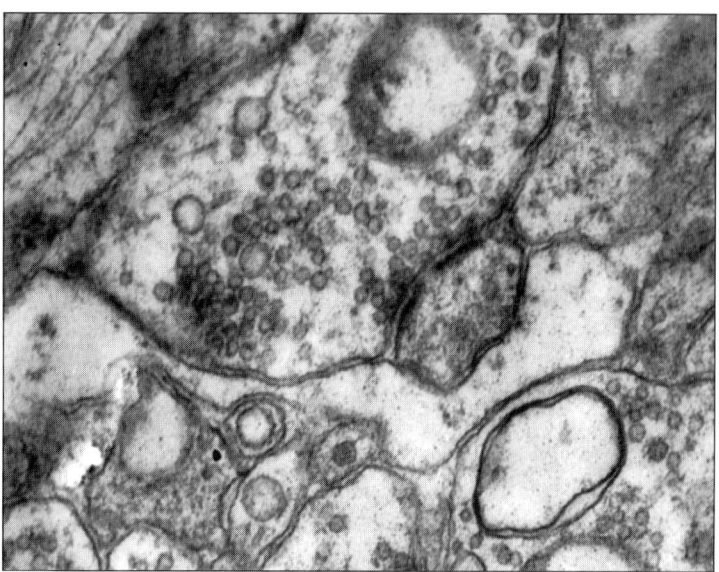

Fig. 5. An axodendritic synapse, × 12,500.

nucleolus composed of granules and filament containing RNA.

The nerve cell has a very intensive metabolism, requiring the supply of oxygen, glucose and other substrates. This activity is related to biosynthesis of proteins and neurotransmitters. It is important to mention that the role of neurotransmitters (acetylcholine, monoamines, neuropeptides and simple amino acids) is not only to mediate the transfer of signals across synapses, but during development, also to act as growth factors modifying neuronal plasticity. More extensive data concerning neuronal metabolism and its histochemical investigations are beyond the scope of this monograph. The great majority of neurons have many dendrites; cells without dendrites are exceptional in the CNS, and those with only one dendrite are also rare. Dendrite growth depends on branching of the growing neurite (Nowakowski et al., 1992). The dendrites could be short or long, but they remain within the structure in which the mother's nerve cell is located.

Synaptogenesis is combined with development of dendrites. The ramifications of dendrites form the so-called dendritic spines (well visualized in Golgi impregnation), which are the site of a great number of synapses. The localization of synapses on dendrites enables dendrites to accomplish their role to receive and transport the impulses to the neuronal perikaryon.

The axon (or neurite), unique for each nerve cell, transports the impulses from the nerve cell to the other cell or to the effector organ. Axons can be very short, with their length measured in micrometers, or as long as one meter when they participate in formation of long nerve pathways. Depending on axonal length, neurons are classified as Golgi type I or type II. The axons are rather poor in organelles, but they include many neurofilaments and neurotubules that are involved in axonal transport. There are mainly three types of synapses in the CNS, depending on the type of contact which they realize: axodendritic, axosomatic and, less often, axoaxonal. Synapses consist of presynaptic and postsynaptic areas, which contact through the presynaptic and postsynaptic membranes, demonstrating a symmetric or asymmetric thickness (Fig. 5).

The membranes are separated only by a synaptic fissure of 15–50 μm in diameter. The presynaptic area, forming the so-called presynaptic bouton, contains vesicles that transport neurotransmitters. Small round vesicles (40–60 μm in diameter) and other larger and dark vesicles are seen. They all belong to the chemical synapses proper for the human CNS. The cell body controls the synapses located at axonal terminals (Jacobson, 1991).

The development of synapses constitutes an important process in CNS maturation. It was found that the first synapses arise very early in development. In Cajal-Retzius cells within cortical layer I, the synapses making contacts with the migrating young cortical neurons arriving first were seen before the end of the second month of development (Larroche et al., 1981). It was found in monkeys that synapses on dendrites may arise even before the formation of boutons (Eckenhoff & Rakic, 1991), which induce the multiplication of synapses. In the majority of structures, synaptogenesis starts when migration of neuroblasts is completed, but in the cerebellum, axons of nerve cells from the external granular layer make synaptic contacts with dendrites of Purkinje cells. Rapid multiplication of synapses was observed and confirmed by morphometric measurement before and after birth, the time during which the CNS is preparing for individual life and contacts with the environment. The processes leading to the formation of synapses on given sites (locations) are not totally clear. In general, it is assumed that synaptogenesis is the result of reciprocal influences between presynaptic and postsynaptic elements. Synaptogenesis appears to be a particular manifestation of trophic interaction between neurons. During the time of development, overproduction of synapses occurs. Examination of synaptogenesis in primates revealed that after a period of low density during fetal life, rapid formation of synapses occurred during the perinatal period in all sensory, motor and associational cortical areas (Bourgeois, 1994). Subsequently, the process of elimination of synapses regulates the final number of synapses, which determines the definitive stabilization of interneuronal contacts. The time of final determination of synaptic number depends on the phylogenetic and ontogenetic age of a particular structure. For example, one may recall that final development of dendritic spines (demonstrating the synaptic number) in respiratory centers was found early after birth (Takashima & Becker, 1986) and that synaptic count in the cortex revealed their elimination during the pre-school years (Huttenlocher, 1984; Michel & Garey, 1984).

Death of neurons is the other event that occurs during normal CNS development. This phenomenon occurs in all developing tissues. In the CNS, it is observed not only in nerve cells, but also in glial cells. The maturation of all regions includes the phase during which some of the previously generated nerve cells die. Cell death may occur after neurons reach their target area. In the spinal cord the adjustment of the motor neuronal population occurs before 25 weeks of fetal development (Forger & Breedlove, 1987), and in the cortex, neuronal death was mostly observed late during gestation (Rabinowicz et al., 1996).

In some animals, up to 50 per cent of neurons die. Looking for a plausible pathomechanism for those regressive events, some investigators suggested that the adjustment of the neuronal population to the function of given structures and the elimination of neurons with erroneously growing axons or changes in some early-formed pathways play a role in this process (Cowan et al., 1984). The 'death of neurons' may involve competitive interaction between nerve cells at the level of their targets. Some correlations observed between the elimination of supernumerary neurons and synapses confirm the theory of adjustment of interneuronal contacts, but such explanations are not sufficient.

In very primitive animal species, cell death appears to be only genetically determined; in vertebrates, it seems to depend on some given external influences. Some factors, the most characteristic of which is NGF, have been found to inhibit neuronal degeneration. It is supposed that neurons need specific survival signals 'suppressing an intrinsic cell suicide program' (Raff et al., 1993), perhaps due to a specific gene. One such gene, Bcl-2, was found in vertebrates. Bcl-2 was the first protein to be recognized as an antidote to cell death by apoptosis in lymphoid tissues, but also in neurons (Le Brun et al., 1993). BAX and ICE are other proteins that control neuronal death. The consecutive increase of reactivity to Bcl-2 and BAX protein in fetal brains appears to correspond to the course of programmed neuronal death (Wiśniewski et al., 1997).

Programmed cell death, or apoptosis, is characterized morphologically by condensation of nuclear chromatin, fragmentation

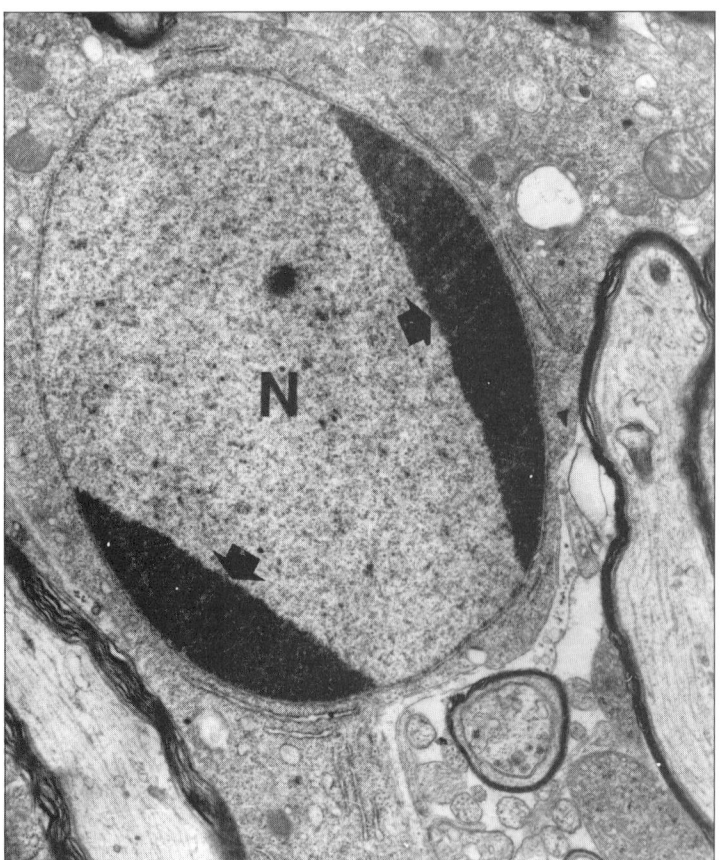

Fig. 6. An apoptotic cell in the CNS. × 18,000. N – nucleus.

of DNA, and formation of encapsulated cell fragments (apoptotic bodies) (Fig. 6). Some authors suggest that other mechanisms of neuronal death must be considered (Bowen, 1993; Maślińska & Muzylak, 1995).

We conclude that neuronal death, which is necessary for the final maturation of connections in the CNS, requires further study. The interaction of all events leading to the creation of the CNS as an active organ is difficult to understand (Guillery & Killackey, 1987).

Myelination is also an important process occurring during maturation of neurons and their axons. The majority of axons in the CNS (and many in the peripheral nervous system) are surrounded by myelin sheaths. Only the initial part and the final peripheral ramifications are free of myelin. In the CNS, myelin sheaths are formed by oligodendroglia; therefore, the whole process of myelination is described as the activity of this cell population.

Neuroglia

The germinal centers located around the central canal, and later in CNS development around cerebral ventricles, not only give rise to nerve cells, but also provide a source of neuroglia for the brain and spinal cord. Ganglionic gangliocytes and Schwann cells constitute the neuronal and glial counterparts in the peripheral nervous system, originating from the neural crest (Berry, 1986).

The process of glial differentiation begins early during development, but the initial stages are barely detectable by routine histological staining. Nevertheless, using such techniques, Roback and Scherer (1935) tried to distinguish between astroglial and oligodendroglial cells among young cells with clear nuclei and observed that the time of glial development differs in various brain structures. Subsequent electron microscopic (EM) observations in animals demonstrated that a proportion of the germinal cells differentiate through spongioblasts into astroglia and oligodendroglia, within the germinal subependymal epithelium, giving rise to neuroglia even postnatally (Caley & Maxwell, 1968). The glial precursors migrate from germinal centers in the periventricular area mostly on the coronal plane, but anterior-posterior migration has also been observed in animals. In ensuing investigations focused on glial development, ultrastructural analyses of glycogen content in glial cells of the developing brain provided additional insight into glial differentiation (Gadisseux & Evrard, 1985), as did the immunohistochemical staining for vimentin, S-100 protein and glial fibrillary acidic protein (GFAP). More recent data obtained by use of retroviral vectors showed that a number of precursor cells arise in the ventricular zone of the CNS (Price et al., 1992), giving rise to neurocytes, astrocytes and oligodendrocytes; one less-defined precursor (N-O) appears to differentiate into neurons and oligodendrocytes.

Astrocytes may also derive from two types of precursors (Noble *et al.*, 1990) A1 and O-A2, the latter giving rise to both astrocytes and oligodendrocytes. From this brief overview of glial origin and differentiation, which will be discussed further in relation to particular types of glial cells, it is clear that studies on glial differentiation are still in progress.

An important finding in glial cell development was the characterization of radial glia as the first glial cells recognizable during CNS development. Radial glia present a special type of cell, extending long processes from germinal periventricular centers to the subpial zone. Such glial fibers serve as corridors for a large proportion of migrating neurons. Radial glia can be identified on the basis of their glycogen content, ultrastructural features and positive reaction for vimentin and GFAP (Choi, 1986; Kadhim *et al.*, 1988; Jacobson, 1991). Neuroglial cells were first identified in the human spinal cord, where at 6 weeks of development, cells with the features of radial glia were detected on light microscopy using impregnational method and at the ultrastructural level. GFAP reactivity was found in glial cells at 7–9 weeks' gestation (WG) (Choi, 1981b; Reske-Nielsen *et al.*, 1987). Observations in the spinal cord revealed that radial glia undergo transformation into astroglia and transitional forms to oligodendroglia (Choi & Kim, 1985). Nevertheless, questions remain about the time and course of glial development in the human brain.

Astroglia

As mentioned above, the successive maturation of glial precursors gives rise to astrocytes. Noble *et al.* (1990) proposed that astrocytes-type 1 (A1) arise first and, later through the production of mitogen growth factor, promote the production of A2 precursors, which differentiate into astrocytes and oligodendrocytes. The processes of A2 cells were shown to be associated with internodes of myelinating axons (Jacobson, 1991). The appearance of astrocytes was observed in different brain structures according to their development rate.

S-100-positive cells, considered to be 'probable astrocytes,' were observed from the ninth week of development, and GFAP-positive astrocytes were seen only after 14–15 weeks in many CNS structures (Roessmann & Gambetti, 1986; Wilkinson *et al.*, 1990). The sequential appearance of various types of astroglial cells depending on the amount of GFAP-positive glial filaments has been examined many times in the cerebral hemispheres. The exhaustion of neuronal migration parallels the formation of astroglia by autophagic disappearance of radial fibers. This process was observed in the cortical plate beginning at week 18 of development and is apparently prolonged in the intermediate zone (Kadhin *et al.*, 1988), consistent with the last phase of neuronal migration (Schmechel & Rakic, 1979a,b).

Nevertheless, the appearance of large and more mature GFAP-positive cells in cerebral hemispheres must be interpreted carefully. The temporal shift of glial cell from the deepest to the most external parts of white matter might reflect astrocyte maturation, but it might also be related to the induction of myelination (Takashima & Becker, 1983). This shift also interferes with the pathological reactions of immature glial cells to hypoxic lesions that often occur in the developing brain (Takashima & Becker, 1983; Takashima *et al.*, 1984). The maturing astroglia differentiate into protoplasmic and fibrous astrocytes and their subtypes, consistent with the multifunctional role of astrocytes in the CNS.

Astroglia are generally characterized by the formation of numerous processes that provide a basic network surrounding the structural elements of the CNS and serve as laminar boundaries between neuroectoder-

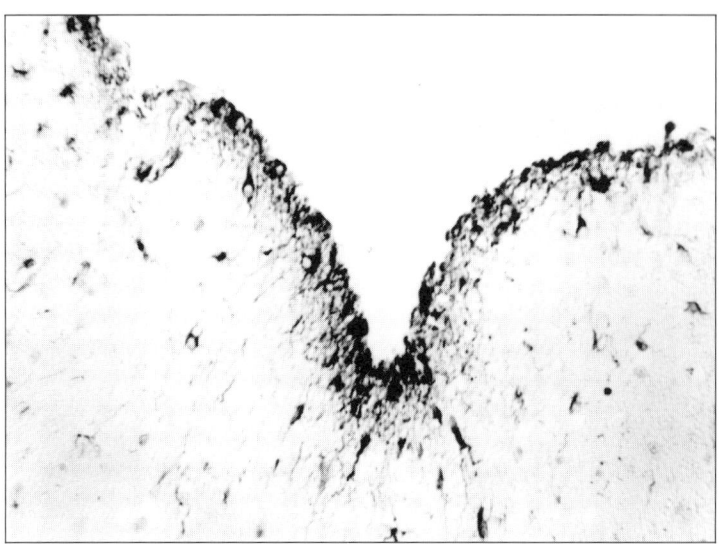

Fig. 7 (above). Membrana gliae limitans. GFAP, × 150.

Fig. 8 (below). Ultrastructural picture of a fibrous astrocyte, × 30,000.

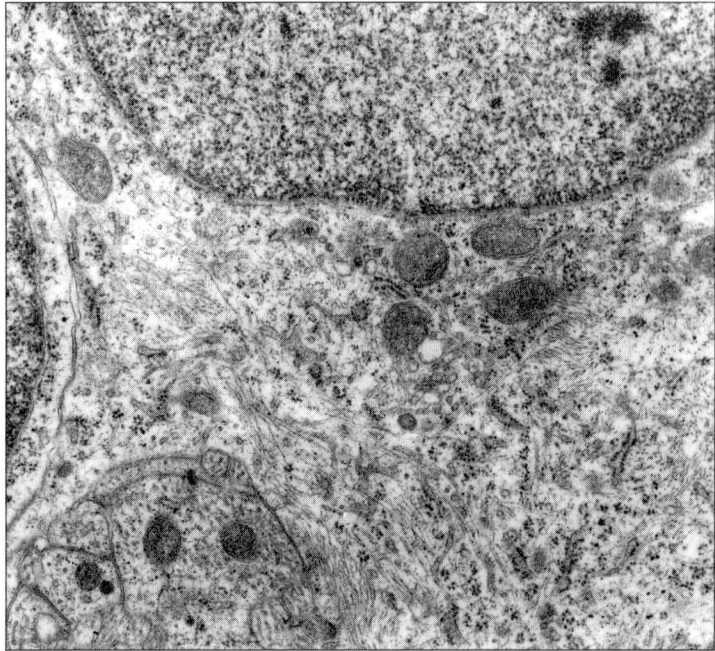

Their name, 'sucker feet,' within the perivascular membrane, is associated with their proposed functional role in the blood–brain barrier (BBB) (Risau & Wolburg, 1990). This hypothesis is discussed further in the content of vessel development and the BBB.

The astrocyte population is roughly divided into its principal types – protoplasmic and fibrous – but an intermediate form is also seen. All astrocytes have a large nucleus with sparse chromatin and a small nucleolus. The nucleus, which is the only organelle visible in routine histological staining, is larger in protoplasmic than in fibrous astrocytes and is probably the largest among glial cells. The perikaryon and processes of astroglial cells can be visualized on light microscopy with gold or silver impregnation techniques or by immunohistochemical reactivities for GFAP. Ultramicroscopic analyses confirm the features of the astroglial nucleus and reveal a rather small perikaryon with a few organelles: mitochondria, endoplasmic reticulum, Golgi apparatus and ribosomes. Only lysosomes are numerous, and glycogen particles are also seen. Gliofilaments are characteristic for astrocytes and their number is the principal difference between the protoplasmic and fibrous types, i.e. gliofilaments are abundant in fibrous astrocytes (Fig. 8) and their long processes and are scarce only in protoplasmic astrocytes. The latter have numerous but short processes, forming special protoplasmic lamellae that shift between surrounding elements.

Protoplasmic astrocytes are distributed in gray matter structures, whereas fibrous ones predominate in the white matter. They are abundant only in some gray matter structures (anterior horn of the spinal cord, inferior olives, globus pallidus, some thalamic nuclei, and molecular layer of the cerebral and cerebellar cortex).

Some special types of astroglia are also observed, including Bergmann glia between Purkinje cells in the cerebellar cortex, Fananas fibers with large processes in

mal tissue and the adjacent formations. Three membranes play such a role: subpial (*membrana gliae limitans superficialis*) (Fig. 7), subependymal (*membrana gliae limitans periventricularis*), and perivascular (*membrana gliae limitans perivascularis*). The membranes are formed by the enlarged endings of astroglia processes.

the molecular layers of the cerebellar cortex, pituicytes in the neural part of the hypophysis, and a special type of glial cell in the retina. Recently, an even more detailed classification of astroglial cells was proposed, based on the recognition of different classes of astrocytes in the mammalian spinal cord. These various astrocyte types may derive from distinct precursor cells at different regions in the developing structure, each with a particular function (Miller *et al.*, 1994). The complexity of morphological types of astroglia is related to their multifunctional role in the structural support and metabolic functions, in structure and function of the BBB, and in repair processes, which until now have not been thoroughly studied.

Oligodendroglia and the formation of myelin sheaths

Oligodendrocytes are the second type of glial cells originating from the germinal neuroectodermal epithelium that lines the CNS ventricular system. This source of oligoglia has been known for many years (Noetzel, 1966; Oksche, 1968), and its differentiation was even analyzed 60 years ago by Roback and Scherer (1935). More recently, it has been hypothesized that the radial-glial cell, the first glial type seen in the human spinal cord, may differentiate not only into astroglia, but also into oligodendroglia cells (Choi & Kim, 1985). Possibly, radial glia represent immature glial cells, which upon completion of their role as a corridor for migrating neurons, give rise to two different types of glia. Studies on the rat optic nerve during development also led Raff *et al.* (1983) to suggest that astrocytes and oligodendrocytes derive from a common progenitor cell. Indeed, further investigations (Noble *et al.*, 1990) on the same experimental model revealed such a common progenitor cell (oligo-type 2 astro = O-A2) that differentiates into both astrocytes and oligodendrocytes (Asou *et al.*, 1995). Price *et al.* (1992) found another precursor cell (N-O), which may differentiate into both nerve and oligodendroglia cells. These authors suggested that such precursors become committed to a differentiation pathway early on. It is also possible that one type of precursor gives rise to oligodendrocytes localized in cortical structures, and another precursor generates the oligodendrocytes in the white matter. Clearly, many questions remain about the differentiation and maturation of oligodendrocytes. The availability of antibodies specific for a cell surface antigen on oligodendrocytic cells (Raff, 1989) provides an important tool to dissect these pathway. The ferritin-positive glial cells found during the second half of gestation in the brain stem and cerebellum suggest their relation to the maturation of oligodendrocytes as well as to the process of myelination (Ozawa *et al.*, 1994). The topographical differences in distribution and particular destination of oligodendroglia cells must be taken into account in further studies, particularly because of their relation with the myelination process.

The oligodendrocytes within the white matter of the CNS are connected in various ways, with myelinated nerve fibers being the myelin forming and maintaining cells. The process of oligodendroglia differentiation appears to be related to the process of myelination.

The number of immature glial cells increases, characterizing the time of pre-myelination. During the period of myelination gliosis (Fig. 9), the number of cells is seven-fold higher than that observed in the mature, well-myelinated capsula interna (Friede, 1961). The proliferation of myelination glia ceases as the myelin sheath begins to form (Jacobson, 1991).

The nuclei of myelination glia become larger and, on light microscopy, appear round, dark or clear, surrounded with some cytoplasm (Roback & Scherer, 1935; Larroche, 1977). In distinguishing between myelination glia with such features and reactive, hypertrophic glial cells that arise

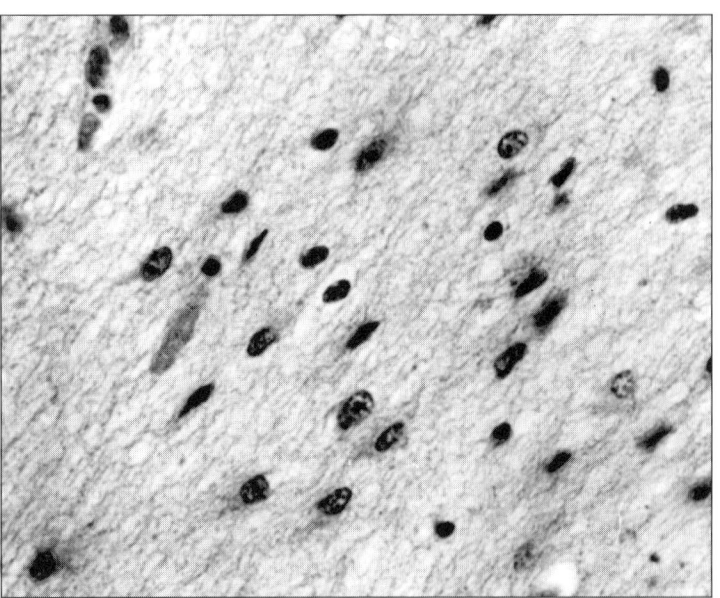

Fig. 9. Myelination glia, with large nucleus and some cytoplasm. HE (hematoxylin-eosin). × 400.

during pathologic processes, it is necessary to consider not only morphological features which may be similar, but also the topography of pathways at the time of premyelination. The significance of the small fat droplets that are often observed within premyelination glial cells has remained unclear until recently. Are they associated with normal glial cell metabolism, or do they reflect some pathologic change? On the basis of comparisons with animal material (Larroche, 1977; Friede, 1989), it appears that these droplets may result from a sequence of preagonal hypoxia. The features of premyelination glia were confirmed and better characterized on ultrastructural examination (Privat, 1975). In times of abundant myelination gliosis, the activity of enzymes such as dehydrogenase, NAD diaphorase and cytochrome oxidase evidently increases (Friede, 1961). The lipids associated with myelin formation appear successively (Chi & Dooling, 1976), and a period of increased lipid synthesis precedes formation of myelin lamellae. Galactocerebrosides appear in the spinal cord up to several weeks before myelination and can be detected on the cell surface of oligodendrocytes (Dickson et al., 1985).

Myelination of an axon begins when oligodendrocytes extend their processes, which wrap around the axon (Asou et al., 1995). The mesaxon becomes longer and loops around the axon many times. During this spiral extension, cytoplasm is deposited around the axon. The proportion between the diameter of nerve fibers and the developing myelin sheath is direct. The growth of the axon, depends on the growth of the nerve cell perikaryon (Martinez & Friede, 1970) and stimulates oligodendrogial cells to further ensheathment (Samorajski & Friede 1968; Friede & Samorajski, 1968). The myelin sheath acquires its definitive features in a series of steps (Fig. 10). During maturation, some cytoplasm is seen within the myelin sheath.

Such uncompacted cytoplasm includes several small vesicles, which are probably involved in the growth of the ensheathment spiral. The cell membranes then fuse totally, forming myelin lamellae, and only the external mesaxon retains some cytoplasm with few organelles. In such compact myelin sheaths, vesicles which were seen previously are no longer present.

Finally, ultrastructural analysis indicates that the myelin sheath is built from alternating dark and clear lamellae derived from the modified membrane of the oligodendrocyte. The myelin sheath in the CNS is divided into segments by short, unmyelinated Ranvier nodes. One process of an oligodendrocyte myelinates one internode, but the processes of one oligodendrocyte may participate in the myelination of many axons. Although estimates differ, it is supposed that one oligodendrocyte may connect with up to 50 myelin sheaths.

The biochemical characteristics of the myelin sheath change during its maturation. The proteins characteristic of myelin lamellae appear and gradually change their proportions (Galas-Zgorzalewicz et al., 1980; Kronquist et al., 1987). The lipids found in the myelin sheath, i.e. phospholipids, glycolipids and cholesterol, are synthesized

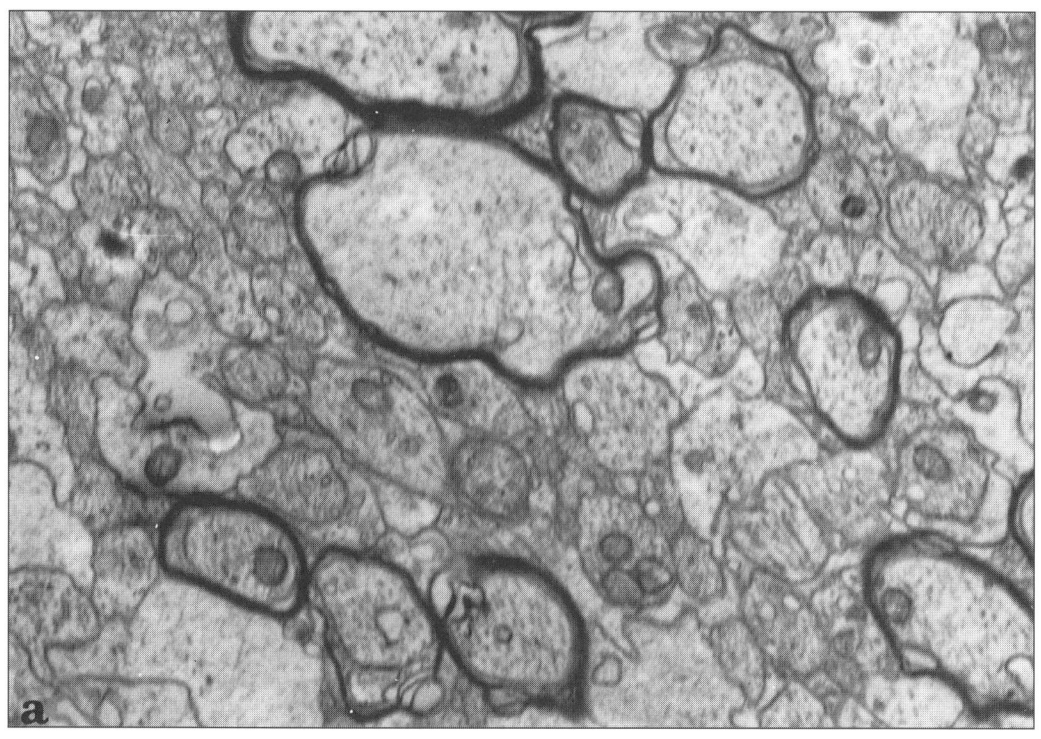
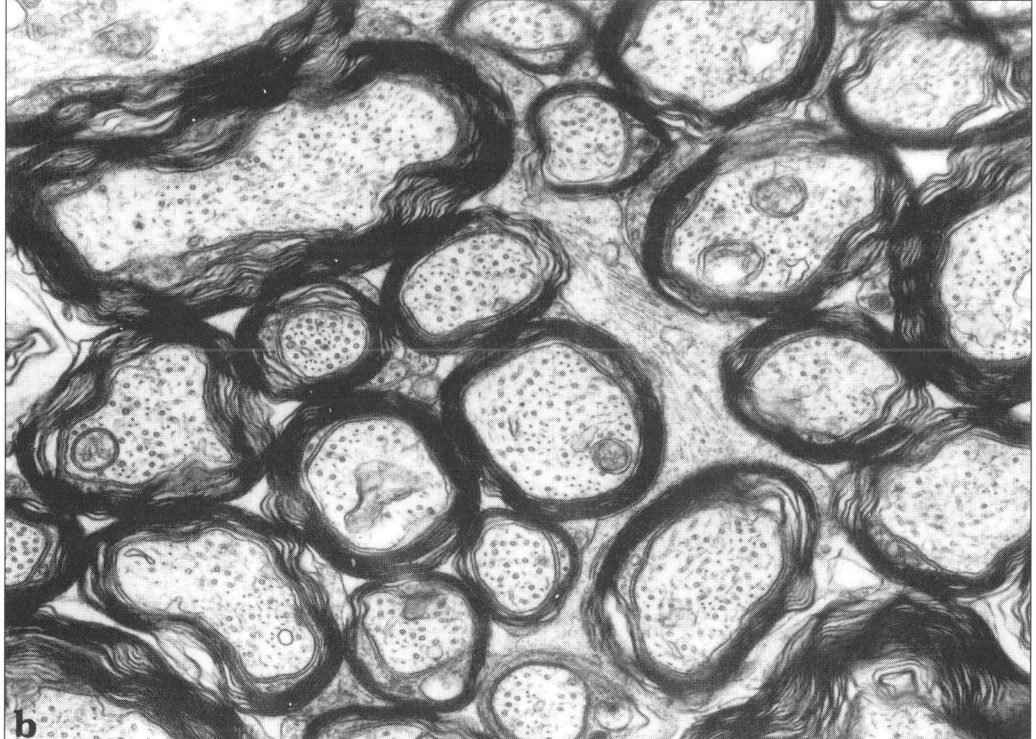

Fig. 10. (a) (above) Myelinating axons within corpus callosum, × 20,000; (b) (below) Myelinated axons within optic nerve, × 30,000.

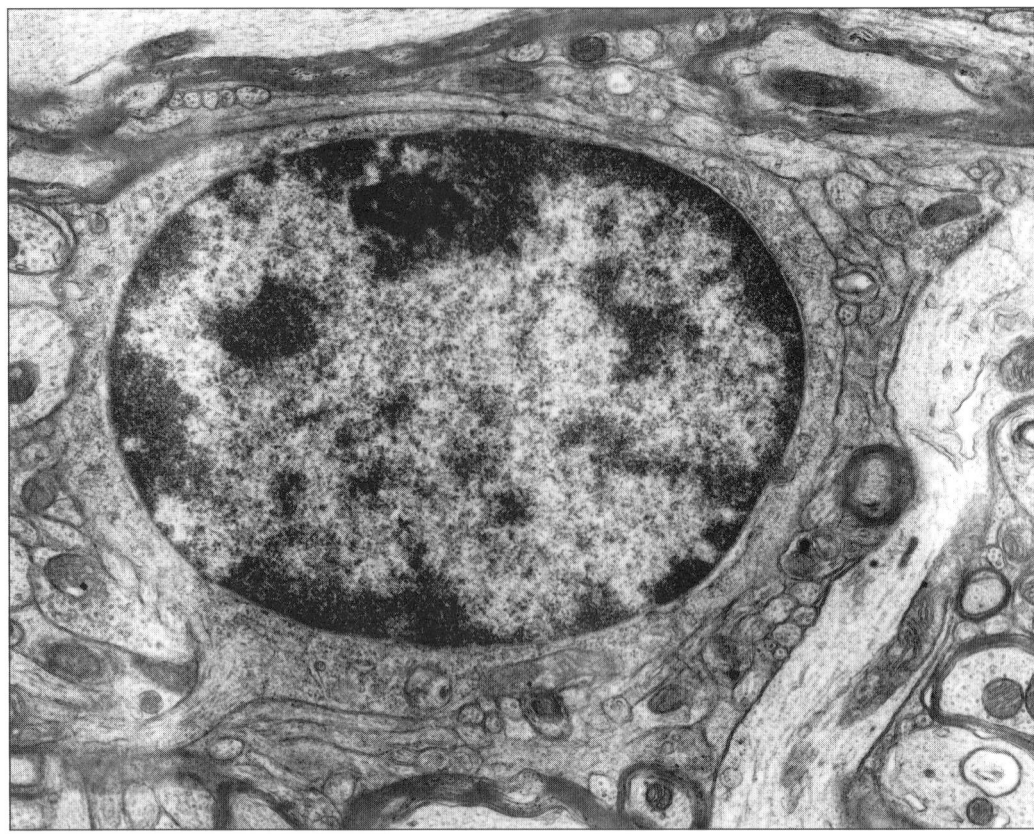

Fig. 11. Ultrastructural picture of an oligodendrocyte, × 18,000.

locally (Jurevics & Morell, 1995) to acquire their adult proportions. The protein and lipid composition demonstrates several correlations with the myelination process (Kinney et al., 1994). Identification of the genes for myelin basic protein (MBP) and proteolipid protein will allow further studies of the molecular mechanisms of myelinogenesis (Knobler, 1995).

The role of myelin sheaths is apparently complex. It is known that sheath development greatly increases (four-fold) the speed of nerve conduction, thus facilitating the complex activity of the CNS (Sarnat, 1992c). The time of onset of myelination differs in particular nerve fibers and in various structures. When myelination begins in axons at least 1.0 nm in diameter is not totally certain. Two morphological events that occur during myelination must be noted. The first is an increase in the vascular network that precedes the formation of myelin sheaths (Sturrock, 1981; 1982). The second is multiplication of astrocytes in myelinating structures (Takashima et al., 1984; Rafałowska & Krajewski, 1991).

The oligodendroglia population is not restricted to cells involved in myelin formation. Fully developed oligodendrocytes are disseminated in both white and gray matter structures. In gray matter, oligodendrocytes appear as satellite cells, named oligo-type I by Rio-Hortega. These cells are seen around neurons, numbering from one to eight cells; around vessels as perivascular satellites, they are present in both gray and white structures. Histological staining of satellite oligodendrocytes reveals a rather small (5–8 nm in diameter), dark nucleus containing a great amount of chromatin. The cells have only a few short processes.

Ultrastructural analysis confirms the abundance of heterochromatin in the oligodendrocyte nucleus, localized mainly within the perinuclear membrane. Cytoplasm is not abundant, but the cell is rich in endoplasmic reticulum and other organelles, including microtubles, although it is deprived of glial filaments (Fig. 11). The metabolic activity of oligodendrocytes is rather high, particularly in perineural satellite cells, since such activity is associated with neighboring nerve cells.

Ependymal cells

Ependymal cells are the last type of cell deriving from the neuroepithelium. At the end stage of maturation, ependymal cells constitute the epithelial layer of the cerebral ventricular system. During development, the ependyma is an active secretory structure involved in cerebral ontogenesis. Its best-known role is to arrest nerve cell multiplication, although there are numerous other important activities. Sarnat (1992a), who reviewed the morphological and functional characteristics of the ependyma in CNS formation and maturation, noted several roles of these cells. For example, the floor plate, a part of the ependyma, establishes polarity and growth gradients of the neural tube. Ependymal cells also arrest neurogenesis in the neuroepithelium, influence guidance of axonal growth cones, affect differentiation of motor neurons, most likely influence maintenance and transformation of radial glial cells, and transport fluids, ions and small molecules between the choroid plexus and cerebrospinal fluid (CSF) and brain tissue.

The part of the ependyma to arise earliest in development, during the fourth WG, is the floor plate, which differentiates from the neuroepithelium upon induction by the notochord. The floor plate extends along the spinal cord and brain stem to the cranial part of the mesencephalon (Van Straaten & Hekking, 1991). At the level of the prosencephalon, it is difficult to find the floor plate, which probably appears only briefly as a derivative of the lamina terminalis. In early development, the floor plate contains the immature neuroepithelial cells, which gradually mature to columnar neuroepithelium. Cells of the floor plate have cytoplasmic processes that reach the basal surface of the spinal cord and brain stem and form the neural median septum. The formation of the ependymal lining of the ventricular walls depends on normal development of the floor plate (Sarnat, 1992b). A special property of the floor plate is its secretion of retinoid acid, which probably plays a key role in inducing the rostrocaudal plan of differentiation of the spinal cord and the brain (Wagner et al., 1990).

Other parts of the ependyma differentiate after the floor plate. The roof plate appears at the sixth week of development. Its most rostral part constitutes the cuboid epithelium of the anterior medullary velum. The cytoplasmic processes of the roof-plate cells projecting to the dorsal part of the developing spinal cord form the dorsal median septum until the 10th WG. Successively, other developing cavities of the CNS acquire their ependymal lining. Within the spinal cord, the ependymal layer forms first at the level of the spinal basal plate, and by about the 10th WG, at the level of the alar plate. Similarly, ependyma forms first in the fourth ventricle and then in the aqueduct.

The formation of an ependymal cushion within the third and particularly the lateral ventricles is strictly associated with neurogenesis in the periventricular germinal matrix. Until the neuroepithelial cells in the ventricular zone remain undifferentiated, they proliferate to furnish a cellular population for newly differentiating structures. As the new cells proliferate and the surface area of the ventricular system increases, the number of nerve cells increases (Smart, 1972). Maturation of ependymal cells stops neuronal generation within the ventricular walls. Therefore, ependymal maturation is most delayed in the telencephalic struc-

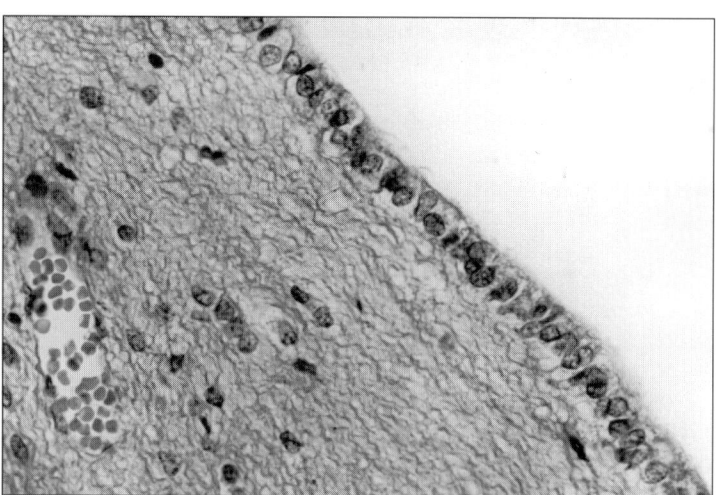

Fig. 12. The ependymal cells lining the ventricular wall. Cresyl violet, × 400.

tures that are ontogenetically the youngest. At 20 WG, the ependyma is well-differentiated in the hippocampal formation, but still undifferentiated in segments corresponding to the neocortex (Sarnat, 1992b). During fetal development and in some areas even after birth, ependymal cells extend processes directed to the CNS surface, but most do not reach this level.

Many of the developmental processes in the CNS appear to depend directly or indirectly on ependymal activity. The presence of the intermediate filaments – vimentin, cytokeratin and GFAP – in ependymal cells during fetal life (Tapscott et al., 1981; Sarnat, 1992b), but the total absence of these proteins in mature ependymal cells strongly suggests their crucial role in developmental processes.

Fetal ependymal cells also have secretory capabilities, producing soluble molecules such as NGF, which is found in ependymal cell processes, and keratin sulfate and N-CAM, which are secreted by the roof plate (Jacobson & Rutishauser, 1986; Linnemann & Bock, 1989; Snow et al., 1990). The chemotropic activity of such molecules, which attract and repel axonal bundles and tracts, guides the axonal growth cones during fetal brain formation (Sarnat, 1992c). Note that the chemotropic role of ependymal cells differs from the structural one of radial glial fibers.

Another diffusible molecule, S-100, is also present in developing but not in mature ependymal cells. This protein is particularly abundant in areas corresponding to the ventral part of the basal plate of the spinal cord and brain stem at 8–11 WG and around the lateral ventricles during the period of neuroblast and glioblast multiplication and migration. The localization of S-100 protein in areas adjacent to the floor plate and at sites of motor neuron development raises the possibility of another role for the ependyma in the generation and maturation of motor neurons at this level. Results of animal studies support this possibility (Sarnat, 1992c).

The last role that may be attributed to ependymal cells during development is their participation in the maintenance and maturation of radial glia. Soluble molecules secreted by ependymal cells may be involved in this process.

The mature ependyma, consisting of simple cuboid epithelium lining the ventricular walls (Fig. 12) and with no secretory activity, plays an important role in the CSF/brain barrier throughout adult life, serving in the selective transport of fluids, ions and small molecules.

Chapter 2

Mesodermal Elements in the CNS

Microglia

Microglia were described by del Rio-Hortega (1919) as a distinct cell type in the CNS, but for many years, the origin of these cells, their relation to other cell types, and their function in normal and pathologic conditions remained unclear. A key question was whether microglial cells shared a neuroectodermal origin with other types of glia, or whether they originated from the mesoderm, deriving from blood elements or from vascular walls.

The first studies on microglia were conducted in animals, and many animal models are still used for investigations. Santha and Juba observed that microglial cells appear concurrently with immature vessels in the developing rat brain (cited after Kershman, 1939). Kershman (1939), in his analysis of representative samples from human brains at 8 to 29 WG using silver carbonate staining, found that microglial cells arise in particular areas or 'fountains' around blood vessels or in points of contact of the choroid plexus with brain structures. He concluded that microglia are of mesenchymal origin and are related to the reticuloendothelial system. Kershman (1939) also described the mature microglial cells as small, with scarce cytoplasm and many thin, highly ramified processes visualized by the silver impregnation method. This form of microglia corresponds to the so-called 'resting' microglia (Fig. 13).

Ultrastructural studies served to distinguish astroglial, oligoglial and microglial cells on the basis of different patterns of silver depositions (Murabe & Sano, 1982). In electron microscopy (EM) studies (Boya, 1975) (Fig. 14), microglial cells appeared small in comparison with other cells, with a relatively large nucleus, scanty cytoplasm and wide cisternae of rough endoplasmic reticulum. Ribosomes were abundant, presenting as a large accumulation of RNA in the cytoplasm, and the Golgi apparatus was not well-developed. Lysosomes and their osmiophilic bodies appeared characteristic for this cell type.

The morphological features of microglia have led some authors to conclusions different from Kerhman's about the origin of this cells. EM studies performed on rat optic nerve identified a possible third type of glia with some features of microglia that were

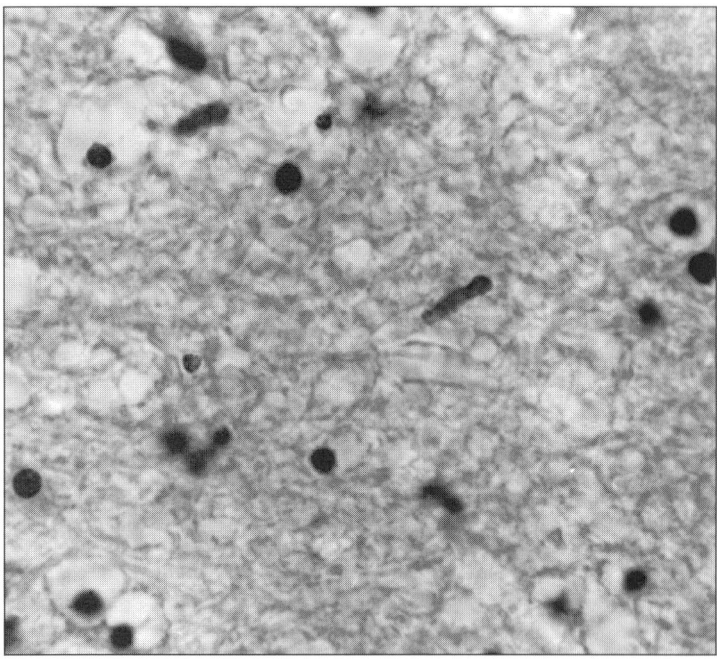

Fig. 13. Microglial cells. HE, × 400.

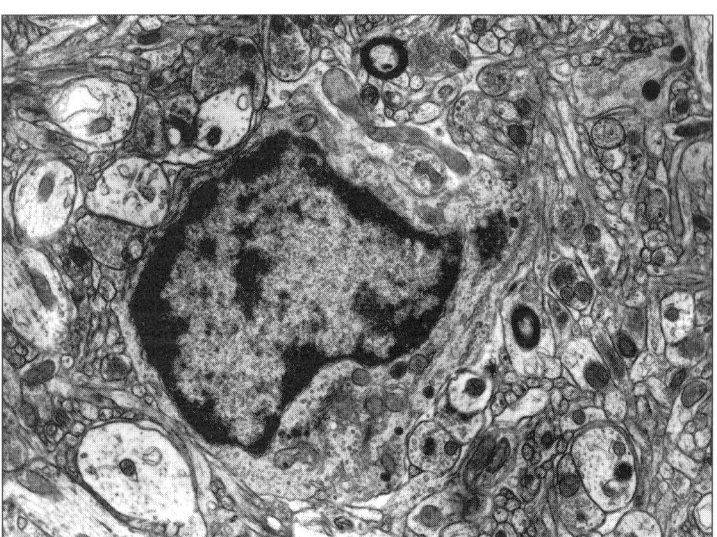

Fig. 14. Ultrastructural picture of microglial cell, × 12,000.

hypothesized to derive from neuroectodermal matrix (Vaughn & Peters, 1968). The autoradiographic studies and immunohistochemical methods, supported this hypothesis, consistent with the results of Fujita and Kitamura (1976) and Kitamura et al. (1984). Hao et al. (1991) identified the macrophage-like cells in cultures of mouse neuroepithelium, obtained from fetal brain before vascularization. Those authors also concluded that these cells correspond to resident microglia of neuroectodermal origin. However, Streit et al. (1989) pointed out that none of those studies demonstrated common markers between glioblasts and mature microglial cells, so that hypotheses about microglial origin were again in doubt. These studies have always been complicated by the peculiar ability of microglia to appear in morphological forms different from mature microglia in normal brain, perhaps due to the different functional states of the cells under study (Murabe & Sano, 1982; Matthews, 1974).

Very important were the studies on the stages of microglial development. Kershman (1939) reported that microglial cells were first detectable even before the eighth week of development in human fetal brain, whereas Choi (1981a) found them at about the 10th week. Apparently, the appearance of microglia has a broad temporal window. After the first abundant 'fountains,' microglial cells appear during the course of brain structure maturation: Kershman (1939) observed developing microglial cells preferentially localized to submeningeal and perivascular sites and near plexus choroideus attachment to brain structures, i.e. all points of contact between neuroectodermal and mesodermal tissue. Microglia at those sites appeared in ameboid form, extending their processes and presenting pseudopodic forms, before obtaining their final mature features.

In studies to determine the major source of such cell precursors invading the brain parenchyma Choi (1981a) proposed hematogenous cells, whereas Imamoto (1981) and Ling (1978) proposed blood monocytes as the main source, a hypothesis strengthened by the observation that intravascular injection of labeled monocytes was followed by the appearance of labeled microglia-like cells in developing rat brains. Streit et al. (1988a) suggested that monocytes may differentiate into microglia during embryonic development, but not in the mature brain. Some authors proposed that perivascular pericytes deriving from monocytes may represent a minor source of microglial cells (Hager, 1975; Baron & Gallego, 1973; Imamoto, 1981). The opinion that microglial cells originate from some 'cousin' of monocytes entering the brain parenchyma directly during development, independently of blood flow, was formulated (Streit & Kinkaid-Colton, 1995).

Observations of microglial cells during all phases of their development demonstrated that they respond to brain tissue injury with the behavior of macrophages, as originally postulated by del Rio-Hortega in 1919. The immature ameboid microglial cells (Giulian & Baker, 1986) were shown to act as phagocytes of neurons during programmed cell death. Mature microglial cells also function as phagocytic macrophages. Immunohistochemical studies confirmed the close relationship between the ameboid and the ramified mature form of microglia (Milligan et al., 1991) and suggested their connections with cells of the monocytic lineage (Chugani et al., 1991; Ling & Wong, 1993). The ever-increasing list of cell surface antigens shared by macrophages and microglia supports the notion that microglia are resident macrophages of the brain (Perry & Gordon, 1988).

It should be noted that other brain macrophages with phenotypes different from those of microglia have been described (Perry & Gordon, 1988). In 1963, Konigsmark and Sidman maintained that they were also blood-derived macrophages, constituting a significant proportion of the macrophagic population in pathologic cases. More recent light and EM studies of acute brain injury in experimental animals confirmed the appearance of macrophages other than microglia deriving from blood monocytes (Schelper & Adrian, 1986). Thus, the evidence suggests that there are two populations of macrophages: one that enters exogenously from blood vessels through a damaged blood–brain barrier and one that derives endogenously, in pathologic conditions from activated microglia.

Microglia not only have a phagocytic role, but also are intimately involved in immunological processes (Hickey & Kimura, 1988). Studies have shown that microglia are able to present antigen to T-cells in a major histocompatibility complex-restricted fashion (Streit et al., 1988a,b; Gehrmann et al., 1993). On the basis of morphology and distribution of microglia in the CNS, Graeber and Streit (1990) postulated that these cells form a network of immunocompetent cells that interact with brain structures. Resting microglia are scattered uniformly through the CNS, but are more concentrated in gray matter than in white structures. Further studies confirmed that resting microglia retain the potential to become activated and can be considered intrinsic brain macrophage precursors. It appears from morphology that resting ramified microglia respond to brain tissue injury by acquiring moderate enlargement of the cells or activated bushy or rod-like forms. The cells might also revert to their resting forms. When necrosis of neuronal elements occurs, each activated cell may change to a phagocytosing, macrophage-like form.

Microglial cell activities are not restricted to a cellular immune response. They are believed to secrete NGF and fibroblast growth factor, which are important for CNS development, and when injury occurs, for protection and repair of damaged tissue (Streit & Kinkaid-Colton, 1995).

On the other hand, excessive amounts of some substances produced by microglia may kill neurons. Such substances include amyloid precursor protein, which is thought to be produced by microglial cells. Thus, these cells may play a role in manufacturing amyloid fibers within senile plaques and indirectly influence the morphological aspects of Alzheimer disease (Wiśniewski et al., 1989). Interleukin-1, other cytokines and reactive oxygen species produced in excess by microglia, i.e. the

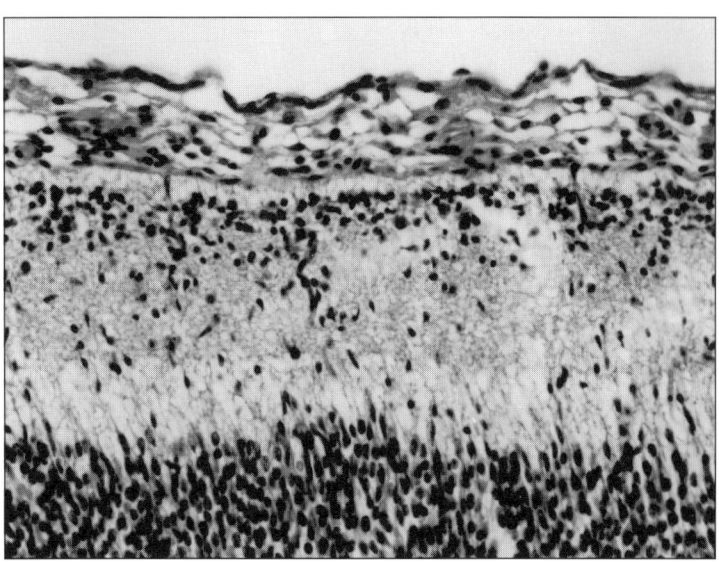

Fig. 15. Thin vessels penetrating the cortex from extra ependymal plexus, × 200.

probable situation in Down's syndrome, may affect the brain tissue of such patients. The human immunodeficiency virus (HIV) type 1 infects microglia (Budka et al., 1987), which produce cytokine messenger molecules at elevated levels and may also be harmful for neurons. During stroke, the overproduction of substances, which in moderate amounts protect damaged nerve tissue, may become dangerous. Such harmful effects have also been postulated in some degenerative diseases of the CNS (Streit & Kinkaid-Colton, 1995).

These negative effects of microglial products were detected in culture in experimental conditions. Presumably, their production in living human brains is controlled by regulatory mechanisms that limit their influence in a given pathologic process.

Vessels

Vascularization of the CNS occurs by way of angiogenesis. Two mechanisms of vessel formation exist in developing organs: (1) vasculogenesis, or the derivation of vessels from endothelial cells (EC) developing from precursor cells that differentiate *in situ* to form channels and a network of primitive vessels, and (2) angiogenesis, or the invasion of extrinsic endothelial sprouts into the developing organ (Parnadaud et al., 1989; Seifert et al., 1992). Which mechanism operates depends on the embryonic origin of the developing organs. The crucial role of the endoderm in the emergence and proliferation of endothelial cell precursors is well known. Thus, in organs originating from the mesoderm associated with the endoderm, the proper cell lineage forms and vasculogenesis proceeds. The endoderm is also important for the development of the hemopoietic cell lineage forming the EC, a cell type endowed with hemangioblastic potential. By contrast, an association between mesoderm and ectoderm in the formation of a given organ does not imply the induction of vasculogenesis (Parnadaud & Deterline-Lièvre 1993). Instead angiogenesis, the penetration of vascular buds into such organs, takes place. This was observed in bone marrow (Jotereau & Donarin 1978), in mouse kidney (Sariola et al., 1983, 1984), and in the CNS (Stewart & Wiley 1981). In some organs with complex structures, both vasculogenesis and angiogenesis can occur (Seifert et al., 1992), but only angiogenesis is observed in the developing brain. The endothelial channels arriving from an extra parenchymal plexus and penetrating the nervous tissue have been well-documented (Fig. 15).

The gradual maturation of the vascular walls, which is associated with the formation of the blood–brain barrier, occurs during fetal life and even after birth, and is associated with the maturation of vascularized structures. This topic is discussed further in Chapter 3, on Vascularization of the CNS (p. 64).

Chapter 3

Consecutive Morphogenesis and Maturation of CNS Structures

Initial stages of CNS development

The first step necessary for the nervous system to originate is the process of neuronal induction. It consists of changes and differentiation of the ectoderm of the embryonic disc into neuroectoderm.

In general, the process of induction means that one group of cells acts as inductor upon another induced group and leads to changes determining their fates. This sequence of events is necessary for formation of the body of a vertebrate (Smith & Slack, 1983). During embryonal development the chordamesoderm arises from the primitive streak and induces the multistep process of neuronal induction (Jacobson & Rutishauser, 1986; Jacobson, 1991). At the beginning of gastrulation, the induction of the brain and sense organs occur and, later, that of more caudal structures. Regional differences in the nervous system come from regionally specified mesoderm. Although specificity of induction belongs to the mesoderm, the ectoderm influences the time and spatial extent of induction. This process, bringing a special cell-to-cell signaling, also includes the activity of hormones, neurotransmitter and growth factors (Jacobson, 1991). The first phases of CNS development are called neurulation and include formation of the neural plate and, subsequently, of the neural tube. These phases occur at 18–30 days' gestation and initiate a long process of growth, differentiation and maturation of CNS structures. The genes controlling the process of neurulation have been identified recently (Papalopulu & Kintner, 1994).

A widely accepted schema of the early stages of CNS formation is the Carnegie system, which defines 23 stages in postovulatory days to 57 (O'Rahilly & Gardner, 1979). These stages appear to be useful in characterizing the consecutive steps of development, when the length of the embryo does not correspond closely to the levels of morphological differentiation.

The Carnegie system is used here to describe primary CNS formation up to closure of the neuronal tube during the first month of development (i.e. 4 weeks). For events occurring in the next month of CNS development, Carnegie stages will only be mentioned (Table 1).

Table 1. Developmental Carnegie stages 1–13 (adapted from O'Rahilly and Müller, 1987)

Stage	Age/days	Pair of somites
1	1	
2	1, 5–3	
3	4	
5	5–6	
6	13	
7	16	
8	18	
9	20	1–3
10	22	4–12
11	24	13–20
12	26	21–29
13	28	30–?
!	!	
!	!	
!	!	
23	57	

Most data presented here on the early developmental events of the CNS come from the precise studies of Müller and O'Rahilly, with complementary information from other investigations.

The first morphologically recognizable primordium of the nervous system, the neural plate (Fig. 16), is detectable at day 18 postovulation, which corresponds to stage 8 of development (O'Rahilly & Müller, 1981), but was seen by autoradiography even earlier, at 16 days (stage 7) (O'Rahilly & Müller, 1987). The subsequent longitudinal invagination of the neural plate results in formation of the neural groove, which at this stage is found in 25 per cent of the embryos examined. The future basal plate, which will be evident in the neural tube as situated more medially, and future alar plate, localized more laterally, are already visible in the neural groove. At stage 8, the accentuated growth of the neural plate anterior part is also observed, and the neural folds are cerebral rather than spinal. Stage 8 is the last presomitic phase of human embryogenesis.

At stage 9, corresponding to postovulatory day 20 and 0.98–1.86 mm of embryonic length, the neural groove represents 71 per cent of this length. This is characterized by the appearance of one to three pairs of somites in the occipital future rhombencephalon, and somite number continues to increase (Müller & O'Rahilly, 1983). Segmentation, which means the appearance along the rostro-caudal axis of serial somites, is an important process in the body plan, occurring secondary to neuronal induction (Sarnat, 1992c). Segmental organization occurs also in the future nervous system. Three major divisions of the future brain, the prosencephalon (forebrain), mesencephalon (midbrain), and rhombencephalon (hindbrain), which later will develop into five can be identified in stage 9 (Streeter, 1927) (Fig. 17). This differentiation occurs in the still open neural groove. The cranial flexure indicating the mesencephalon and four subdivisions of rhombencephalon (the upper one representing the hypoglossal region) are also detectable. Caudally to the rhombencephalon, the future spinal cord occupies no more than 30 per cent of the total length of the neural groove (Müller & O'Rahilly, 1983). In some embryos at this stage, even elements of the neural crest, the most external part of the neural groove, are distinguishable (O'Rahilly, 1965). In the context of general embryonic development, note that the heart is often already present at postovulatory day 20.

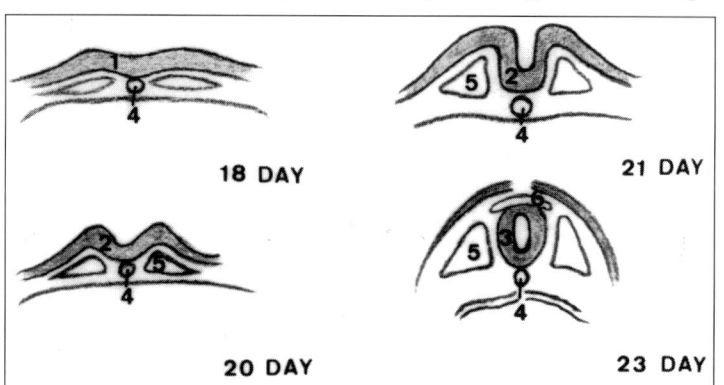

Fig. 16. Consecutive stages of neural tube formation:
1. Neural plate
2. Neural groove
3. Neural tube
4. Notochord
5. Somite
6. Neural crest.

Formation of the neuronal tube begins at about day 22 (Fig. 18), corresponding to stage 10, characterized by 4–12 pairs of somites and an embryonic length of 1.3–3.3 mm (Müller & O'Rahilly 1985). The neural groove begins to close when about six pairs of somites are seen at the border between the cervical and rhombencephalic levels and they progress caudally and rostrally. This model of neural tube formation was confirmed by O'Rahilly and Müller (1994), when it was called into question by Van Allen et al. (1993). On the basis of animal studies, Van Allen proposed the multi-site closure of the neural tube. Similar multi-site, but only anterior neural tube closure was suggested by Golden and Chernoff (1995).

The anterior part corresponding to the future brain is also changing at this stage. The first telencephalic structure, the *lamina terminalis*, appears, and the first diencephalic subdivision, the future site of optic primordia and thalamus, differentiates within the prosencephalon, which increases in length (O'Rahilly & Müller, 1994). The mesencephalic flexure changes its angle from 150°–104°, and the rhombencephalon becomes shorter relative to other parts of the CNS, especially compared with the future spinal cord, which increases five-fold. During this period, mitotic figures within the neural groove are most frequent at the spinal level.

Neural crest formation also progresses. Its cells derive from the open neural groove, the neural tube, and perhaps also the special surface ectoderm. It was even suggested that some mesenchymal cells are intermixed in the formation of this structure (Sidman & Rakic, 1982), but the neural ectoderm is the main source of neuronal crest cells (O'Rahilly & Müller, 1994). Derivatives of the neural crest are later dispersed in the peripheral nervous system where they contribute to the formation of eyes, meninges, and spinal and cranial nerve sensory ganglia (Sidman & Rakic, 1982; O'Rahilly & Müller, 1987). A review of recent investigations of neural crest development (Gershon, 1993) suggests that the destiny of neural crest cells is not finally determined before their migration to target points and that the microenvironment might ultimately determine their fate. At stage 10, the material for ganglia of cranial nerves V, VII, IX and X, is already available.

During this stage, the pulmonary primordium, arteries and veins are the principal morphological features of general embryonic development. Blood circulation also begins at this stage as the sequelae of the first cardiac contractions.

Stage 11 corresponds to postovulatory day 24, 13–20 pairs of somites, and 1.6–4.3 mm of embryonic length. This stage is characterized by closure of the rostral neuropore (Müller & O'Rahilly, 1986), when 20 pairs of somites are already present (O'Rahilly & Müller, 1994). Closure of the neural tube in its anterior part progresses rostrally from the mesencephalon and caudally from the

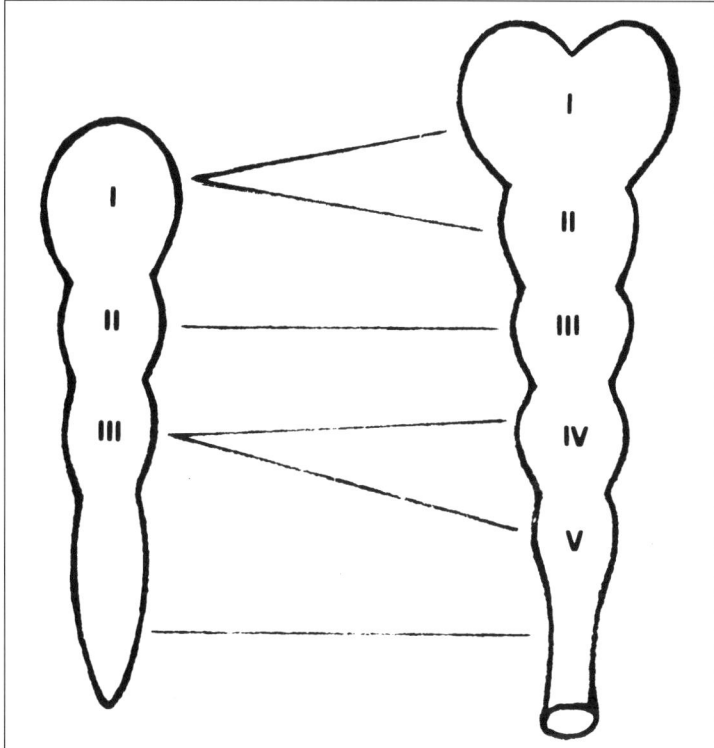

Fig. 17. Subdivisions of the future brain:

A B
I prosencephalon I telencephalon
II mesencephalon II diencephalon
III rhombencephalon III mesencephalon
IV metencephalon
V myelencephalon.

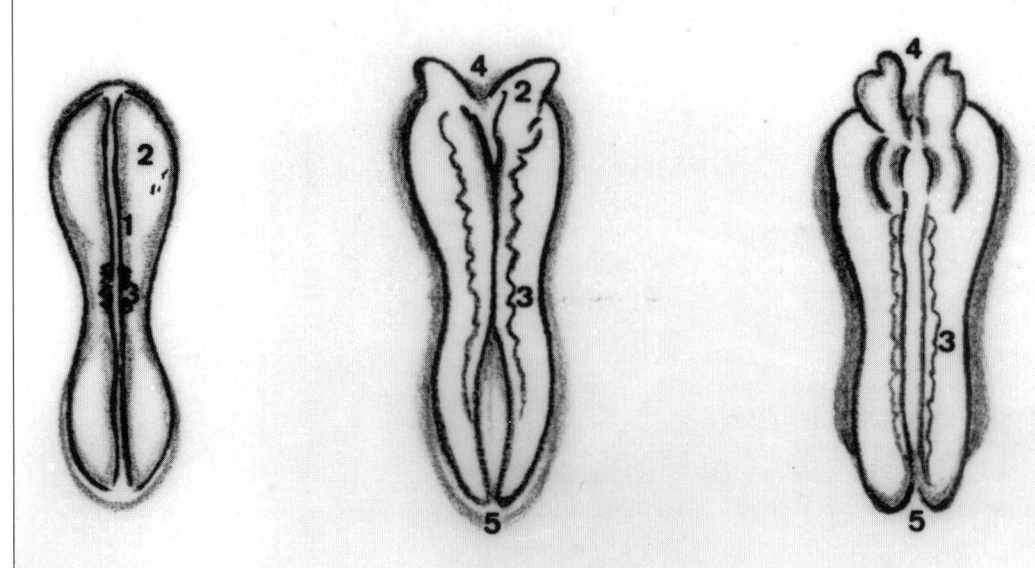

Fig. 18. Closure of the neural tube:

1. Neural groove
2. Neural fold
3. Somite
4. Anterior neuropore
5. Posterior neuropore

lamina terminalis, which arises from the medial closure of the terminal lip. It may be important for the pathomechanism of dysraphic states that at the dorsal lip of the closing neuropore the fusion of the neural epithelium occurs later than that of the surface epithelium. For this reason, this area is less resistant to lesions than the terminal lip (O'Rahilly & Müller, 1994). The process of anterior neuropore closure is very rapid. The lamina terminalis, which begins to differentiate around day 22, appears as the structure closing the anterior neuropore at day 24. In the adult brain, only remnants of this structure are visible within the anterior wall of the third ventricle.

During development, within its dorsal part (the commisural plate) prosencephalic commissures will originate and the ventral part of the optic chiasm. During this stage, the neural tube progressively elongates, but the caudal neuropore remains open. Neuromeres, which are serial swellings of the neural tube, are seen at all levels of the future brain. At the end of this stage, the optic vesicles (described below) appear, and the buds of mammillary bodies and neurohypophysial components are identifiable. Finally, an event occurs that is important for the initial internal cellular and functional organization of the CNS — the formation of the primordial plexiform layer (marginal zone), a cell-sparse external layer, including neuroectodermal cell processes in the future spinal cord and rhombencephalon. The pia mater appears at the rhombencephalic level.

Stage 12 occurs on day 26 and is characterized by 21–29 pairs of somites and an embryonic length reaching 3–5 mm. At this stage, the commissural plate is seen at the site of the former rostral neuropore, and the closure of the caudal neuropore occurs when 25 pairs of somites are seen (Müller & O'Rahilly, 1987; O'Rahilly & Müller, 1994) at the future second sacral vertebral level and future somite 31. The caudal eminence (end-bud), which is the thickening located caudally to the newly closed neuropore and present as mass of pluripotential tissue, is very visible. It will give rise to caudal somites and the neural cord. In the future brain, only an enlargement of the telencephalon medium occurs. An important event is the appearance of neurofibrils in neuroblasts and their processes within the rhombencephalon (in the nucleus of the lateral longitudinal tract). A marginal layer

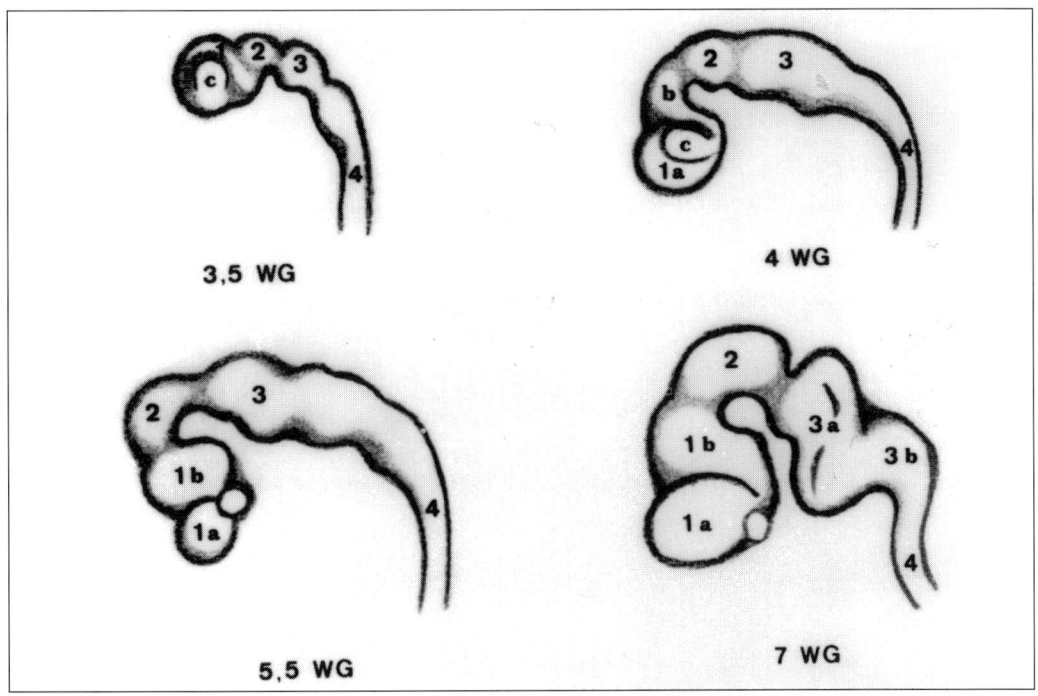

Fig. 19. Growth of primitive brain

1. Prosencephalon
(a) Telencephalon
(b) Diencephalon
(c) Optic vesicle

2. Mesencephalon

3. Rhombencephalon
(a) Metencephalon
(pons + cerebellum)
(b) Myelencephalon

4. Spinal cord

appears at the mesencephalic level. The neural crest develops in a caudal direction, and its cells continue to form the pia mater. The general development of the embryo progresses, as upper and then lower limb buds appear.

Stage 13 occurs at day 28 in an embryo with more than 30, and even with a final number of 40 pairs of somites and 4–5.5 mm in length (Ostertag, 1956; Müller & O'Rahilly, 1988a). The neural tube is already closed, and 'primary neurulation' is complete (Fig. 18).

Nevertheless, the caudal eminence differentiates, providing cellular material for the notochord, somites (32–40), and for the neural cord from which the nervous system of the caudal part of the body arises. The central canal extends into the neural cord. This process of 'secondary neurulation' continues to the seventh week. Thus, the CNS derives not only from the neural plate, but also from this most caudal formation (Müller & O'Rahilly, 1988a). With the closure of the neural tube, its internal cavity is separated from the amniotic fluid. This cavity is still filled with fluid probably produced by lining cells and termed 'ependymal fluid'.

At this stage, the brain becomes enlarged dorsoventrally, with the infundibular area, chiasmatic plate, *lamina terminalis* and commissural plate clearly visible. Within the optic vesicles, retinal cells and the lens disc appear. Three layers can be distinguished in the internal structure of the wall of the neural tube: ependymal, intermediate and marginal. In the spinal cord, the ventral roots start to develop, and spinal ganglia form from the neural crest. In the future brain, the first indication of a developing cerebellum appears as a narrowing between the most anterior part of the rhombencephalon and the isthmus of the mesencephalon. The fourth ventricle is already visible. At the end of 4 weeks (stage 13), the period of CNS development that proceeds with rostro-caudal symmetry, the so-called phase of primitive CNS formation (Ostertag, 1956), comes to a close (Fig. 19).

Although the embryonic period (8 weeks of development) is not yet over, we think that a summary of the processes occurring in particular brain structures might provide a clearer picture of CNS morphogenesis and maturation.

Spinal cord

The fundamental plan of embryonic CNS development is best reflected in the spinal cord, as observed by Sidman and Rakic (1982). At the end of the phase of CNS primitive formation during the first gestational month, the spinal cord presents its basic features. The ependymal, mantle (or intermediate), and marginal layers are quite distinguishable around the central canal. The walls of the spinal cord increase in volume, leading to compression of the central canal in vertical shape. The roof and floor plates remain thin. The cells lining the roof plate will become well-differentiated ependymal cells (Sarnat, 1992c). The cells of floor plate examined in 4–7 week-old embryos (stages 14–20) present microvilli and cilia on their apical surface and contain numerous endoplasmic organelles including multi-vesicular structures. This picture suggests the secretory activity of floor plate cells during embryonic development (Tanaka et al., 1988). Most important are recent studies attributing a particular role to the floor plate in induction of CNS development (Sarnat, 1992c), as discussed in the chapter on ependymal development. The immature neuroepithelial cells lining the lateral walls of the central canal divide, producing the population of neuroblasts that provide the material necessary for the spinal cord neuronal structures. Later, these cells differentiate into ependymal cells (Sarnat, 1992c). The mitotic activity of cells in the spinal cord is intensive during the first trimester of gestation (Sidman & Rakic, 1982).

Within the thick walls of the spinal cord, the sulcus limitans divide the mantel layer into two parts during week five of development (stages 14, 15). The ventral part, forming the basal plate that gives rise to the anterior spinal horn, becomes more voluminous than alar plate. This is due to differentiation of large neurons within the basal plate. The development of the spinal cord structures progresses in rostro-caudal direction. During this process, maturation at the cervical level is more advanced than at the lumbar level. Already during week 5, the motor cells in the upper level of the spinal cord are located ventrolaterally and emit their axons ventrally to form the roots (Sidman & Rakic, 1982). They will start to form the brachial and lumbosacral plexus (Sarnat, 1992c). The roots arising from sensory spinal ganglia enter the spinal cord at the cervical and lumbar levels. The first synapses within the motor nucleus of the spinal cord are also found at this stage of development (Milokhin, 1983).

Spinal cord development continues during the next 6–8 weeks (stages 16–23). The anterior and posterior horns and the marginal layer are well-demarcated. The volume of those still immature structures is initially similar at all levels of the spinal cord. During further development, this volume begins to differ at the cervical, thoracic and lumbar levels as a result of programmed cell death. The subsequent maturation of neurons is reflected in the appearance of axodendritic synapses (Wozniak et al., 1980). The seven-fold increase in the number of synapses at the cervical level was observed during the week 8 of gestation (Flower, 1985). The marginal zone of the spinal cord also reveals features of maturation. EM examination indicated the presence of some organelles in cytoplasm of young nerve cells and formation of synapses (Rizvi et al., 1986).

All of these developmental events leading to the activity of CNS result in the first movements of the 6–7-week-old embryo and to the first reflexes at seven and a half weeks (Flower, 1985). The development of glia parallels to the maturation of neuronal structures. The first GFAP-positive cells arising within the intermediate zone are detectable at seven WG (Reske-Nielsen et al., 1987).

By the end of week 8, corresponding to the last Carnegie stage of development (stage 23), when the embryo reaches 30 mm in length four well-defined concentric layers have replaced the three primitive layers of the spinal cord. These concentric layers include (1) the ventricular layer, with mitotic activity of neuroepithelial cells, (2) the subventricular zone, characterized by high proliferative activity of further glia and only some groups of neurons, (3) the intermediate zone, comprising post mitotic neuroblasts, and (4) the marginal zone, located at the surface of the spinal cord (Angevine, 1970; Sarnat, 1992c). At this stage, morphological differentiation and functional development of the spinal cord is sufficiently advanced to consider the CNS as an active organ.

Throughout fetal life, all parameters reflecting spinal cord maturation change sequentially. The progress of morphological maturation of neurons, within the marginal zone, was documented by EM observations (Rizvi et al., 1986) at 18 and 25 weeks of development. The four-fold increase in the number of synapses by 11 WG correlates with neuronal maturation (Flower, 1985). By the end of the first trimester the structural development of the spinal cord is definitive (Ostertag, 1956). Until this time, the increase in volume of both basal plates leads to the formation of ventral fissure of the spinal cord. The medial expansion of alar plates results in the final compression of the dorsal portion of the central canal and finally in the formation of the posterior medial septum named also raphe posterior, which involves processes of roof plate cells and is complete by 10 WG. The growth of posterior columns during the second half of fetal life results in maturation of this boundary between them, presenting the features deserving the last name 'raphe' (Parkinson & del Bizio, 1996).

The maturation process in the glial population is well documented. Immunohistochemical staining for GFAP and vimentin identified radial glial cells at 15 weeks and loss of vimentin reactivity as these cells differentiate into mature astrocytes during the next weeks (Kamada et al., 1984). At similar time (15–16 weeks), GFAP-positive staining is seen in cells that will present ultrastructural features of oligodendrocytes, concurrent with the onset of myelin sheath formation. GFAP staining in these cells is no longer seen at 17–18 weeks, being characteristic only for early stages of their development (Choi & Kim, 1984). The first myelin sheaths are seen in the spinal cord at 22–24 weeks in embryos 66 mm of length. This important process, which begins at the middle of prenatal life, will continue until adulthood. At 22 weeks, myelin sheaths appear around anterior roots and shortly thereafter around the posterior roots; at 25 weeks, myelin sheaths are visible in fasciculus cuneatus. The sequence of the spinal cord pathway myelination, as it relates to the other levels of the CNS, is discussed in this Chapter on CNS myelination of the CNS structure (p. 60).

Macroscopically, spinal cord growth differs from that of the spinal canal, a difference that begins at the end of the first trimester and is visible by midgestation (Ostertag, 1956). Between weeks 25 and 33, the spinal cord terminates at around the third lumbar vertebra (Hawass et al., 1987) and, at birth, at the lower border of the first lumbar vertebra, i.e. at the adult level (Govender et al., 1989).

Brain stem

The components derived from the rhombencephalon, i.e. the medulla oblongata and pons, together with the mesencephalon, give rise to the brain stem. The isthmus should also be mentioned as a particular segment joining the mesencephalon and rhombencephalon, which is observed only during a given period of development (the

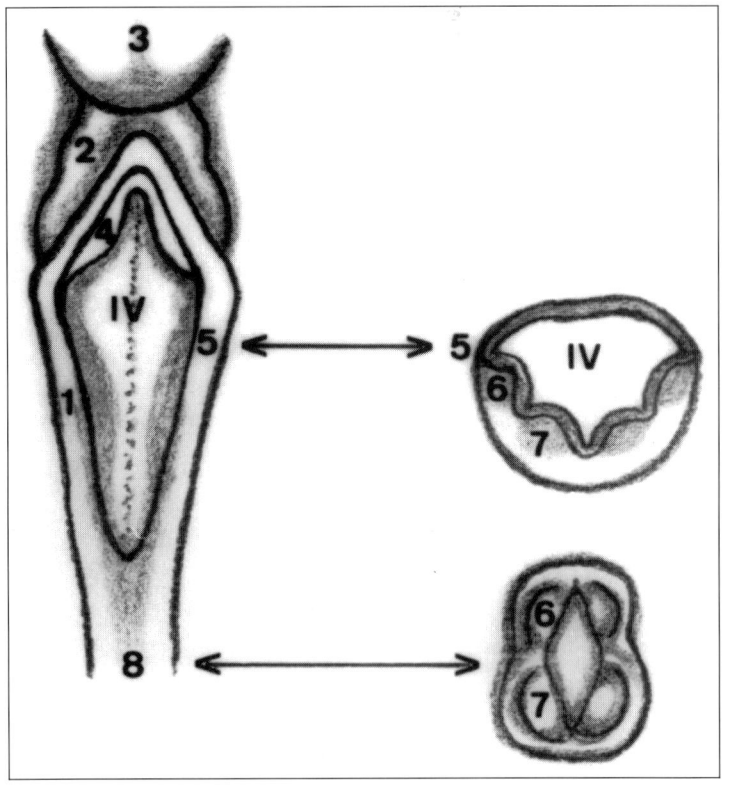

Fig. 20. Development of the IV ventricle

1. Myelencephalon
2. Metencephalon
3. Mesencephalon
4. Rhombic lip
5. Roof plate and its attachment
6. Alar plate
7. Basal plate
8. Spinal cord

second month) as a constriction between those parts of the neural tube. The isthmus is also involved in formation of the primordium cerebelli (Müller & O'Rahilly, 1988a). The appearance of the isthmus obscures some of the internal relationships between the rhombencephalon and mesencephalon (Sidman & Rakic, 1982). The boundary between them becomes indistinct; the nucleus of the fourth cranial nerve develops in the isthmus and, in adult brain, it is considered to belong to the mesencephalon.

The most caudal part of the brain stem, the future medulla oblongata, undergoes structural changes early in development that serve to distinguish it clearly from the spinal cord. The changes start before the end of the formative phase and include rotation of its lateral walls 'comparable to opening of a book' as it was described many years ago by Langman (1963) (Fig. 20).

Subsequently, the extended roof plate, the future inferior medullary velum, presents only a layer of ependymal cells attached to both lateral walls. The floor plate remains as this of the fourth ventricle. The internal structure of the lateral walls is similar to that of the spinal cord, but the topographical relationship between the columns of nerve cells that give rise to brain stem nuclei changes. The basal plate of the myelencephalon, occupying both sides of the median sulcus, divides into the median group, including somatic efferent nuclei, and the lateral group for the visceral efferent center. The still visible sulcus limitans separates the basal from the alar plate, which becomes subdivided into a medial and a lateral part. Those intrinsic topographical relationships within the nerve tube structures are also seen at the tegmental level within the ventral part of the metencephalon, the future pons.

During week 5 (stage 14), the motor nuclei of cranial nerves III to XII appear in both the ventromedial and ventrolateral columns along all parts of the brain stem, including the mesencephalon, pons and medulla. Their axons form the motor roots. At the same time, the sensory ganglia give rise to the roots of cranial nerves V, VII, VIII, IX and X, with differentiation of neurons in sensory columns occurring later than in motor columns.

The external relationships between myelencephalic and metencephalic derivatives are modified during the next 5–7 weeks (developmental stages 14, 16 and 17) because of changes in brain stem flexures. The mesencephalic flexure forms an acute angle, while the opposite pontine flexure appears at the level of the isthmus, and the cervical flexure between the myelencephalon and the spinal cord forms a right angle. Those events lead to the enlargement of the fourth ventricle and to an approach of anterior and posterior lateral walls at 6–8 weeks of development. The anterior part 'bends over' the posterior part (Figs. 19 and 21). It is the first step in the process by which the growing cerebellum obtains (week 14) its position over the roof of the fourth ventricle (Sidman & Rakic, 1982). The formation of the fourth ventricle correlates with the appearance of the choroid plexus at about the end of 6 weeks of development (French, 1983). The median aperture (foramen of Magendie) of the fourth ventricle opens before the end of the second month or even the fourth month (Gardner, 1973; Sarnat, 1992c). The lateral apertures open some time later (Gardner, 1973), preparing the pathways of CSF circulation. More details on the development of CSF pathways are presented in the chapter on the entire ventricular system.

At this time, the mesencephalon is the most prominent part of the brain stem (Fig. 21), with internal differentiation of its structures correlating with that in other parts of the brain stem. Such internal differentiation within the brain stem progresses during the second part of the second developmental month.

Between the sixth and seventh week (stages 16, 17), the motor nerve nuclei reach their final positions. The changes in their final localization appear to occur in a passive way. The displacement of cell aggregates is apparently due to the formation of other cellular structures and to the changes in configuration of the brain stem (Sidman & Rakic, 1982). At this stage, the nucleus ambiguous is finally formed, and the eighth cranial nerve has both vestibular and cochlear components. Axons of the nerve cells start to form the brain stem pathways, including the medial longitudinal fascicles, and the cerebro-bulbar and tecto-bulbar tracts. According to Sidman and Rakic (1982), the developmental events by the end of week 7 place the 'principal neuronal system' for rhombencephalic reflexes in 'definitive' positions.

In addition to the existing principal cranial nerve nuclei, new neuronal formations appear successively just before the end of the second developmental month. The salivatory nuclei and locus coeruleus appear in the medulla oblongata, whereas the red nucleus and substantia nigra emerge in the mesencephalon. The end of the second month also brings the appearance of pyramidal tract decussation.

By the end of this month, the cellular source in the ventricular zone of the fourth ventricle is depleted, but a new source of nerve cells is present in the rhombic lip. The rhombic lip, from which the corpus ponto-bulbare originates (Sarnat, 1992c), represents a special area of the subventricular zone (Sidman & Rakic, 1982) located at the lateral part of the brain stem along the line of attachment of the roof of the fourth ventricle. It is a major source of cells that will migrate to several target points into the brain stem, both superficially through the subpial marginal zone and more centrally through the intermediate zone. It also provides the cells for the cerebellar external granular layer, which will be described later in a separate chapter. This cellular migration is ongoing at stage 23 of development (Müller & O'Rahilly, 1990b). Neurons migrating through superficial pathways provide the cellular material for the inferior olivary nuclei, arcuate nuclei and basal pontine nuclei. Mitotic activity in the rhombic lip and migration of its derivatives lasts until the beginning of the sixth month of development, when the corpus ponto-bulbare disappears.

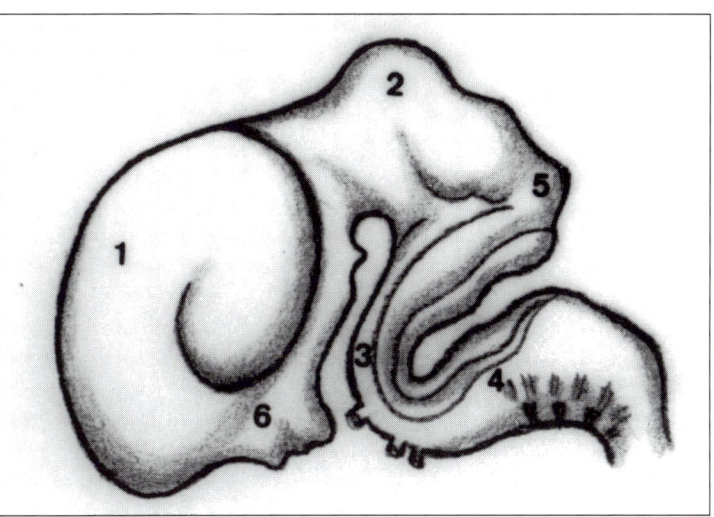

Fig. 21. Lateral view of brain stem flexure at 8.5 WG.

1. Cerebral hemispheres
2. Mesencephalon
3. Pons
4. Medulla
5. Isthmus
6. Diencephalon

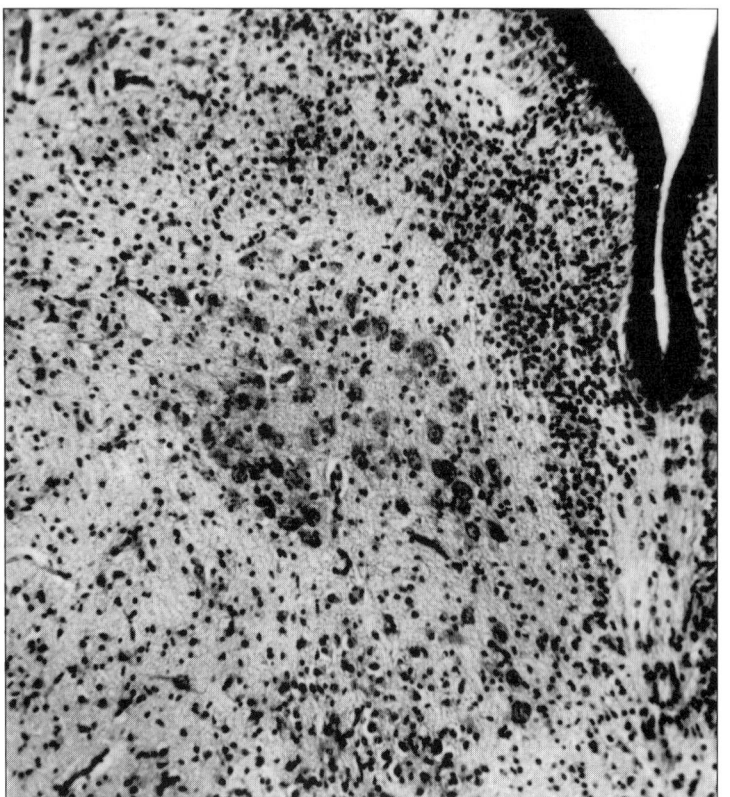

Fig. 22. Tegmental part of medulla with hypoglossal nucleus at midgestation. Cresyl violet, × 160.

During this period, other important events occur at the level of the mesencephalon. In the course of the third month, the nuclei of the oculomotor complex, i.e. nucleus of Perlia and of Westfall-Edinger, appear, but this complex acquires its final structure after midgestation.

The red nucleus, which arises from the basal plate during the second month, develops considerably during the third month. Populations of small and large neurons are still seen within this nucleus, but they differentiate until the fifth month. This nucleus takes on its final shape no sooner than within five postnatal years.

The substantia nigra also has a long period of differentiation and maturation. This complex structure arises during week 7, and grows during the next weeks, to extend from the pons to the subthalamic area. Although the cells demonstrate the first pigment granules at about the sixth postnatal month, the final form and pigmentation of the substantia nigra is not complete until the fifth postnatal year.

By midgestation, the quadrigeminal plate, which begins to form during the second month but is very visible during the third month, is complete. The growth of all structures of the mesencephalon tegmental region leads to the diminution and narrowing of the mesencephalic ventricle, ultimately forming the aqueduct of Sylvius. When the intrinsic structure of the brain stem is complete, the ensuing developmental events include maturation of nerve cells (Fig. 22) and their processes and elaboration of synaptic contacts. Takashima and Becker (1986) performed a detailed morphometric evaluation of those contacts, using Golgi impregnation techniques. They documented that medullary respiratory centers demonstrate maturation, resulting in the final number of dendritic spines during the first postnatal year.

In this overview of brain stem development, reticular formation was omitted, because this phylogenetically very old, diffuse structure presents particular difficulties in observing the appearance of its elements and is thus insufficiently characterized in its early phases of development.

Cerebellum

The tuberculum cerebelli, or the cerebellar primordium, appears at the end of formative phase (week 4) of CNS development, but it is more evident in the middle of next week (stages 14, 15). This structure arise from the dorsolateral part of the alar plate of the rhombencephalon anterior segment and from the isthmic segment (Müller & O'Rahilly, 1989a) rostrally from the anterior roof of the fourth ventricle. Sidman and Rakic (1982) described its shape as an inverted letter 'V.' The considerable development of symmetric structures in the lateral walls of the fourth ventricle results in their fusion at about 7 weeks of development

(Sarnat 1992c). Sidman and Rakic (1982) described the cerebellum not as the fusion product of two components of a paired organ, but rather as an unpaired structure with different rates of development of its central and lateral components.

The growth of cerebellar primordium is so conspicuous during the early phase, that between the fifth and sixth week of development (stages 16, 17) the cerebellar plate is wider than the telencephalon (measuring the diagonal diameter of both hemispheres together), (Müller & O'Rahilly, 1989a,b). At this stage, the cerebellar primordium is growing downward into the lumen of the fourth ventricle, which is enlarged as a sequel of the formation of the pontine flexure (French, 1983) (Fig. 23).

The roof plate of the ventricle attached to the growing organ corresponds to a line that demarcates the ventricular and outer surface of the cerebellum. During the next weeks, the cerebellum expands also in an outer direction, forming its extraventricular part. The area representing flocculonodular lobe and primordium of corpus cerebelli including further vermis and cerebellar hemispheres, is recognizable even at weeks 5–6 of development (Müller & O'Rahilly, 1989a).

During the early stages of cerebellar development, the immature neuroepithelial cells, that give rise to its structures, derive from the ventricular zone of the anterior part of the fourth ventricle. The cerebellar wall presents three distinct layers: ventricular, intermediate and marginal. Starting at 8 weeks (stage 23), the layers of the cerebellar primordium change because of formation of the external granular layer. A unique aspect of cerebellar development is the availability of two germinal plates as sources of immature neuroepithelial cells. The first germinal plate, i.e. the primitive ventricular layer, provides the precursors of Purkinje cells, Golgi II and basket cells, and cells of the cerebellar nuclei (Sarnat, 1992c). The second germinal plate, i.e. the

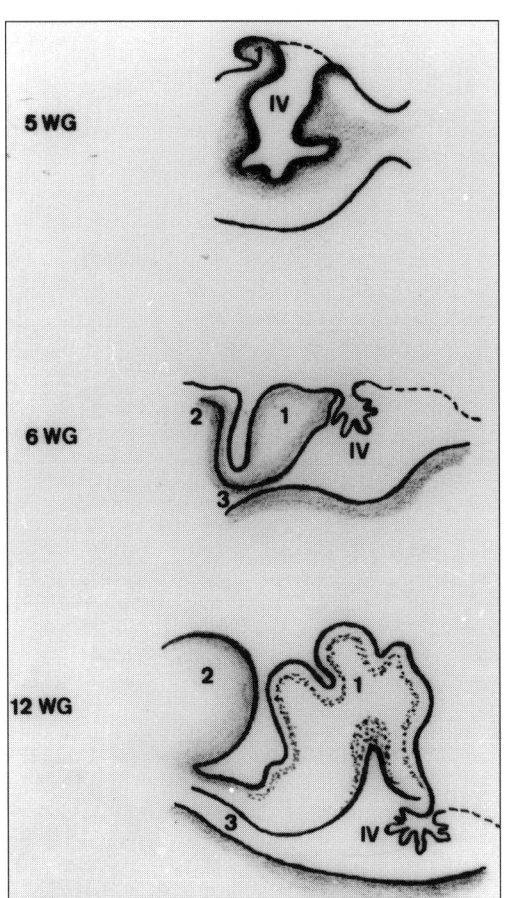

Fig. 23. Formation of cerebellar primordium (sagittal view).

1. Cerebellum
2. Mesencephalon
3. Aqueduct

external granular layer, consists of cells arriving from the lateral surface of the fourth ventricle (the rhombic lip). These cells multiply and migrate over the external subpial surface of the cerebellar primordium. They finally form the external granular layer, recognizable at 8 weeks, which will give rise to small neurons that migrate inwards and form the granular layer of the cerebellar cortex.

The sequence of cell multiplication and migration from both germinal plates overlaps such that the external and internal features of the cerebellum form gradually. Within the ventricular zone, the cells destined for the cerebellar nuclei appear first. At weeks 9–10, Purkinje cells arise (Müller & O'Rahilly, 1987) and finally Golgi II and basket cells. After long debates, it was fi-

Fig. 24. Formation of Purkinje cell layer in cerebellar hemisphere.

(a) at 20 WG, × 200;

(b) at 26 WG, × 200;

(c) at 32 WG, × 200.

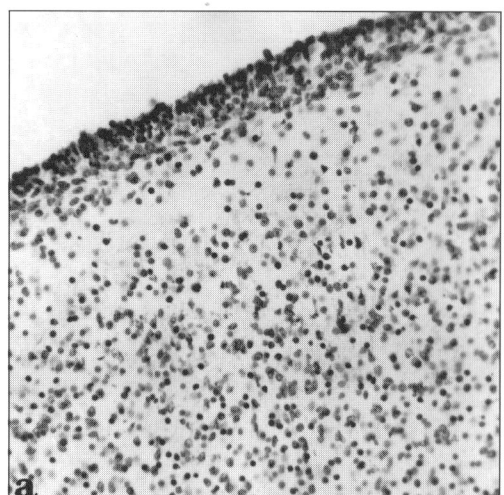
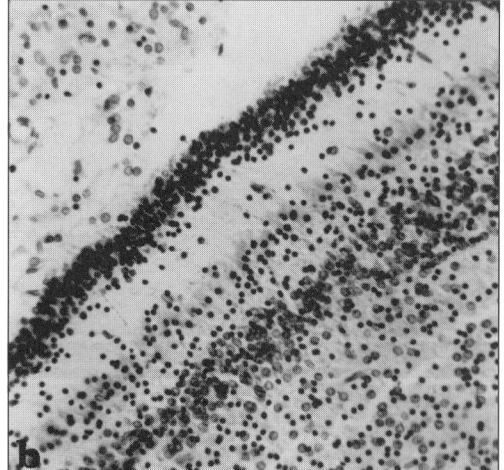
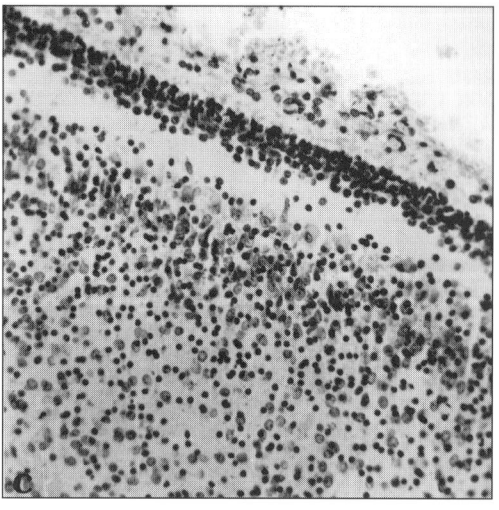

nally confirmed that most of the small neurons destined for the molecular layer arise from the ventricular zone (Hallonet et al., 1990). The Purkinje cells, still small, migrate through the cell-sparse future granular layer and reach their final site, indicating the line of the cerebellar cortex. They remain very immature and bipolar, but at 13 weeks (Sidman & Rakic, 1982), their layer can be well visualized. The groups of cells representing the deep cerebellar nuclei are also seen at this time. This appears to coincide with the end of cell multiplication in the cerebellar ventricular zone. After this phase, the cerebellum increases in volume, and cerebellar fissures begin to form at week 12. The postero-lateral fissure appears first, separating the nodulus and flocculus from the cerebellum proper, followed by other fissures in the vermis and then in the cerebellar hemispheres (Larsell, 1947). At 16 weeks, the cerebellum completely covers the fourth ventricle and appears as a well-formed structure. Advanced differentiation of the cerebellar internal structures is represented at this time by the cerebellar nuclei, which acquire their final form of fastiglial, emboliform and globose nuclei. Only the dentate nuclei require a lengthy developmental period, reaching final form after the fifth month of gestation (Sidman & Rakic, 1982). The extremely thick external granular layer seen at the eighth week gives rise to the future granular nerve cells about 3 months later. They migrate inward, through molecular layer and Purkinje cells layer to the internal granular layer. This process is accomplished with the help of Bergmann glia processes which serve as guides in the way between Purkinje and other cells. The migrating cells progressively occupy more external positions and finally form the granular layer. The migration of neuroblasts is similar to that of the telencephalic cortex. Cells proliferation within the external granular layer continues after birth. This layer begin to disappear shortly before birth, but is still visible postnatally for 7–9 months. The cerebellar cortex presents particular features in the second half of intrauterine development. The Purkinje cells, generated so early, remain 'dormant' for several weeks; but at 21 weeks of development, they already have many processes and at 22 weeks they even appear to form the first synapses (Fig. 24).

Between the 20th and 30th week, the developing cerebellar cortex presents a five-layered structure, containing the external granular, molecular, Purkinje cells layers as well as the lamina dissecans and internal granular layer. The cell-sparse lamina dissecans contains a great number of afferent axons when the target structure, i.e. the internal granular layer, is not ready to make appropriate contacts. Later, at about 30–32 weeks, the lamina dissecans disappears, and the wall of the cerebellar cortex is four-layered until the external granular layer is exhausted (Fig. 25).

Note that the developmental and maturation processes within the cerebellar structures occur approximately 2 weeks earlier in the archi- than in neocerebellar structures. This difference is reflected in the rate of extinction of the lamina dissecans (Larroche, 1977) and in exhaustion of the external granular layer. The maturation rate of Purkinje cells and their dendrites also evidences regional differences (Goodlett et al., 1990). During the maturation process, the cerebellum increases in volume, and the fissures develop (Fig. 26) such that the surface area of the cerebellum increases 2,000-fold by the seventh postnatal month. The myelination of cerebellar pathways is discussed in a separate section on Myelination of all CNS pathways (p. 60).

Prosencephalon (forebrain)

The forebrain comprises the telencephalon and the diencephalon, each forming paired structures. It includes all derivatives of the first primitive vesicle of the future brain, which can be identified together with the two other vesicles still in an open neural tube at about day 20 of development (stage 9) (Müller & O'Rahilly, 1983). They arise and develop successively after the closure of the anterior neuropore by the lamina terminalis at 24 days. During further development, the lamina terminalis will form the anterior wall of the future third ventricle and, as will be later discussed, participates in the formation of prosencephalic commissures; ventrally the formation of the optic chiasm will occur. The origin and role of the lamina terminalis are mentioned here in the light of recent suggestions that this structure participates in early stages of development and plays a particular role in the

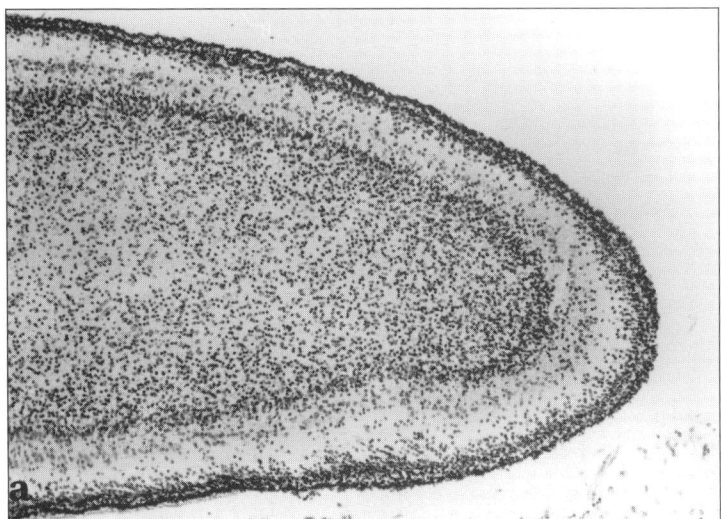
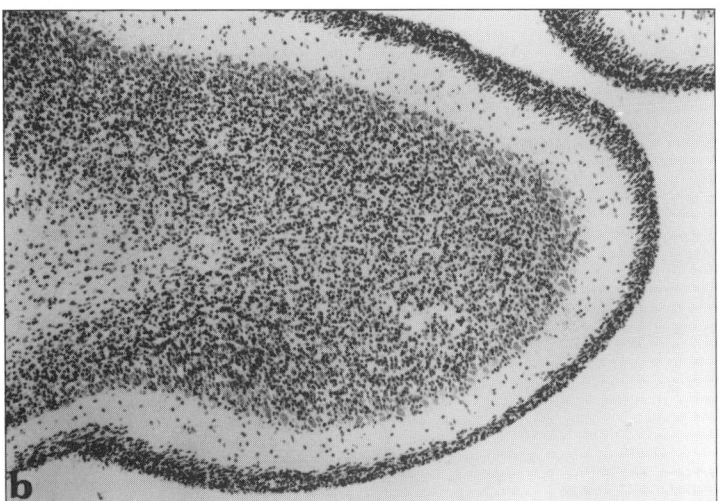

Fig. 25. Organization of cerebellar cortex.

(a) at 28 WG, × 120;

(b) at 40 WG, × 120.

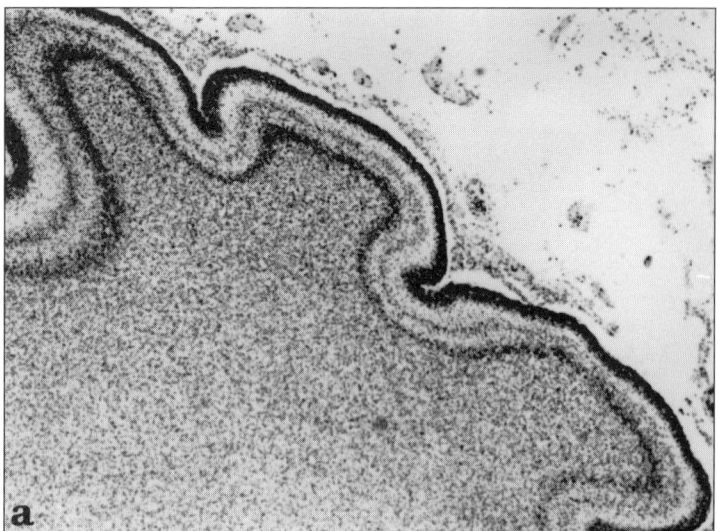

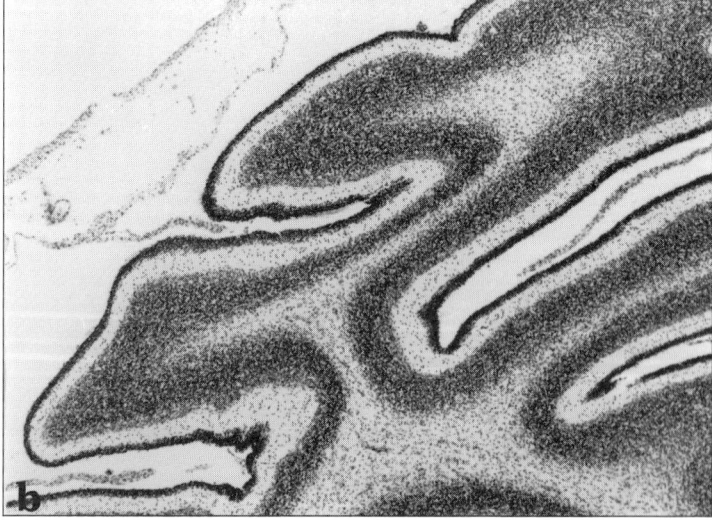

Fig. 26.
Development of cerebellar fissures.

(a) at 32 WG, × 80;

(b) at 40 WG, × 80.

origin of all prosencephalic structures (Müller & O'Rahilly, 1988a, 1989a; Sarnat, 1992c).

The derivatives of each half of the neural tube at the diencephalic level become tightly connected with telencephalic components, resulting in the formation of two symmetrical complexes of gray structures located in the deep periventricular area or at the basal surface of the brain. Finally, in current descriptions of the adult brain, the telencephalic and diencephalic derivatives are collectively called the brain hemispheres (Paxinos, 1990).

Diencephalic structures

Differentiation of the diencephalon is signaled by the focal symmetrical thickening of the ventricular wall, which contains the germinal material. The first lateral thickening appears at day 32 (stage 14), and another medial thickening arises at day 33 (stage 15). Müller and O'Rahilly (1988b,c) termed these structures 'ventricular eminences' instead of 'ganglionic eminences', the name used by the Boulder Committee (1970), or the older term, 'ridge'. After previous misinterpretations, these structures were finally recognized as the lateral eminence, being telencephalic and giving rise to the corpus striatum, and the medial eminence, which will provide cellular material to components of the diencephalon. The eminences, despite the developmental history of this part of the brain, are separated only by the sulcus strio-thalamicus (sulcus terminalis), which will contain the choroid plexus, and by the third month of development, the vena terminalis.

Diencephalic derivatives start to arise at the beginning of the second gestational month, which is characterized by evagination of the cerebral vesicles (Müller & O'Rahilly, 1988a) and formation of the future hemispheres, introducing the bilateral symmetry of the CNS. After this early stage, five subdivisions of the diencephalon can be recognized as longitudinal zones corresponding, respectively, to the future hypothalamus, subthalamus, ventral thalamus, epithalamus and dorsal thalamus (Kahle, 1956; Müller & O'Rahilly, 1988c, 1989a). All these structures are well visible at day 37 (stage 16). Starting with the hypothalamus, differentiation of all parts of the diencephalon occurs, in a partly sequential and partly simultaneous manner.

Development in the five zones of the diencephalon, which start to appear at 33–37 days of development (stages 15, 16), are described according to the time when they differentiate (Fig. 27).

Hypothalamus

The hypothalamus includes the mammillary bodies, which are the first hypothalamic subdivisions to appear during the sixth week of development (stages 16, 17), and its connections, the mamillo-tegmental and mamillo-thalamic tracts, which arise during the ensuing weeks (Sidman & Rakic, 1982). The hypothalamus *sensu stricto* develops much later. It includes vegetative centers, i.e. preoptic, supraoptic, paraventricular, ventro-medial and dorso-medial nuclei, which appear sequentially. The preoptic nucleus is seen at about 6 weeks (stage 17) of development (Müller & O'Rahilly, 1989b). The supraoptic and paraventricular nuclei can be identified at 12 weeks, and their secretory activity is detected at 18 weeks (Vladimirov & Altukhova, 1983). All hypothalamic nuclei are discernible at the third month of development. Within this region, neuronal migration is observed (Kahle, 1956) between the end of the second and the beginning of the third months, when an appropriate ventricular germinal zone becomes exhausted. Afferent fibers grow into the hypothalamic structure, participating in its final differentiation. Maturation of this area probably continues even after birth because the volume of the hypothalamus in newborns is small compared with that in adult brains.

Subthalamus

The subthalamus is an important part of the diencephalon because it comprises among other components (e.g. fields of Forel), nuclei belonging to the extrapyramidal system: the globus pallidus, endopeduncular nucleus and subthalamic nucleus (of Luys).

The derivation of the globus palladium from this part of the CNS was recognized first by Spatz (1924, 1925) and later confirmed by Kahle (1956) and Müller and O'Rahilly (1989a). The structure begins its development at the sixth week of fetal life (stage 16). At the seventh week (stages 18–20), the external parts of the globus pallidus and other components of the hypothalamus form their predominant features. Kahle (1956) noted that their formation is rapid, after an early exhaustion of germinal centers. Further development results in a situation whereby the globus pallidus occupies a lateral position between subthalamic components and is localized in the hemisphere. Thereafter, it is incorporated into the telencephalon between the 10th and 14th weeks, first the lateral and then the medial portion (Sidman & Rakic, 1982). The subthalamic nucleus arises on day 37 (stage 16) (Fig. 28).

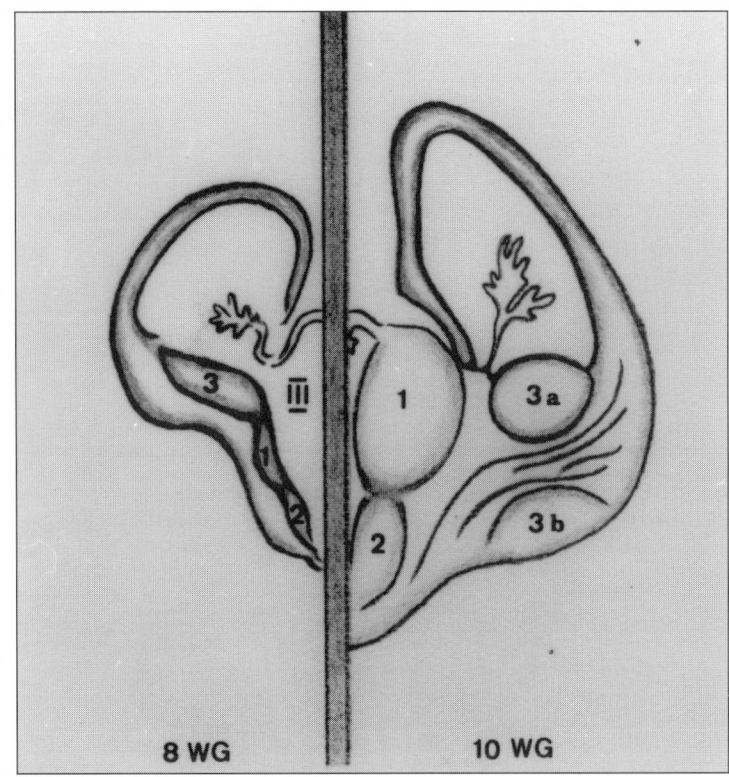

Fig. 27.
Development of diencephalon and striatum
1. Thalamus
2. Hypothalamus
3. Striatum
(a) caudate nucleus
(b) lentiform nucleus

Ventral thalamus

This zone is recognized as a part of the diencephalon when the subthalamus is definitely considered as a separate part, and constitutes the dominant part of the diencephalon at the beginning of the third month. During consecutive differentiation,

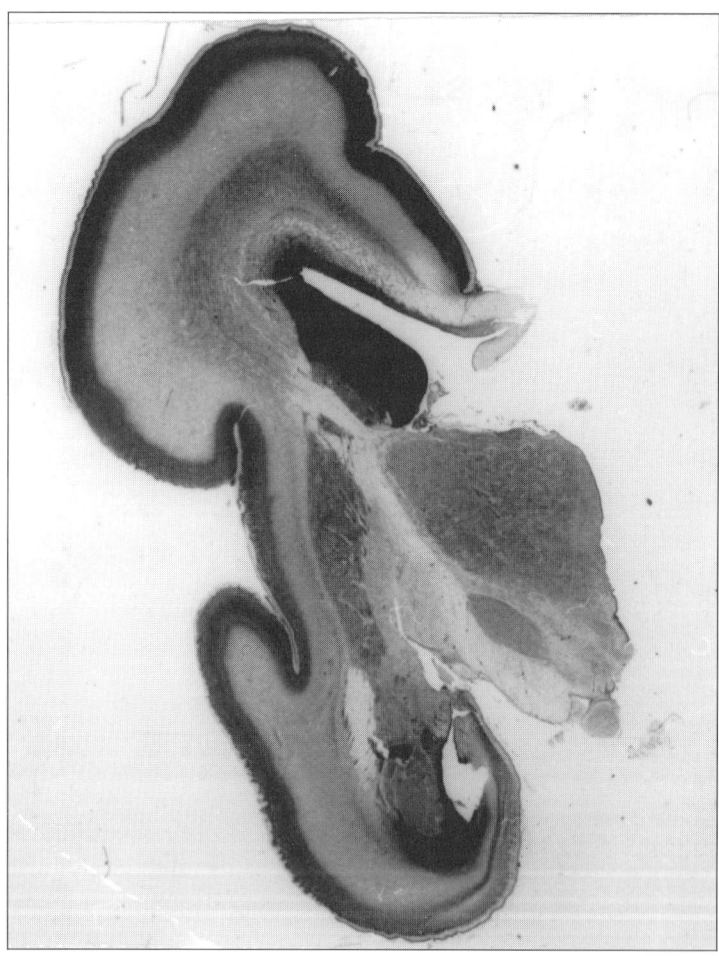

Fig. 28. Coronal section of cerebral hemisphere at middle of gestation including diencephalic derivates. Cresyl violet, × 3.

the zone incerta, the reticular nucleus, and the ventral part of the corpus geniculatum laterale can be recognized as compounds of the ventral thalamus.

Epithalamus

The epithalamus corresponds to the habenular structures, with the primordium of habenulae appearing at week 6–7 of development (stages 17–19) and the habenular commissure forming at week 9.

Dorsal thalamus

The dorsal thalamus is the last of the diencephalic components to develop (Fig. 28). The ventricular zone of the dorsal thalamus is very thick between the eighth and 12th week of development, providing an abundance of cellular material in a rather short time. Exhaustion of this zone starts during the second half of the third month. In the part destined to become the pulvinar, germinal material remains until the first week of the fourth month. The pulvinar arises during the 16th and 34th week. The fascicles of nerve fibers entering and passing through the thalamus play an important role in its differentiation. The intensive growth of the *pars dorsalis thalami* influences the final position of the ventral thalamus and the epithalamus. Sidman and Rakic (1982) proposed the following course of thalamic development. The differentiation of specific sensory nuclei (visual, auditory, tactile) is followed by nonspecific thalamo-striatal and other connections and finally by the appearance of the last associative nuclei. Note that the projections from the thalamus to the telencephalon arise earlier than the topographic organization of the telencephalic cortex.

The lateral geniculate nuclei, including in part derivatives of the ventral thalamus, becomes demarcated from the thalamus at week 8 and present their laminated structure at 22 weeks of development (Sidman & Rakic, 1982).

The simultaneous enlargement of diencephalic derivatives and cerebral vesicles, combined with the increase in axons and in interaxonal connection, leads to the striato-thalamic junction during the third month of development. This junction results in the formation of a macroscopically uniform mass of subcortical gray structures.

In the fourth month of development, the growth of the thalamus results in the formation of the massa intermedia, which produces a partial fusion of thalami of both hemispheres.

Besides the five diencephalon components, we will mention three diencephalic derivatives that either are not connected or belong only partially to this portion of the CNS in the adult brain. All three appear early during development.

Eyes. The optic primordia appear at 22 days (Sarnat 1992c), or occur according to O'Rahilly and Müller (1994) at day 24 (stage 10) at the rostral end of the neural plate before closure of the neural tube. Eyes appear at 28–32 days of development (stages 13, 14), when the optic cup and lens are observed. Growth of retinal elements is evidenced at 5–6 weeks (stage 15–17), when optic vesicles are pushed ventrally and rostrally, reaching their final position and developing during the next months. At the seventh month, the retina is nearly mature and at 8 months, can respond to light impulses (Sidman & Rakic, 1982).

Amygdaloid complex. Its primordium appears during the fifth week of development (stages 14, 15) (Müller & O'Rahilly, 1988b,c). The origin of this nuclear group named 'the basal ganglion of temporal lobe' (Sidman & Rakic, 1982), was very controversial and for a long time was attributed mainly to the telencephalon (Kahle, 1969; Sidman & Rakic, 1982). More recent investigations indicate that the early stages of amygdaloid body formation derive from the medial diencephalic eminence (Müller & O'Rahilly, 1988c). Since day 37 (stage 16) the medial eminence includes a telencephalic component and its relation with the amygdaloid complex could also be taken into account (Müller & O'Rahilly, 1989a). The amygdaloid complex develops intensively during the sixth to seventh week, when four nuclei – basal, central, lateral and cortical – can be identified (stages 18–20) (Müller & O'Rahilly, 1990a). These nuclei are well-differentiated by the fourth month. The cyto-architectural development in the amygdala also reveals some transient cell units. Nikolic and Kostovic (1986) found such transient cell clusters in the fetal lateral amygdaloid nucleus at 11–24 weeks of development, during final differentiation of this structure.

Hypophysis. During development of the floor plate at the level of the hypothalamus, the adenohypophysis, the ectodermal derivative closely associated with the infundibulum, forms at about 32 days (stage 14). During the fifth WG (stages 16, 17), the neurohypophysis appears (Müller & O'Rahilly, 1988a,b). It reveals neurosecretory granules after 10 WG (Vladimirov & Altukhova, 1983).

Telencephalic structures

Pallium

The formation and maturation of the entire cortical mantle, i.e. pallium, might represent one of most important processes in CNS ontogeny and phylogeny. It is also one of the longest processes in CNS development, beginning with the emergence of the primordium of hemispheric vesicles, which heralds the bilateral symmetry of the brain. Cortical maturation, resulting in final organization of the brain as an active organ and the coordination of all human activity is completed several years after birth. The gray matter that covers the cerebral hemispheres as pallium is a heterogeneous formation. Differences in the three parts of the pallium are demonstrated by (a) the time and rate of development, (b) the proportion of formation of the ventral surface of hemispheres, and (c) the cytoarchitecture of each part of the cortex. The different parts of the pallium include (1) paleocortex, the most primitive, (2) the archicortex, and (3) the neocortex, the most developed in humans. All of these parts appear very early in ontogeny. Recent comparative studies show that even the mammals that are phylogenetically earliest, have a six-layered cortex. Northcutt and Kaas (1995) proposed to change the designation neocortex, archicortex and paleocortex for isocortex, hippocampal and olfactory cortex respectively. Nevertheless, the particular histogenetic characteristics and the degree of differentiation in species at various levels

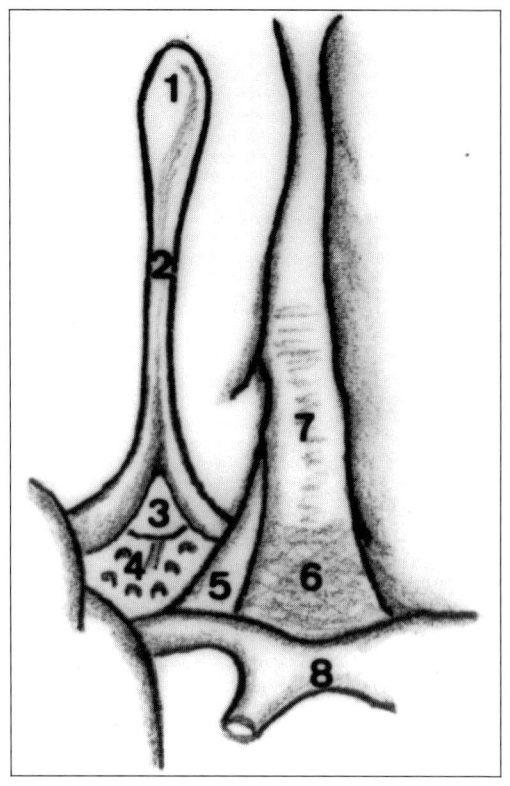

Fig. 29. The peripheral part of the rhinencephalon.

1. Olfactory bulb
2. Olfactory tract
3. Olfactory tubercle
4. Anterior perforate substance
5. Diagonal band
6. Lamina terminalis
7. Corpus callosum
8. Optic chiasm

Both the paleocortex and archicortex belong to the allocortex, (Filimonov, 1947; Vogt & Vogt, 1919), which never presents as the six-layered structure characteristic of the neocortex. Sidman and Rakic (1982), adopting the view of earlier neuroanatomists (Filimonov, 1947; Feremutsch, 1962), separated the third transitional type of the cortex, the periallocortex or mesocortex. The periallocortex is located between some allopallial and neopallial structures, and the periarchicortex portion borders archicortical structures. Other authors, such as Kahle (1969), do not accept this classification, including the mesocortical structures as paleopallium and archipallium, but a more detailed classification appears to better reflect the complexity of the cortex covering the human pallium (Table 2).

We describe below the consecutive development of all three components of the hemispheric pallium. It will become clear that the allocortical structures, particularly the paleocortex, present several still unsolved problems.

of development suggest the use of the traditional designation.

The paleocortex (olfactory cortex) is the most primitive component of the cerebral

Table 2. Division of cortical mantel (according to Sidman & Rakic, 1982)

Division of cortical mantel (according to Sidman, Rakic, 1982)

I Allocortex

1) Paleocortex
  - olfactory
  - ant. perforate
  - periamygdal cortex
  - septal area

2) Archicortex
  Hippocampal formation
  - Hippocampus
  - Subiculum
  - Dentate gyrus

  Periarchiocortex
  - entorhinal cortex
  - presubiculum
  - parasubiculum

Peripaleocortex
  - insular cortex
  - prepirifom area (rostral part)

II Mesocortex = periallcortex
  - Claustrum

III Isocortex = Neocortex

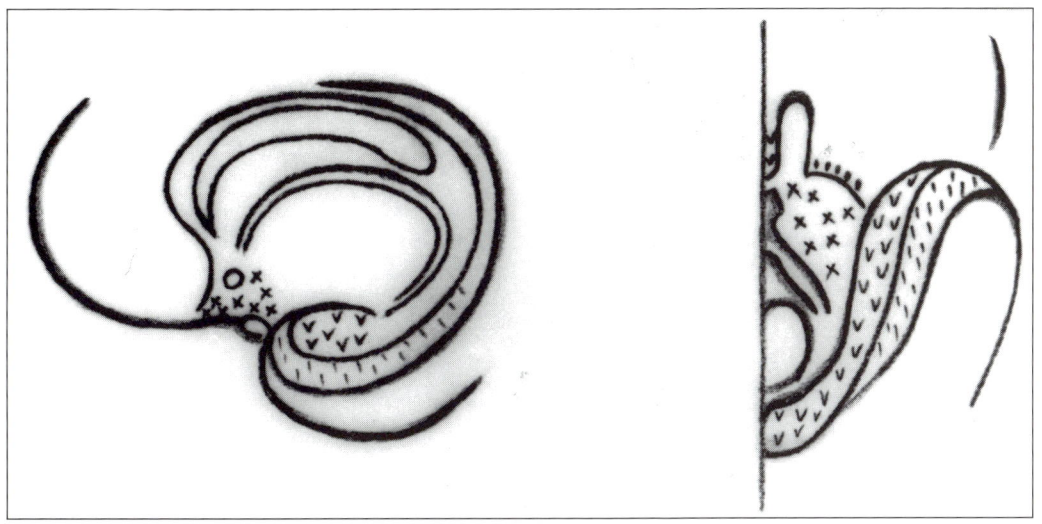

Fig. 30. Area occupied by the allocortex at 4–5 months' of fetal life.

**** Peripaleocortex
++++ Paleocortex
vvvv Archicortex
////// Periarchicortex

pallium and, in large part, it is intimately associated with olfactory function (the peripheral part of the rhinencephalon) (Fig. 29). The paleocortex is localized on the basal surface of the brain and does not change position during development, although the relative participation of its components on the surface of the hemispheric wall changes considerably.

During the early stages of development, the primitive paleocortex occupies most of this surface. This proportional preponderance continues through the third to fourth month, but later, the growth of the neopallium changes those relations (Fig. 30). In adult brains, the paleocortex is restricted to a small area, in part not well visible behind the pole of temporal lobe. It should be mentioned that during the fourth and fifth months of gestation, the development of the corpus callosum (CC) and positional changes in the hippocampus make the topography of the paleocortical region less clear, and the participation of this region in the total area of the hemispheric surface gradually diminishes.

Note that paleocortical structures differ enough from all other cortical areas to raise questions about their inclusion in the cerebral cortex. Nevertheless, they constitute a part of pallium that covers a segment of the antero-ventral surface of the telencephalon.

The paleocortex arises very early in development. Müller and O'Rahilly (1988b) observed the primordium of olfactory area at the 32nd day of development (stage 14). Kahle (1969) noted that each part of gray matter of the hemispheres (cortex, nuclei) receives nerve cells from a precisely delineated segment of matrix, lining the ventricular wall. During early development, this relationship is visualized even in routine morphological staining by the topography of matrix centers and the migration of neuroblasts to target areas. The synchronous events of development – the exhaustion of germinal cells and the formation of proper structures – confirm this sequence of events. The germinal cells destined to become part of the paleocortex originate from the matrix centers localized in the floor of the lateral ventricle.

All parts of the paleocortex develop gradually during the second and fourth month, acquiring their final architectonic features, and mature further during the fifth month. The topographical connections between matrix segments and their paleocortical derivatives continue to exist during the third month of development, but gradually disappear during the fourth month. This is due to outgrowth of the striatum, which protrudes between the germinal layer and targets paleocortical areas into the anterior horn of the lateral ventricle. The topographical relations in this region change, and the rest of the germinal layers for the paleocortex become limited to the medial part of the ganglionic eminence and the ventricular angle. Considering the very early beginning of paleocortical development, it is somewhat surprising that its matrix is not totally exhausted until the seventh month, when only ependymal cells line this segment of the ventricular wall (Kahle, 1969). During the maturation of the paleocortex, some cytoarchitectonic characteristics appear. The pallium of the olfactory tubercle assumes a cortex-like appearance, but none of the paleocortex components acquire the features of a true cortex.

Kahle (1969) noted slow migration of neuroblasts from the matrix centers to paleocortical structures beginning in the second developmental month and lasting for a long period. During migration, a continuous mass of neurons is seen between the germinal layer and target areas. These cells never form a true cortical plate characteristic for development of the neocortex (Filimonov, 1947; Macchi 1951). At about day 41 (stage 17) of development (Müller and O'Rahilly, 1989b), the future paleocortex, archicortex and neocortex are easily distinguishable. The development of paleocortical structures including olfactory bulbs, anterior perforate substance, periamygdaloid cortex and septal area progress since this early period.

The olfactory bulb. The olfactory bulb, which was described over 100 years ago by His (1889), is considered an evagination of the paleocortex appearing at the end of the sixth week and continuing to develop until the 13th week, when the olfactory ventricle is well formed. The internal histological differentiation of the olfactory bulb occurs between 8 and 13 weeks, when olfactory cell layers are well formed. The olfactory nerve fibers arise from the olfactory placode fibers form the external layer (which has a peripheral origin), even before the formation of the olfactory bulb. At about 18 weeks, the olfactory nerve fibers from the external layer of the olfactory bulb (Sidman & Rakic, 1982). The anterior olfactory nucleus develops at about the end of the second month around the caudal end of olfactory ventricle. During further maturation, all acquired features of the olfactory bulb regress somewhat. The olfactory ventricle disappears around 18.5 weeks in most cases, a process that exemplifies the regression of some structures and functions in humans in comparison with species that are phylogenetically more primitive (Crosby et al., 1961).

The anterior perforate substance. The anterior perforate substance, comprising the prepiriform area, and the olfactory tubercle located posteriorly to the olfactory bulb also begin their development very early. The olfactory tubercle was observed by Humphrey (1967) at the beginning of the sixth week, before the appearance of the olfactory bulb. This was confirmed by O'Rahilly et al. (1987), who described its appearance at the 37th day (stage 16).

The periamygdaloid cortex. The periamygdaloid cortex is considered by Sidman and Rakic (1982) as a component of the paleocortex. It also appears at the middle of the second month, during the third and fourth months of development, it is divided progressively into three and finally four subdivisions, and until the end of fetal life is rotated in the medial direction within the temporal lobe.

The area of the prosencephalic septum. The most anterior and medial parts of the developing prosencephalon, arise from the ventricular layer of the antero-medial hemispheric wall. The prosencephalic septum has similar close developmental relationships not only with paleocortical, but also diencephalic hypothalamic components. It is located in the medial part of the paleocortex, anteriorly to the lamina terminalis (Fig. 31) and should be distinguished from the septum pellucidum, which, according to Sidman and Rakic (1982), derives from the archicortex. The decussation of anterior commissure fibers passes through the septal area.

The first structural features of the septal nucleus are noted at day 41 of development (stage 17) (Müller & O'Rahilly, 1989b). The primordium of the nucleus of the diagonal band (of Broca) appears and is well-visible together with the medial septal nucleus at 6–7 WG (stages 18–20) (Müller & O'Rahilly, 1990a). Other nuclei appear subsequently, together with the nucleus accumbens septi, whose inclusion in the septal area is still being debated. At 15–16 WG, the lateral zone of the septal area already shows extensive differentiation, and during the first postnatal months, the entire formation becomes well differentiated (Brown, 1983). That author suggested a role for septal connections in the organization of the limbic system. The septal area, together with the nucleus basalis complex (nucleus of Meynert), is known for its cholinergic activity. The cholinergic system is detectable in the nucleus of Meynert during the first trimester of prenatal development (Candy et al., 1985). Kostovic (1986) showed that histochemical differentiation starts here at the ninth week of development, increases 2 weeks later, and at 15 weeks, acetylcholinesterase (AChE)-reactive cells are seen in the already well-differentiated nuclei, i.e. basal, diagonal and medial septal. During further development, until the 35th week, fibers with AChE-reactivity extend to the subplate zone of all neocortical regions. The connections of the septal nuclei suggest their importance in behavioral and cognitive functions (Müller & O'Rahilly, 1990a).

According to several neuroanatomists (Rose, 1926; Filimonov, 1947), the peripaleocortex is comprised of an insular and a prepiriform region. It may be well delineated during the third month of development. The segments of the peripaleocortex

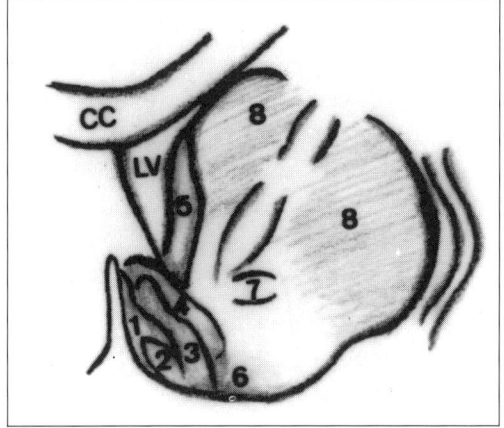

differentiate during maturation, and ultimately four segments present a gradient from the paleocortex to the neocortex to which peripaleocortex is connected with no demarcation.

Archicortex (hippocampal complex)

The archicortical structures including the dentate gyrus, Ammon's horn and subicu-

Fig. 31. Area of prosencephalic septum:

CC – Corpus callosum
LV – Lateral ventricle
1 – Medial septal nucleus
2 – Nucleus of the diagonal band
3 – Islands of Caleja
4 – Nucleus accumbens septi
5 – Lateral septal nucleus
6 – Olfactory tubercle
7 – Anterior commissure
8 – Striatum

Fig. 32. Early stages of archicortex formation.

AC – archicortex
V – ventricle

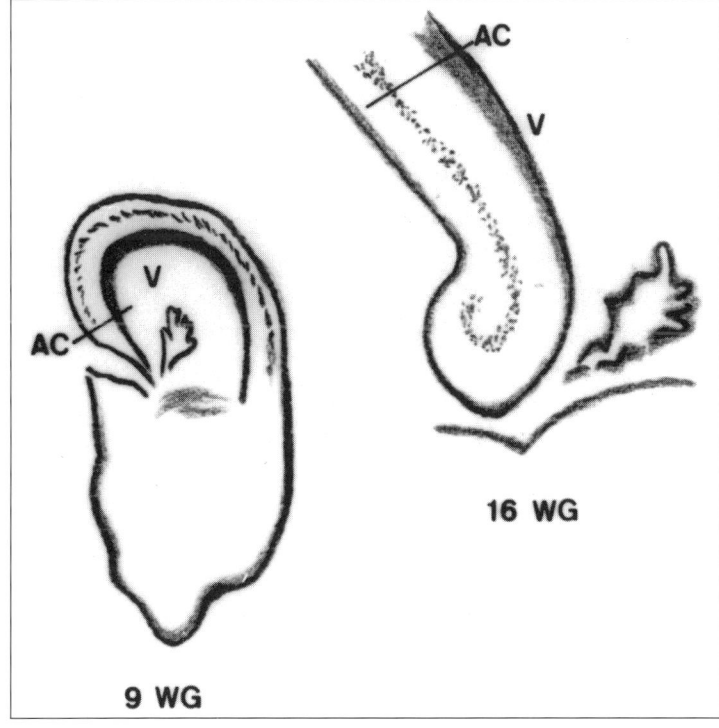

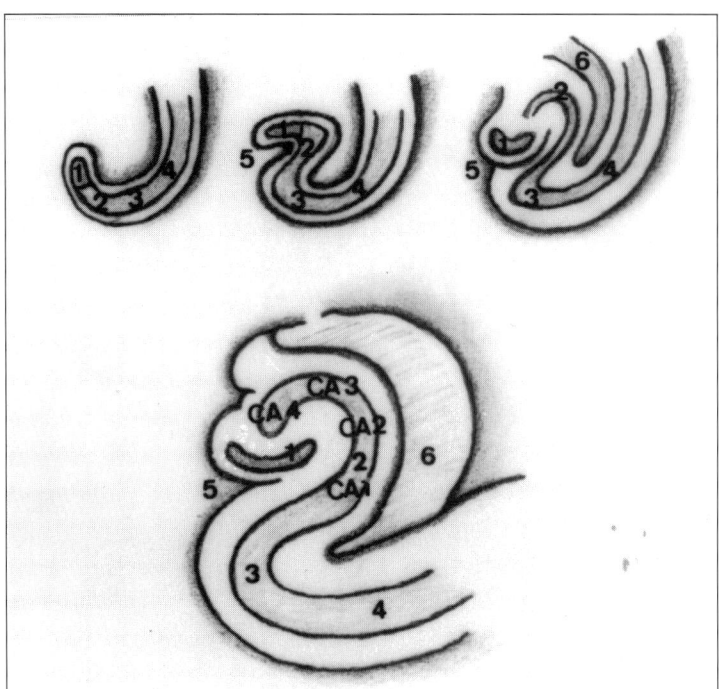

Fig. 33. Rolling out of archicortex stripe:

1. Dentate gyrus
2. Ammon's horn
3. Subiculum
4. Entorhinal cortex
5. Hippocampal sulcus
6. Ventricle

lum, form the hippocampal formation (Sidman & Rakic, 1982).

The hippocampal region is localized when telencephalic vesicles arise at the medial part of each of them (Fig. 32), occupying a large portion of these vesicles during the early stages of development (Kahle, 1969). From the 10th–16th week of development, the position of the hippocampal region changes, and by the end of the fourth month, its anterior part extends as only a thin taenia tecta above the CC and as rudimental grey tissue together with the septum pellucidum below the CC. More posteriorly, the archicortical structures form the characteristic Ammon's horn with the adjacent periarchicortex. The related developmental processes play a role in the final formation and localization of hippocampal region.

The formation of telencephalon, or 'rotation' as described by Kahle (1969), consists of extensive growth of telencephalic vesicles in the anterior, upper and lateral directions in respect to centrally located basal ganglia. This results in gradually progressing formation of hemispheric lobes, when the archicortex remains at its primary parasagittal position. The development of the CC alters the topography of growing archicortical structures, inducing their distention in the antero-posterior direction. This results in extreme thinning of their anterior part (indusium griseum, tenia tecta) and more caudal localization of the hippocampal formation. The formation of hemispheric lobes is followed by the formation of three horns of lateral ventricles. The rolling out (Fig. 33) of the archicortical stripe results in a final modeling of Ammon's horn and the protrusion of the eminence of Ammon's horn into the inferior horn of the lateral ventricle.

Archicortical structures begin to develop early on. The primordium of the hippocampus appears at day 32 of development (stage 14) (Müller & O'Rahilly, 1988a) as a thickening of the dorso-medial wall of the telencephalic vesicle. It is more clearly identifiable at day 33 (stage 15) (Müller & O'Rahilly, 1988b). The germinal layer destined for the archicortex occupies a relatively large part of the ventricular wall, dorsally to the choroidal fissure and deep in the interhemispheric fissure. This segment is well-demarcated and characterized by a rather thin matrix. At day 42 (stage 17) (Müller & O'Rahilly, 1989b), the wall of the cerebral hemispheres reveals the features in its marginal layer that distinguish segments corresponding to the future paleocortex, archicortex and neocortex, but neuronal migration to the archicortex has not yet begun. At those early developmental stages (around the seventh week of development) before differentiation of archicortical structures, the cell population that appears anteriorly to the hippocampal primordium migrates tangentially over the telencephalic surface, giving rise to the subpial granular layer seen during neocortical development (Rakic & Yakovlev, 1968).

Neuronal migration to the archicortex from the ventricular zone begins during the third month of development, first to Ammon's horn and then to the dentate gyrus (Angevine, 1975). Both of those structures are recognizable at the 10th week of development. The lack of the cortical plate (Kahle, 1969) distinguishes archicortical from neocortical formations. Neuronal migration to Ammon's horn proceeds from the inside to the outside, the first cells populating the internal and the last, the external levels of the cortical structure which is normal for the entire cortical mantle. Neurons destined for dentate gyrus arrive in the sequence of outside to inside, arising along the inner margin of the granular layer and then are simply displaced outward (Angevine, 1975). Only during the early phase (about 13 weeks) does the dentate gyrus have a cortex-like appearance (Sidman & Rakic, 1982). The process of neuronal migration to hippocampal areas becomes intensive at 10–12 weeks of development. At the end of week 12, the border between the hippocampus and the subiculum is clearly visible.

Within Ammon's horn, parts of the cortical stripe, i.e. sectors CA1, CA2 and CA3, are identifiable at 13–14 weeks and area CA2 remains from this time the most differentiated (the CA4 sector is not taken into account by this author) (Angevine, 1965) (Fig. 34).

The events associated with neuronal migration and differentiation lead to different growth patterns in Ammon's horn and the dentate gyrus, which results in 'rotation' of the structures and formation of the hippocampal fissure (Fig. 33). According to Humphrey (1967a), 'the definitive hippocampal fissure first appears when differences in growth rate of the gyrus dentatus and the cornu Ammonis result in a thicker telencephalic wall in the dentate gyrus'. Between the 10th and 16th weeks, the hippocampal fissure shifts, progressively separating the granular layer of the dentate gyrus from the hippocampal pyramidal layer. The fissure extends to the surface close to the junction of Ammon's horn and the subiculum. During 18–20 weeks, the hippocampal fissure continues to shift, and at the end of structural development, it lies between the granular layer of the dentate gyrus and the entorhinal area. Further growth of archicortical structures ultimately obliterates the hippocampal fissure. Efferent fibers of the entorhinal area reach the external layer of archicortical structures (dentate gyrus), crossing this fused fissure. These efferent fibers are involved in the formation of the wide *lamina zonalis* of the

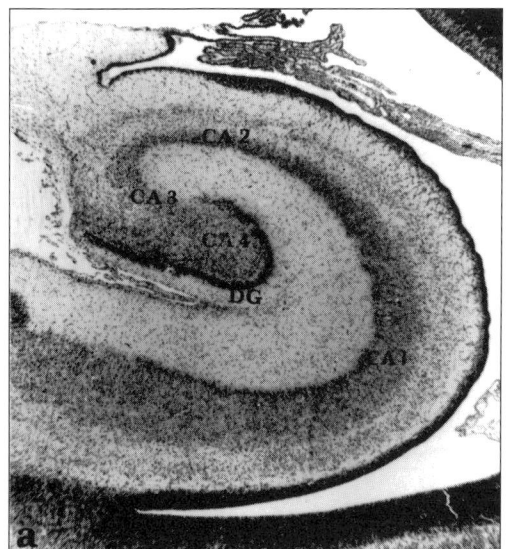

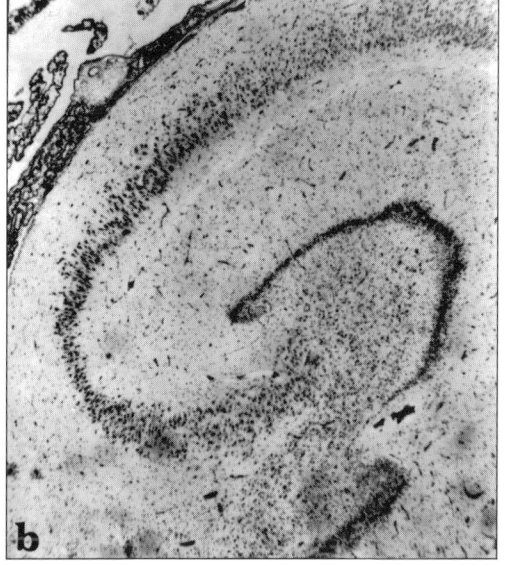

Fig. 34. Maturation of hippocampus.

(a) 32 WG. Sectors CA1, CA2, CA3, CA4. DG – Dentate gyrus

(b) 40 WG. Cresyl violet, × 10.

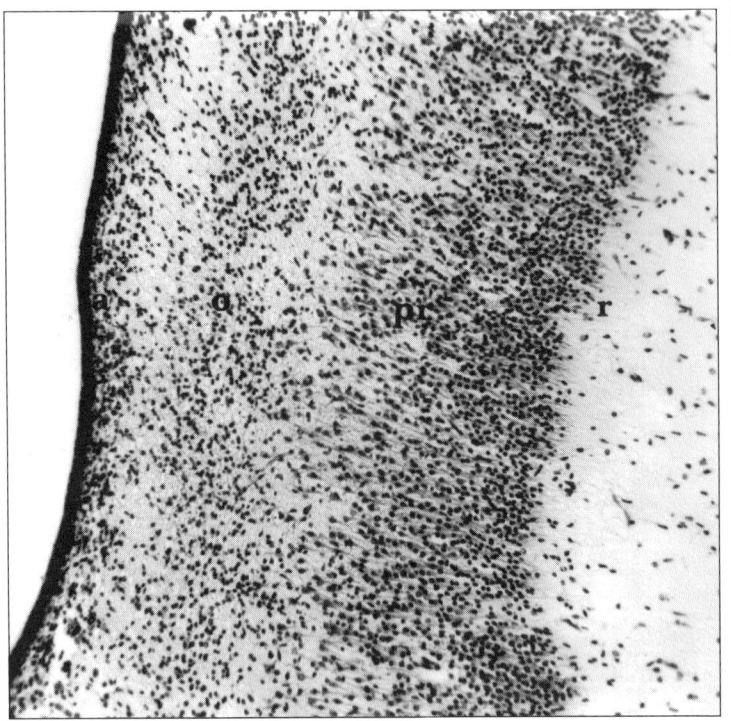

Fig. 35. The structure of CA2 sector of hippocampal cortex at 32 WG. Cresyl violet, × 100.

a – alveus
o – stratum oriens
pr – stratum pyramidale
r – stratum radiatum of the hippocampus

the migratory phase from the germinal layer seems inconsistent with the development of this phylogenetically old structure, this is compensated for the intensity of this process, which enables the archicortical structures to arise rapidly – at the end of the fourth month, the appropriate matrix centers are nearly exhausted.

During the fifth and sixth months, the rate of Ammon's horn development (Figs. 34 and 35), and of differentiation of archicortical neurons, is also rapid. At birth, the hippocampal region is well-differentiated, although with great density of neurons, reflecting the immaturity of sectors CA1 and CA4 (Kuchna, 1994). Filimonov (1965) noted that histogenesis of the archicortex begins later than in the neocortex, but its neurons mature earlier with different rates in particular sectors (Fig. 36). The more rapid maturation of the archicortex confirms the comparison of several processes occurring during maturation of the frontal and hippocampal regions: (1) serotonin-2 binding sites in the human hippocampus reach nearly adult levels earlier than in the frontal cortex (Marcusson et al., 1984), and (2) in newborn rabbits, synapses in hippocampus mature more rapidly than in the frontal cortex (Dąmbska & Maślińska, 1982). The reciprocal entorhinal-hippocampal connections were also found as developing prior to neocortical pathways (Hevner & Kinney, 1996).

archicortical area. Finally, at about the 30th week of development, the hippocampal fissure appears only as a shallow indentation of the surface between dentate and entorhinal areas (Sidman & Rakic, 1982).

The temporal development of the fornix with the hippocampal commissure and of the CC parallels that of Ammon's horn. These structures begin to develop in 11–12 WG, when a protrusion-like shift of the CC occurs between the archicortex and the remnants of its matrix. Because of this shift, only the thin taenia tecta (indusium griseum) persists above the CC during further growth. The subcallosal gray rudiment, which later joins the olfactory paleocortex and the septum pellucidum (Sidman & Rakic, 1982), remains below the commisural magna. Ammon's horn, the principal part of the archicortex, reaches its more posterior/inferior position as the neopallium grows. The principal formative events in the hippocampal formation occur during the third and fourth gestational months. Although the relatively late beginning of

The periarchicortex

The periarchicortex is, according to Sidman and Rakic (1982), interposed between the neocortex and archicortex and includes three parts: presubiculum, parasubiculum and entorhinal cortex. The periarchicortex is recognizable at the beginning of the third month of development and precedes the appearance of the archicortex. During the sixth month of development, the part of periarchicortex adjacent to the archicortex is discernible as the presubiculum, and the part adjacent to neocortex, as the entorhinal area. The formation of the lamina dissecans brings a very characteristic feature to the periarchicortex. Its cell-sparse layer formed by a split of middle layer divides the cortex into two cellular layers. The developmental origin of the lamina dissecans is not clear, but underlines the character of this cortex as an intermediate formation between unilayered archicortex and the six-layered neocortex. Within the presubiculum, the lamina dissecans is seen between week 13 and 14 of development, and within the enthorhinal area, at about 15–16 weeks. The rate of the maturation process proceeds from the archicortex through the presubiculum and entorhinal cortex. Within the entorhinal area, a thin additional lamina dissecans appears late in the fifth month. The neurons within the entorhinal area mature as in the hippocampal formation, evidently earlier than in the neocortex area (Sidman & Rakic, 1982).

Neocortex (isocortex). The development of the neocortex starts within the thin wall of the lateral vesicles, operating at 32–33 days (stages 14, 15) (Marin-Padilla, 1988) which later will develop into the cerebral hemispheres.

Migration of neuroblasts

The neuroblasts destined for the neocortex multiply within the periventricular matrix (ventricular zone) (Fig. 37), many of them in segments corresponding to the parts of the future neocortical mantle (Kahle, 1969). After the last division, the neuroblasts start their migration. The migration along the processes of radial glia, which serve as guides to the target areas of neocortical stripe, is responsible for the columnar arrangement of neurons deriving from given matrix segments. This process has been studied and described exhaustively (Sidman & Rakic, 1973; Kadhim et al., 1988; Choi, 1986). Nevertheless, the fate of an additional group of dividing cells localized in the subventricular zone (Sidman & Rakic, 1982) has not been finally determined. The young neuroepithelial cells capable of differentiating into both neurons and glia reveal at this very early stage of development the positive immunohistochemical reaction for vimentin. Stagaard and Mollgard

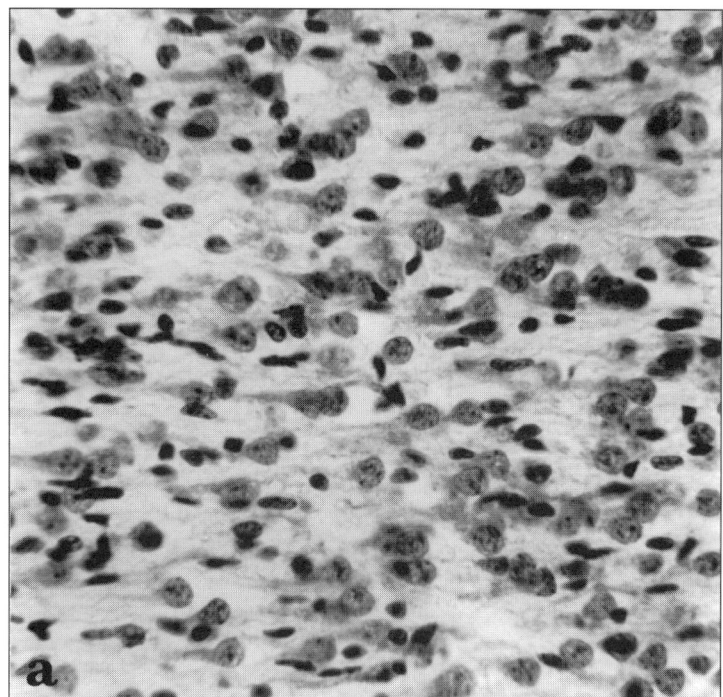
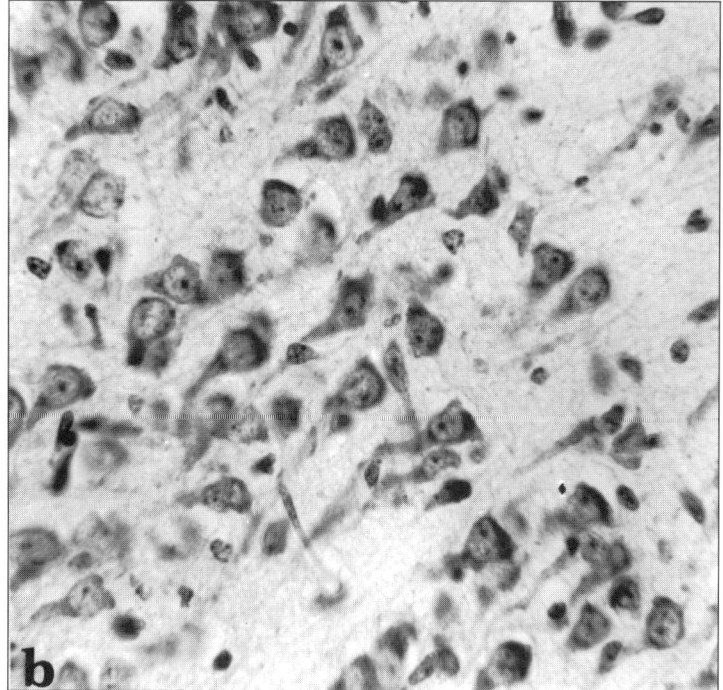

Fig. 36. Different levels of maturation at 40 WG. (a) sector CA1; b) sector CA2;

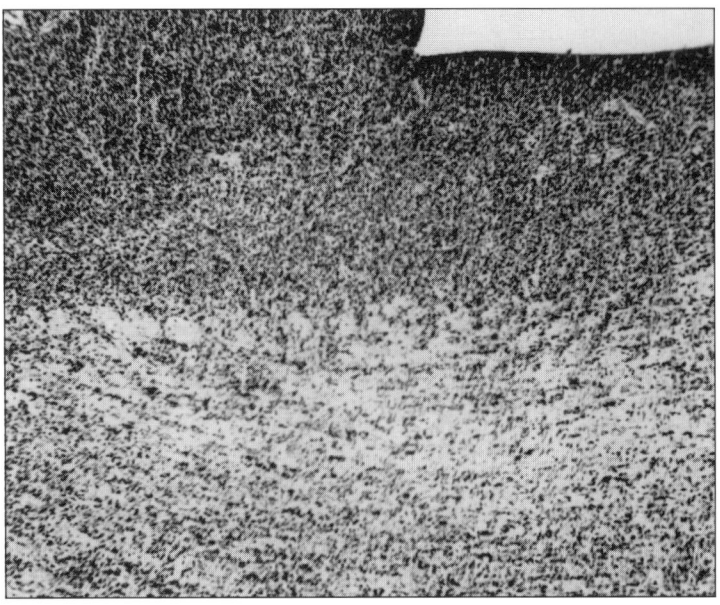

Fig. 37 (above). Neuroblasts within the ventricular zone at 10 WG. Cresyl violet, × 100.

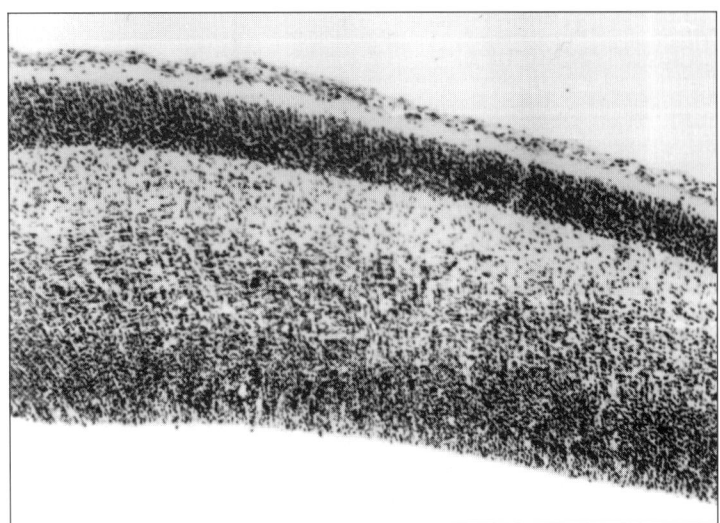

Fig. 38 (below). The hemispheric wall in 10 week-old embryos with waves of migrating nerve cell. Cresyl violet, × 80.

(1989) suggest that this substance may have a functional role in cellular movements.

The most recent data allow us to recognize that despite and even before the radial migration of neurons, young nerve cells move tangentially. It has been suggested that at the beginning of the migratory process, some cells shift in the ventricular area in a tangential plane. Later, at the final phase of radial migration, other cells also migrate tangentially before reaching the way to the cortex (Tan & Breen, 1993; O'Rourke et al., 1992; Fishell et al., 1993; Herrup & Silver, 1994). Finally, although this type of migration has until now not been sufficiently understood, it seems that both radial and tangential migration play a role in formation of the cortex. Most recent investigations looking for signals guiding immature neurons to their final destination in the cerebral cortex allowed us to find some particular genes expressed in migrating cells. We believe that they are not the last to be discovered (Barinaga, 1996).

The process of neuronal migration to the future neocortex consists of abundant waves with numerous immature nerve cells (Fig. 38), lasts during the main part of intrauterine development (Fig. 39), and even extends beyond birth. Five months of age can be considered the stage at which the movements of young neurons to their final position are in great part completed. Two regulations are imposed upon this process: (1) the sequence of neuronal migration to relevant cortical layers, and (2) the duration and timing of migration to various parts of the neocortical mantle.

The first cells found in the marginal layer of the hemispheric cortex are the Cajal-Retzius (C-R) cells. Correlative studies give evidence of the early maturation of those cells around the sixth to seventh WG. EM studies revealed the first synapses on C-R cell somas and processes as early as 7 WG (Marin-Padilla, 1983; Larroche, 1981; Larroche et al., 1981; Milokhin & Iakushova, 1988; Choi, 1988). At this phase of development – at the end of 6 WG – some fibers, probably ascending from the midbrain, that belong to the primitive internal capsule were observed to reach the superficial zone of the developing cerebral cortex (Marin-Padilla, 1983). These fibers participate in the organization of the primordial plexiform lamina (the external subpial white matter), which together with C-R cells and a few less-defined cellular elements, were considered by Marin-Padilla to be phylogenetically primitive 'premammalian' cortex.

The C-R cells presenting polymorphic forms are only a transient population; they disappear after the 24th week of development (Meyer & Gonzalez-Hernandez, 1993). This early maturation of cortical layer I coincides with the development of the glia limitans and the formation of the glial-pial barrier (Choi, 1988).

At this time, the ventricular zone containing neuroepithelial undifferentiated cells is covered by the primordial plexiform layer. Afterwards, the subventricular zone can be distinguished (Mollgard & Jacobsen, 1984). A few days later, on or around 7.5 WG, the neuroblasts migrating toward the future neocortex give rise to the cortical plate (Marin-Padilla, 1983, 1995; Choi, 1988). The cortical plate is formed within the primordial plexiform layer, dividing it into an outer marginal zone and an inner subplate zone.

The latter is separated from the subventricular zone by the intermediate zone. Finally, during migration, the following zones can be distinguished in the wall: (1) ventricular zone, (2) subventricular, (3) intermediate, (4) subplate, (5) cortical, and (6) outer marginal (Mollgard & Jacobsen, 1984). The fact that at this stage of development, some plasma proteins were detected not only in a single cell type, but also in different types of nerve cells and even glial cells in the developing hemisphere (Mollgard & Jacobsen, 1984) supports their common origin.

The sequence of neuronal migration to the future cortex was initially studied in animals. Using autoradiographic methods, Angevine and Sidman (1961) observed in mice that the migration to the cortex follows the inside-out sequence. Their observations were confirmed in humans (Sidman & Rakic, 1973): neuroblasts settle down consecutively in the VI, V, IV, III, and finally, the II cortical layer. Migration to the neocortex starts at the end of the second month of gestation. As was previously mentioned, the thin layer of neuroblasts in the

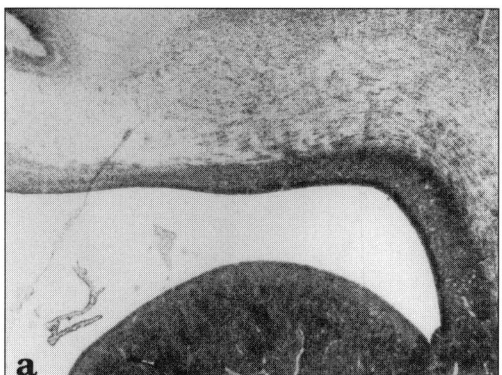
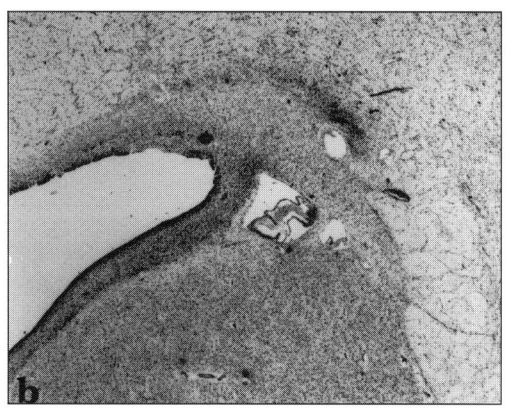
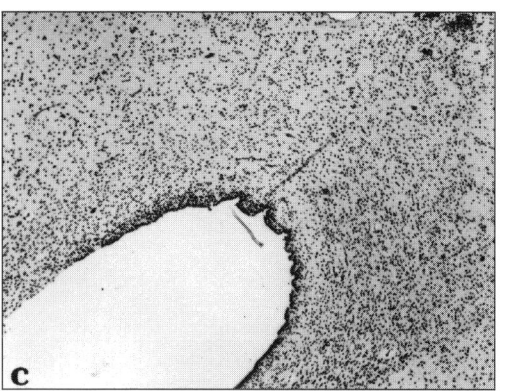

Fig. 39. The periventricular matrix at the level of anterior horn consecutively exhausted during neuroectodermal cell migration.

(a) at 20 WG;

(b) at 34 WG;

(c) at 40 WG. Cresyl violet, × 100.

cortical plate is observed at this time. Sidman and Rakic (1982) found two great consecutive waves of migrating cells, the first during the third month, and the second during the fourth month of gestation. Between these two waves, the cortical plate appears to be divided into two laminae. The activity of this process is highest during this period, diminishes during the fifth month (Fig. 40), and is nearly completed by around

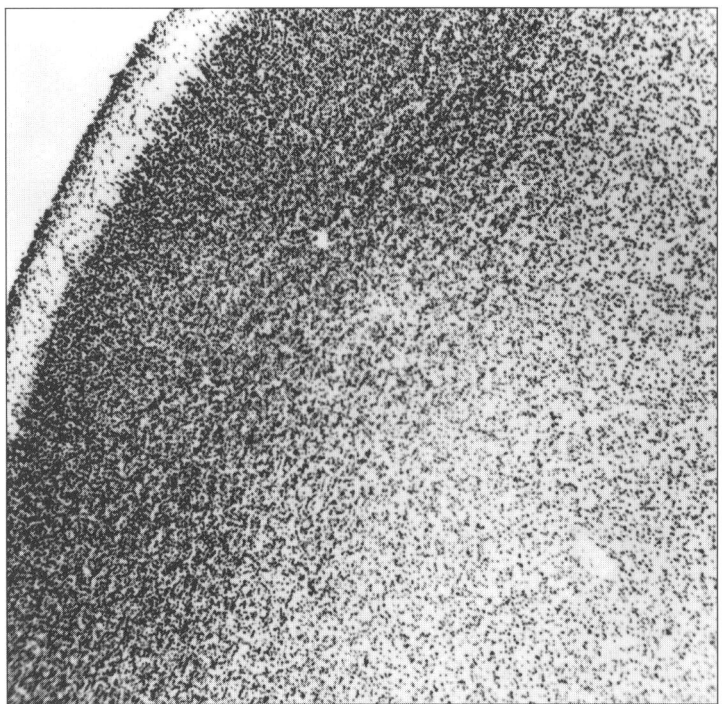

Fig. 40. The frontal cortex at 18 WG. Cresyl violet, × 80.

The questions of how far and when the destination of migrating cells is determined has already been mentioned when neuronal development was discussed. Studies concerning cortical development demonstrated that the neuronal fates are determined progressively. The first determination is for cells destined to mesocortex and neocortex (limbic and non-limbic phenotype) (Ferri & Levitt, 1993). Then, very early, the destination of neurons to given layers is specified (McConnell, 1992). Experimental studies on rats confirm that the destination of neurons with future long or short projection is specified even before the neuronal migration to given cortical layers (Koester & O'Leary, 1993). Experiments with transplantation suggest that the definite destination among neocortical areas is determined later (McConnell, 1992).

the middle of the seventh month. However, a few young nerve cells may reach the cortex even after birth (Kahle, 1969; Evrard et al., 1989; Kostovic et al., 1989), and the migratory process and passive neuronal displacement (Norman et al., 1995) can be considered complete at 5 months after birth (Sarnat, 1992c).

When differentiation of the neuroepithelium arrests its mitotic activity, and the neurons destined for the cortex leave the periventricular germinal centers, the ventricular wall becomes finally lined with ependymal cells only (Sarnat, 1992a,b). The subventricular zone, representing at this stage the germinal layer, still contains only the last remaining nerve cells and a majority of glial precursors. The glial differentiation in those centers was visualized

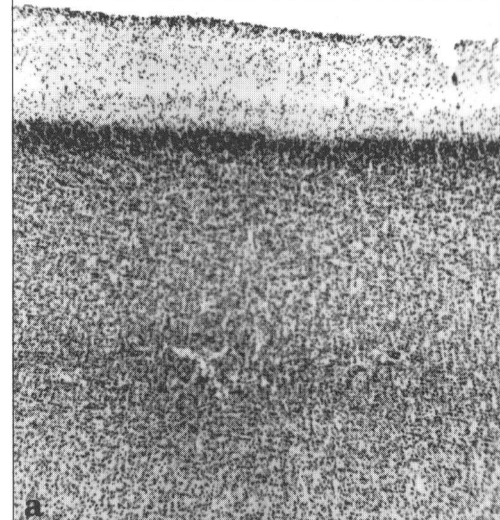
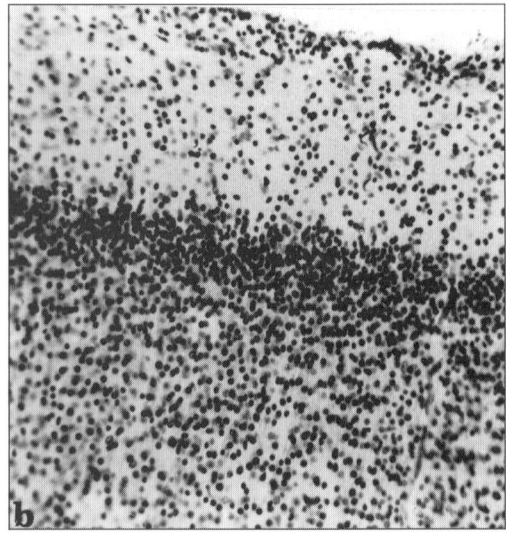

Fig. 41. The parietal cortex at 28 weeks of development. Cresyl violet. (a) the cortical layering still visible, × 80. (b) the external layers with immature cells, × 160.

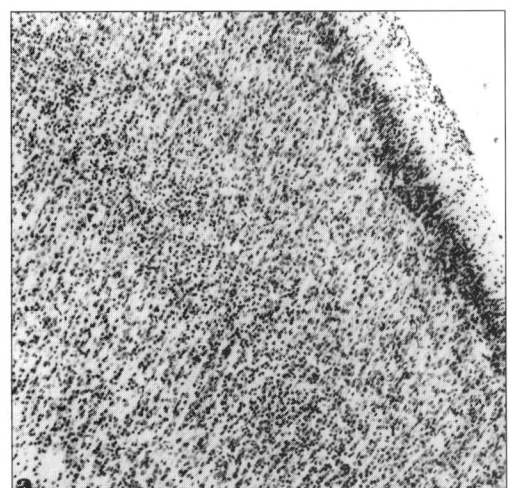
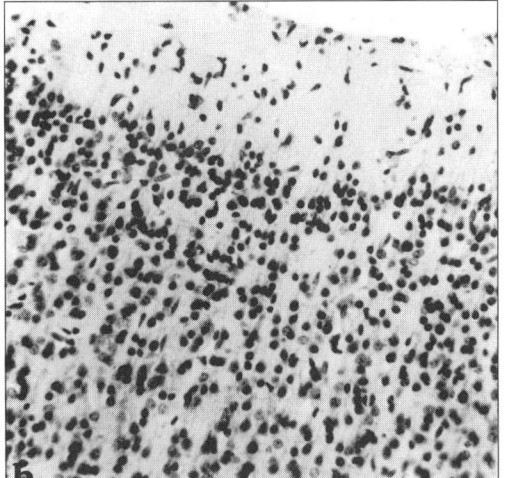

Fig. 42. The parietal cortex at 34 WG. Cresyl violet.

(a) general view, × 80; (b) maturing external layers, × 160.

around the middle of gestation, by using the reaction for glial fibrillary acidic proteins (GFAP) (Gould & Howard, 1987). When the germinative zone diminishes and has nearly vanished, the perivascular cuffs of matrix cells still exist in the territory of the former germinal centers. Larroche (1977) speculated that this observation suggests that migration occurs via the perivascular spaces.

Maturation of cortical ribbon

When neuroblasts reach layer II and the process of migration is almost entirely accomplished, the cortex presents as a dense, uniform mass of neuroblasts, although their laminar segregation still exists. This situation is quite visible consecutively in various cortical areas after midgestation. Apart from subpial layer I, only layer II can be distinguished as particularly immature and more dense than deeper parts of the cortical ribbon. From this stage, the morphological differentiation of cortical layering and the maturation of cortical structure starts (Figs. 41, 42 and 43).

Observation of the process of neuronal migration and exhaustion of germinal centers allows the postulation that structural development is not simultaneous in the entire

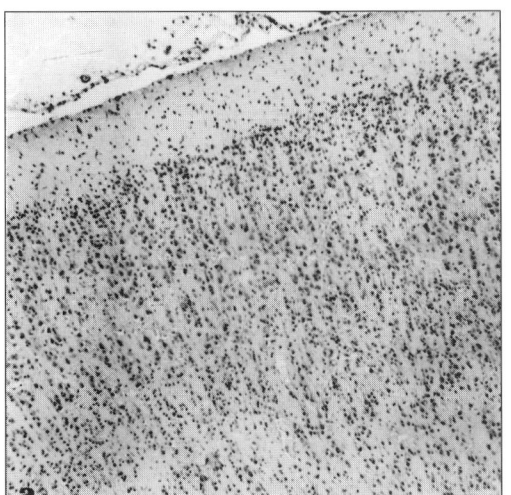
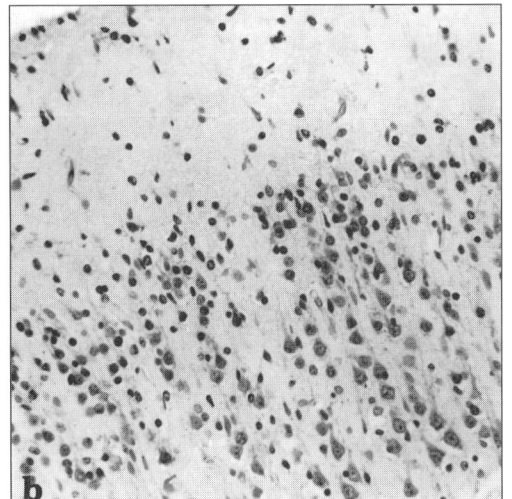

Fig. 43. The parietal cortex of a mature newborn. Cresyl violet.

(a) general view, × 80; (b) external layers with advanced neuronal maturation, × 160.

neocortex. The comprehensive morphological study of Kahle (1969) presents very well the differences in timing of neuronal migration to various parts of the neocortex and the narrowing of the appropriate segments of the germinal layer. He observed that the onset of migration from areas close to the archipallial segments, although delayed, concludes earlier than in other neocortical parts of the ventricular walls. This sequence of events is visible in the development of the area calcarina and resembles the timing observed in the archipallial cortex.

The most prolonged migration takes place from the wall of the anterior horn and is not yet finished at the time of birth.

A particular phenomenon that occurs during the development of the neocortex must be mentioned. At about 13th–14th WG, a thin, superficial accessory layer of Ranke including matrix cells, appears underneath the meninges. These cells seem to originate within the olfactory matrix, or anteriorly to the hippocampal primordium (Rakic & Yakovlev, 1965), and they cover the entire convexity of hemispheres at about 18 WG (Gadisseaux et al., 1992). Then the granular layer successively disappears so that these cells are no longer visible over the precentral cortex at 30–32 WG, over the calcarine at 33 WG, and over the frontal cortex in nearly mature newborns. Only a few such cells survive during the whole life (Meyer & Gonzalez-Hernandez, 1993).

It has been proposed that the majority of cells of the subpial layer are glial cells and that they contribute to the formation of the glial-pial barrier, participating in an arrest of excessive neuronal migration (Sarnat 1991). Brun (1965) suggested that this layer is important for some cortical malformations. Its role in the formation of glioneuronal heterotopia has also been emphasized (Dąmbska et al., 1986; Sarnat, 1991). Nevertheless, it was also reported that within this layer exist several neuronal cells that contribute to transient early innervation of the developing cortical plate (Meyer & Gonzalez-Hernandez, 1993).

The further development of the cortex includes several processes. The basic one is maturation of nerve cells, consisting morphologically of the growth of the cell body, acquisition of the organelles, and growth of the cellular processes, axons and dendrites. The nerve cells progressively acquire their final mature features that are characteristic for each cortical layer, in a given cortical area, as a general rule of this process. Sidman and Rakic (1982) emphasized that the neurons that migrate earlier and those that are connected with long cortico-subcortical pathways mature earlier. Later, other mature neurons connect with cortico-cortical associative tracts. At the same time, the number of efferent and afferent fibers (to the cortex) increases. The population of glial cells increases as well, along with their size, and the capillaries vascularizing the cortex develop their network. All these processes lead to the decrease in cell density. The cortex becomes larger and gradually divides into six well-differentiated layers during the seventh month of development (Figs. 41, 42 and 43). Elimination of a large portion of neurons by so-called 'cell death' is another mechanism occurring in cortical maturation which is in relation to the elaboration of interneural connections (see Chapter 1, on Neurons (p. 3)). Recent morphometric investigation demonstrated that particularly great number of cortical neurons disappear during the last quarter of pregnancy (Rabinowicz et al., 1996).

The formation of synapses is an important event that is essential to the assembly of the cortical circuits and to maturation of the cortex as an organ endowed with cognitive function. The first synapses other than those in layer I appear after week 8.5 of development and then (Norman et al., 1995) in fetal life; the dynamics of the appearance of synapses is different in various parts of the cortex. Gruner (1970) observed that desmosome-like structures are visible in the electron microscope, earlier than the axo-dendritic, axo-somatic, dendro-somatic, and near-term dendro-dendritic synapses. The production of synapses progresses, and their number reaches the maximum after birth, and then it decreases and attains the value typical for a particular cortical area. The functional and anatomical studies of Goldman-Rakic (1987) in non-human primates suggest that the phase of the greatest number of synapses correlates with the development of cognitive function, but the mature cortex as an organ requires the elimination of any excess of synapses.

During the morphological development of the cortex, its metabolic processes mature; for example, the oxidative metabolism in the frontal cortex increases three times during the second half of gestation. Bioenzymatic and histoenzymatic studies of oxydo-reductive mitochondrial enzyme activities demonstrated that these activities are observed first in the earlier-developing cortical layers; in the motor cortex, they originate from layer V, and in the sensory cortex, from layer IV. Finally, these enzymatic activities appear in layers connected with associative cortico-cortical tracts. Metabolic development has its own proper rate in the motor, visual and associative cortex. This process is prolonged in motor and associative centers until 11 years of age (Farkas-Bargeton et al., 1984). The cortical cholinergic function also starts early in development – during the second trimester of gestation (Perry et al., 1986).

Regional development. The sequence of various maturation processes was studied separately in different cortical areas, providing new data concerning the parameters examined. A short review of some of these parameters may help to understand the characteristic features and topographic differences occurring during cortical maturation.

The visual cortex, in particular, was examined often. The early appearance of the calcarine fissure, at about the 16th week of development, suggests the early maturation of this cortical area. Its marginal layer was studied by Zheng et al. (1989). They demonstrated that at 13 WG, the C-R cells, already endowed with synapses, dominate in the structure of this layer. At weeks 21–23, layer I is well developed, but it is still changing at weeks 26–32, during which time it is characterized by a prominent plexiform lamina. During the sixth gestational month, the undifferentiated cortical plate under this layer develops gradually in the same sequence as in the previous migration. The layers develop from VI through II, although it appears that layer IV differentiates first, because of dissection into two sublayers by a light lamina – the stria of Gennari. Evaluation of the maturation of the visual cortex by measuring neuropil proportion and the thickness of layers in area 17 (primary) and area 18 (secondary) revealed that area 18 reaches its adult volume two months before area 17, which reaches this stage at about four months after birth (Zilles et al., 1986; Garey & de Courten, 1983). Prenatal and postnatal development of the cortical layers in the visual cortex was also studied by Becker et al. (1984), by evaluating the length of dendritic branching in layers V and III. They found that dendritic branching occurs earlier in layer V than in layer III and that these layers reach 65 per cent and 35 per cent, respectively, of their maximum dendritic tree before birth. Using the method of Golgi impregnation and counting of spines, they found that synaptogenesis begins in fetal life which is in agreement with former ultrastructural observations of Gruner (1970). Counting of apical dendrites demonstrated that the number of spines increased from the late fetal period through the fifth month after birth, during which the maximum number of spines was observed (Michel & Garey, 1984). Synaptogenesis in the entire area 17 was estimated as reaching its maximum value around the eighth month, after which loss of synapses was observed until

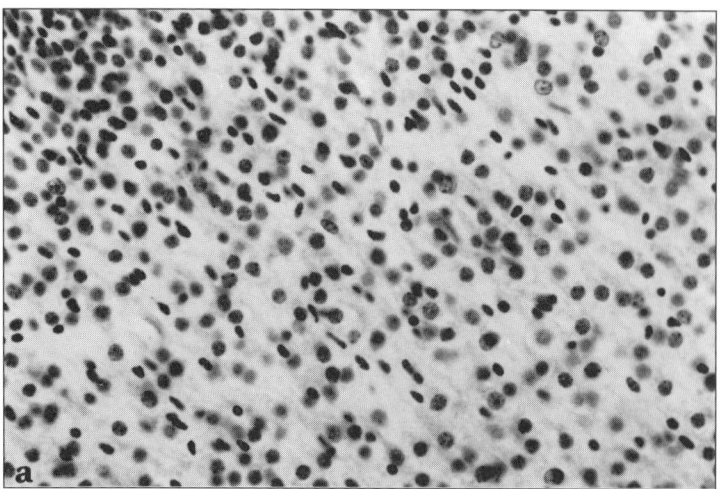

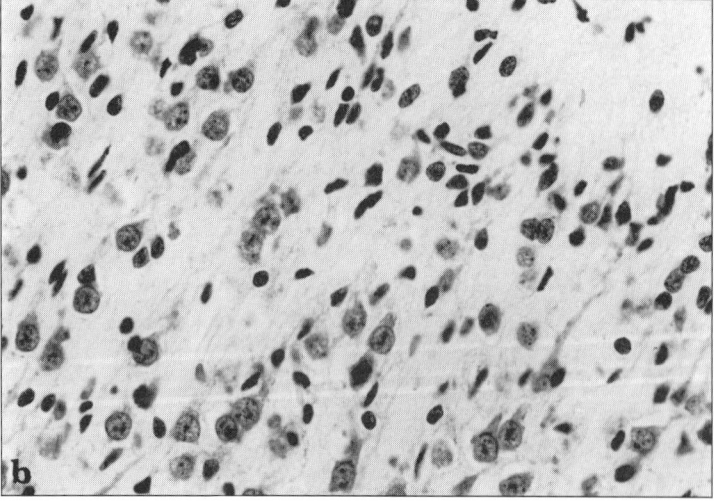

Fig. 44. Pyramidal neurons of layer III of precentral cortex.

(a) 28 WG, × 400;
(b) 36 WG × 400

11 years of age, when the definite synaptic density of about 60 per cent of its maximum is present (Garey & de Courten, 1983). The arrival of afferent fibers at the maturing visual cortex was also examined. Kostovic and Rakic (1984) demonstrated by cholinesterase reaction (ChE) that afferent fibers originating from the pulvinar (the principal area of subcortical projections to the prestriate cortex) penetrate at midgestation to the subplate zone. They accumulate in this zone before reaching their targets in the prestriatal visual cortex during the second half of gestation.

The development of temporal cortex was also studied in the auditory cortex. Cortical afferens were examined by using acetylcholinesterase (AChE) histochemistry in 10–28-week-old fetal brains. It was found that AChE-positive fibers emerge from the ventroposterior thalamic territory as early as at about the 10.5 weeks of development, but such fibers penetrate the subplate zone of the auditory cortex at the 16th–18th week, finally reaching the immature cortex at weeks 22–28 (Krmpotic-Nemanic et al., 1983). Those results were confirmed more recently by observation of the role of subplate neurons in the process of formation of the connections between thalamus and neocortex (Ghosh & Shatz, 1993). In this period, the stratification of the temporal cortex gradually progresses (Kahle, 1969). The superior temporal gyri are formed first, and then the middle and inferior are formed (Chi et al., 1977). The prolonged cortical development of this area has been well documented. Krmpotic-Nemanic et al. (1988) examined the cytoarchitectonic parameters of the associative auditory cortex and found that in this region, the subplate zone disappears gradually until the third month after birth and that the associative auditory cortex itself contains some immature nerve cells (until the postnatal period).

Motor cortex development appears to start in approximately the same period described above. The central sulcus appears during the sixth month of gestation, when the future motor cortex is composed of small, packed nerve cells without cytoplasm. Layer V is the first one identifiable – during the seventh gestational month. This sequence of maturation is in agreement with the previously mentioned priority in mitochondrial enzyme maturation in this layer (Farkas-Bargeton et al., 1984). The Betz cells demonstrate identifiable Nissl bodies on light microscopy, earlier than any other cells – at the end of the ninth month of gestation. The cell density decreases with maturation of consecutive cortical layers, although it is very high during the entire intrauterine life (Fig. 44) (Rabinowicz, 1964; Larroche, 1977). One month before birth, the cell density of layer V is four times higher than in a full-term newborn, and of layer II is approximately seven times higher.

During the seventh gestational month, the gyri and sulci in the frontal lobe also develop, but other parameters of maturation of the frontal cortex testify that this process is long-lasting. A Golgi study performed of the prefrontal cortex revealed that all six layers can be recognized between weeks 26 and 29. Further data concerning neuronal maturation, dendritic differentiation, and formation of spines between 26 and 34 WG testify that these processes coincide with the ingrowth of afferent fibers to the cortex. Before this ingrowth occurs, differentiation of neurons in the subplate zone, where the fibers arrive before entering the cortex, takes place. It was suggested recently that a particularly wide frontal subplate zone is important for cortico-cortical connections (Rakic, 1995). Those observations led to the conclusion that cortical neuronal differentiation is determined by formation of different types of connections (Mrzljak *et al.*, 1988). Consideration of the other parameters of maturation of the frontal cortex allow the conclusion that this process is particularly prolonged. The AChE staining revealed the development of activity of the frontal cortex after the first postnatal year and prolongation until young adulthood (Kostovic *et al.*, 1988).

The fates of the subplate zone in this late-developing cortical area are also significant. The subplate zone appears and can be clearly distinguished before 15 WG. At this time, it contains more mature neurons, especially polymorphous ones, than have been observed in the cortical plate. During further development, the intense differentiation of the subplate zone neurons, including formation of synapses, coincides with the presence of afferent cortical fibers in this zone (Mrzljak *et al.*, 1988). The subplate zone observed in the premotor and prefrontal cortex reveals a developmental peak between 20 and 34 WG, and afterwards

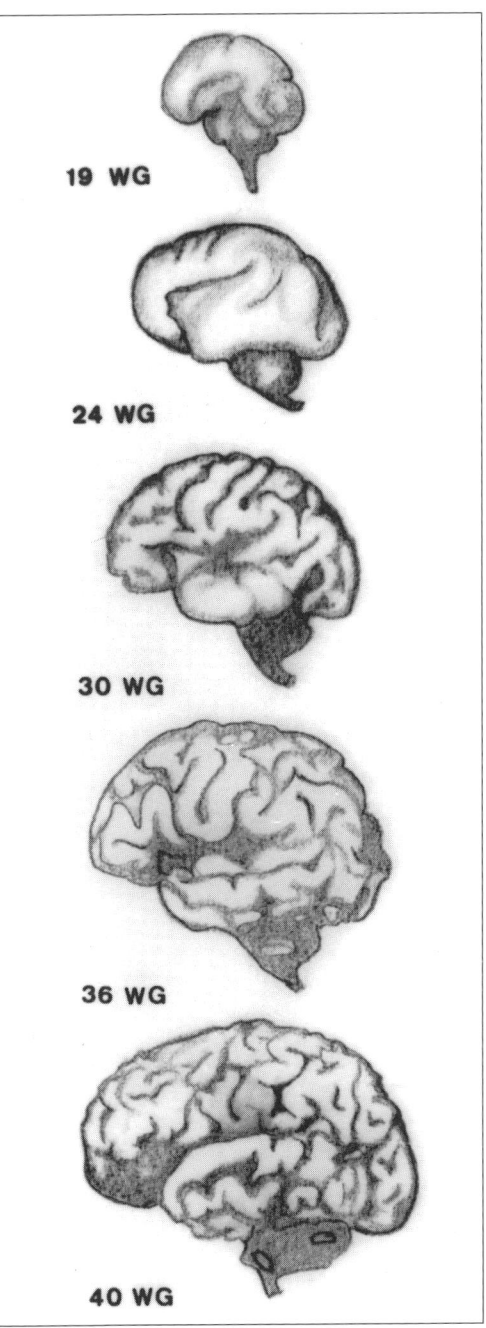

Fig. 45. The overview of cortical folding.

it gradually disappears except for single neurons, until the sixth month after birth. Kostovic *et al.* (1989) propose that those 'waiting' neurons may participate in structural and functional plasticity of the cortex after perinatal brain lesions.

Finally the development of the cortical ribbon leads to its folding, expressed by the formation of gyri and sulci, characteristic for the general view of cerebral hemispheres (Fig. 45). The mechanism of this process necessary for the final modeling of the CNS and its embracing by the cranial vault is difficult to understand. A specialized process of gyrification was required to explain the topography of gyrification, being asymmetrical for each hemisphere (Armstrong et al., 1995). Most recently, van Essen (1997) presented a tension-based theory of morphogenetic mechanism acting during the CNS development. According to this hypothesis, the tension along axons, dendrites and glial processes may play an important role determining the shape of given brain regions. The cortical axons migrate outward looking for compatible targets. When the connection is made, the tension along axons may explain the formation of folding of the cortical ribbon.

Finally, we would like to review the formation of cortical sulci, on the basis of our own experience, the observations of Kahle (1969), and the particularly elaborate data of Chi & Dooling, 1976; Chi et al. (1977) and van der Knaap et al. (1996), the last based on MR images.

The following describes the most important data on pallial folding during intrauterine life:

Month of gestation (1 month/4 weeks)	Formation of sulci
IV	Sylvian fissure
V	Parieto-occipital fissure Cingulate sulcus
VI	Central sulcus Temporal sup. sulcus
VII	Temporal middle. sulcus Frontal superior -"- Interparietal -"- Frontal middle -"-
VIII	Temporal inferior -"- Frontal inferior -"-
IX–X	Secondary sulci
Birth	Tertiary sulci

During its maturation, the neopallium receives its blood supply from developing vessels. The endothelial channels begin to penetrate the telencephalon from the primitive leptomeningeal plexus after the seventh WG. The increase in the volume of the cerebral hemisphere and particularly of the cortical stripe coincides with the formation of gyri and probably induces the growth of short penetrating vessels (Kuban & Gilles, 1985). These vessels follow the law of parallel maturation of structure and appropriate vascularization (Farkas-Bargeton & Thieffry, 1967) (see Chapter 2, on Vessels (p. 22), and Chapter 3, on Vascularization of the CNS (p. 64)).

The development of the neopallium starts at the second month of gestation. The neopallium becomes a functional part of the neuraxis after midgestation (Flower, 1985), but cortical maturation continues to a late postnatal age. Some parameters become stabilized in late childhood or even in young adulthood. Finally, the human neocortex reaches its adult volume in early postnatal life (Caviness et al., 1996). All processes are concentrated around the formation of this principal organ of human cognitive function.

Insular cortex

A complete review of cortical mantle development must include mention of the insular region, which has often been regarded as a particular type of cortex. Rose (1926) used the term 'cortex begemitus' because of difficulties in defining a single ventricular area for its origin. Kahle (1969) also did not consider the insular cortex part of the neocortex, noting that the migration and exhaustion phases of its germinal centers and cortical differentiation occur earlier than in the neocortex. The cortical phase appears within the future insula at 7–8 weeks (Müller & O'Rahilly, 1990b), but already during the third gestational month, the relationship between the appropriate ventricular area and this plate is successively disrupted because of development of the striatum. Some authors (Filimonov 1947; Kahle 1969) considered the insular region a transitional form between allocortex and neocortex (mesocortex – cortex intermedius – periallocortex). Sidman and Rakic (1982) agree that this classification is appropriate for the basal part of the insula.

Other telencephalic derivatives

Claustrum

This is another structure whose origin is still unclear. It arises at 9 weeks of development, but is distinguishable even before the beginning of the fourth developmental month (Sidman & Rakic, 1982) as a narrow stripe of neurons separated from the insular cortex by the external capsule and from the putamen by the internal capsule. Close ontogenic connections of the claustrum with the insular cortex have been suggested (Rose, 1926; Filmonov, 1965). Kahle (1969) did not find such connections, but did find those between the claustrum and the putamen. Nevertheless, the claustrum has been considered a component of the basal ganglia originating from the lateral eminence (Landau, 1923; Hewitt, 1958, 1959). Müller and O'Rahilly (1990b) identified developmental relationships between the claustrum and the olfactory area at 78 weeks (stages 21–23). However, recent comparisons of animal material with human CNS suggest the cortical origin of the claustrum (Morys et al., 1993).

The striatum is the last part of the telencephalon that does not belong to the cortical structures prevailing in this part of the brain, but it participates in the formation of basal ganglia. Its development starts at the end of the first gestational month (stages 14, 15) (Sidman & Rakic, 1982; Müller & O'Rahilly, 1988b). During the first half of the second month, the telencephalic vesicles grow and the lateral ventricular eminence is clearly visible, providing the source of striatal neurons. The striatum displays a mitotic activity that progresses

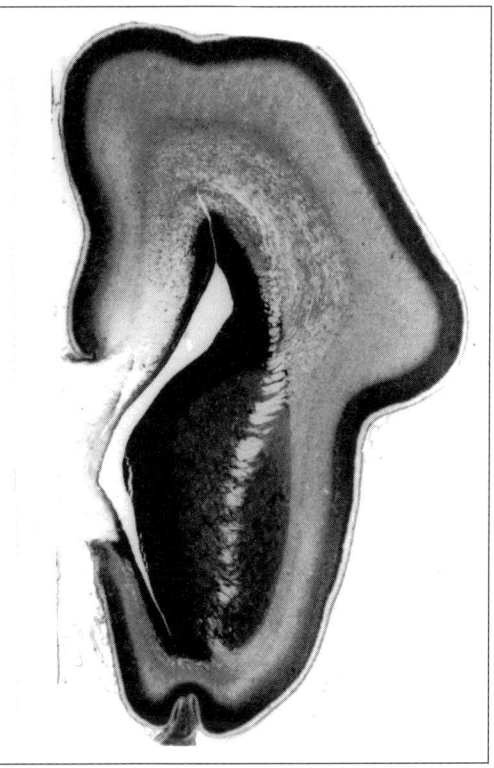

Fig. 46. Anterior part of striatum and internal capsule at the middle of gestation. Cresyl violet, × 4.

in the caudo-oral direction and is not exhausted in the head of the nucleus caudatus until at least the seventh month of development (Kahle, 1969). Some cells may generate even after birth (Sidman & Rakic, 1982). The capsula interna, which arises during the eigth week, divides the striatum into the caudatum and the putamen. The whole structure grows, and the shape of the caudatum is dependent on the formation of the ventricular system (Fig. 46). Its intrinsic structure containing small and large neurons differentiate definitively between the third and fourth month of development.

Globus pallidus

This structure adjoins the striatum and is anatomically included with basal ganglia, deriving ontogenetically from the diencephalon; its development is described with other diencephalic derivatives.

The ventricular system of the brain hemispheres includes the cavity of the di-

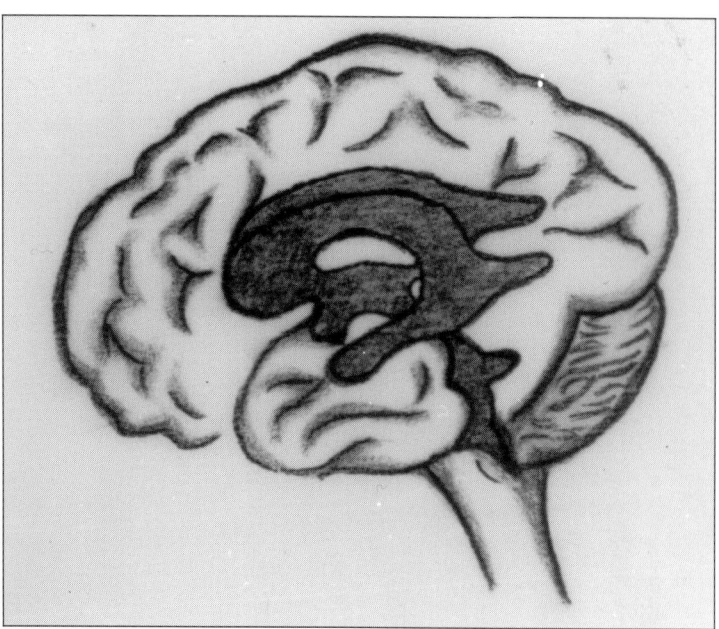

Fig. 47. Overview of ventricular system.

encephalon (i.e. the third ventricle), cavities of the telencephlon (i.e. the lateral ventricles), and the temporary midline cavities (Fig. 47). The ventricles appear after the closure of the anterior, and the posterior neuropores at days 24 and 25 of development, respectively. At this stage, the central canal, which loses contact with its surroundings, is large and still not further divided.

About 32 days (stage 14) of development, the forming hemispheric vesicles communicate with the third ventricle and form a common space. This space is successively enlarged because of the intensive growth of cerebral vesicles. The formation of compact masses of gray subcortical structures, including the insular region, together with the enlargement of the pallium leads to differentiation of the third and lateral ventricles. The shape of the third ventricle becomes more or less defined by about 37 days (stage 16). At this stage, the interventricular foramina connecting the prosencephalic ventricular system are still wide open. They become better defined at day 41 (stage 17) (Müller & O'Rahilly, 1988a, 1989b). The particular shape of the lateral ventricles, including three ventricular horns, corresponds to the newly forming pallial lobes. The form of the ventricular horns is well defined by 12 weeks of development (O'Rahilly & Müller, 1987). Kahle (1969), who analyzed the dynamics of hemispheric development, suggested that the correlation between growth of hemispheres, subcortical structures and cortical pallium results in their 'rotation'. The frontal horn may arise as a simple sequel to the growth of frontal lobe. On the other hand, the formation of the occipital horn may be the result of deformation of the basal hemispheric wall by the growing cerebellum. This horn develops relatively late, i.e. at about 18 weeks (O'Rahilly & Müller, 1987), and presents a clear variability in shape. Sarnat (1992a) observed that only 25 per cent of normal brains have symmetrical occipital horns. This information may be important for evaluation of computed tomography (CT) and magnetic resonance imaging (MRI) studies.

Another morphological event important for the final shape of the lateral ventricles is the development of CC, which will be discussed below, together with other components of the commissural system.

Choroid plexus and cerebrospinal fluid (CSF) circulation

Ventricular development is also correlated with the origin and circulation of the cerebrospinal fluid, since the shape of the ventricles is in part influenced by the pressure inside its space. The closure of the neuropore isolates the central canal from the surroundings such that the canal contains only fluid, secreted probably by epithelial cells (Sidman & Rakic, 1982). It is not clear whether during early development some connection exists between the ventricular system and the subarachnoidal space at the level of the fourth ventricle across the very thin roof. The adult relationship between the ventricular system and the meningeal space begins with the development of the choroid plexuses. Within the fourth ventricle, it appears at days 41–43 of development (stages 17, 18), protruding from its roof and is well visible at days 46–47 (stage 19) (French, 1983; Otani & Tanaka, 1988). The foramen Magendie and Luschka develop later and are thought to open between the second to fourth month of development (see p. 31). The choroid plexus of the lateral ventricles arises by invagination of the medial wall through the choroid fissure formed between the diencephalic and telencephalic derivatives. The epithelium of the invaginating ventricular zone undergoes changes that lead to the appearance of primary villi of the plexus at its surface. Mesenchymal tissue and vessels penetrate into the plexus from the interhemispheric space. The choroid plexus of the lateral ventricles arises by days 45–46 of development (stage 19) (French, 1983), is evident at 47–48 days (stage 20) (Otani & Tanaka, 1988), but acquires the adult form only during the last trimester of gestation (Sidman & Rakic, 1982). Within the third ventricle, the choroid plexus appears at the latest at days 48–49 of development (stage 21) (French, 1983). Nearly half of the circulating CSF is produced by the choroid plexus; the other half comes from the extracellular space within neural tissue (Gross & Goldberg, 1995). As noted by Friede (1989), the intimate contact between the CSF and the surrounding brain structures and their extracellular space assumes the important continuous exchange between them, known as the 'sink action' of the CSF. The circulation of the CSF occurs from the lateral ventricles through the foramina of Monroe, then into the third and fourth ventricles, and through the cerebellar foramina (of Magendie & Luschka) into the meningeal space. There, the developmental process consists of the gradual transformation of the small-meshed meningeal parenchyma into the mature subarachnoidal space, a process that begins as early as about day 44 of development (O'Rahilly & Müller, 1986). Within the subarachnoidal space, the CSF is reabsorbed chiefly at arachnoid granulations (Davson, 1967) and then enters the cerebral venous system.

Several midline cavities arise that are later obliterated during brain development. *Cavum septi pellucidi*, this space between two walls of the septum pellucidum is lined by glial cells and appears between 10 and 11 weeks of development in correlation with growth of CC. It is normally obliterated after birth, in some fetuses, even before birth. The cavum septi pellucidi is seen in 82 per cent of full-term newborns and in a few cases, may persist even to adulthood (Larroche & Baudey, 1961; Sarnat, 1992a).

Cavum vergae, which lies posterior to the cavum septi pellucidi and communicates with it (Shaw & Alvord, 1969), develops around 10–11 weeks and is usually obliterated after birth.

The *cavum veli interpositi* is normally the only potential space between the splenium of the CC and the roof of the mesencephalon. It contains only leptomeningeal, not glial, elements. This potential space is visualized on CT and MRI and therefore warrants special attention to avoid eventual misinterpretation.

Forebrain commissures enable the connections between brain hemispheres. The first to arise is the posterior commissure, which is observed at the fifth to sixth week of development (stages 15–17), followed by the habenular commissure.

At the anterior part of the prosencephalon, the first crossing of fibers arising from both hemispheres occurs within the lamina reuniens of His at about the sixth week of development (stage 18). At 7.5 weeks (stage 22), differentiation within the lamina terminalis take place. The commissural plate forms a bed for the anterior commissure, which is identified at 9–10 weeks of development; the fornix with hippocampal commissure, which presents the connections of the archicortical structures and appears at 10–11 weeks of development; and the neocortical CC, which develops last, since 12 weeks. It has been observed for a long time that the growth of the CC progresses in a rostro-caudal direction, and rostrum, corpus and splenium successively appear, because fibers cross anteriorly first and then more posteriorly. Nevertheless, the mechanism of CC formation has not, until now, been known (Norman et al., 1995). It has only been observed that all its parts are seen by week 30 of development. However, the developmental processes within the forebrain commissures continue throughout the fetal period along with the formation of interstructural connections.

Myelination of the CNS structures

The nerve fibers within the CNS acquire myelin sheaths gradually. From the second half of gestation until the third to fourth year of life, myelination can be observed on light microscopy by routine histologic staining. More recently, the early stages of myelination have been examined ultrastructurally and biochemically. The protein and lipid composition of myelin was studied by using extraction as well as immunohistochemical methods (Weidenheim et al., 1992; Hasegawa et al., 1992; Kinney et al., 1994; Bodhireddy et al., 1994; Tanaka et al., 1995). Measurement of the area of myelin staining also appears to be helpful in estimating the extent of myelination (Benes et al., 1994). Those studies indicate that the early stages of myelin formation occur somewhat earlier and the maturation of myelin somewhat later than estimated by routine histochemical methods. Nevertheless, the sequence of myelination within the CNS principal tracts and areas was established on the basis of morphological studies performed on a large series of fetal and infant brains (Yakovlev & Lecours, 1967; Rorke & Riggs, 1969; Larroche, 1977; Gilles et al., 1983; Brody et al., 1987; Kinney et al., 1988). Myelination in the brain and spinal cord appeared as a progressive process, despite its temporal association with regressive events such as programmed neuronal death and axonal loss (Brody et al., 1987). It has been well established that some pathways within the CNS become myelinated very rapidly, whereas others myelinate slowly, and the rate of myelination does not depend on the time of its onset. It has been observed that phylogenetically older tracts of the spinal cord and brain stem acquire the first myelin sheaths and that myelination progresses in most instances in a caudo-cephalic direction (Larroche, 1977). Ascending tracts of the spinal cord follow this sequence and in newborns are more myelinated at the caudal level. On the other hand, the descending tracts at the same age are better myelinated at the upper spinal level (Rorke & Riggs, 1969), according to the prevailing rule that myelination follows the direction of impulse production. The observations of Flechsig (1920) also suggested that in general, sensory tracts appear to be myelinated earlier than motor tracts, and projectory connections are myelinated before associative connections.

Myelination, seen on light microscopy by routine staining, begins around midgestation in the spinal cord. The further course of this process has been variably estimated (Yakovlev & Lecours, 1967; Rorke & Riggs, 1969; Larroche, 1977; Gilles et al., 1983; Brody et al., 1987; Kinney et al., 1988; Dambska & Laure-Kamionowska, 1990; Sarnat, 1992c), depending on the material used for study and the methods for myelin staining. In most of these studies, the samples have not been grouped according to neuropathological diagnosis, except for severe pathology, which together with possible differences in gestational age estimations, may explain the differences in evaluations of myelination stages in particular groups. Despite such possible differences in evaluation of myelination, those studies demonstrated very similar final results with respect to the progress and sequence of myelination within particular structures and provide an overview of the general course of myelin sheaths formation within the CNS. Below, we describe some trends in, and events of this process in the principal structures of the CNS, on the basis of histological examination and taking into consideration the corrections brought by more sensitive methods. Analysis of myelin basic protein (MBP), considered particularly sensitive was used most often (Bodhireddy et al., 1994).

Spinal cord

It is generally accepted that myelination begins in the spinal cord at midgestation, but ultrastructural observations and immunohistochemical analysis of myelin-associated gene expression reveal the earliest signs of myelination in the lumbo-sacral area at 12–13 WG, as well as the appearance of myelin in all cord areas examined (except for corticospinal tracts) at 24 weeks (Weidenheim et al., 1992). The first pathway in the spinal cord to become myelinated is the median longitudinal fasciculus. Histological analysis indicates that this process progresses in this tract after midgestation, and at term, it is well-myelinated. Except for corticospinal tracts, other pathways begin myelination shortly thereafter, but the process occurs more slowly. Newborns at term have myelin sheaths in all spinal cord pathways, but the degree of myelination is evidently variable. This variability indicates that myelination continues after birth. The first signs of corticospinal tract myelination appear shortly before birth (Gilles et al., 1983; Larroche 1977; Dąmbska, Laure-Kamionowska 1991). Analysis of this process using MBP immunohistochemistry generally supports this estimation (Tanaka et al., 1995).

Brain stem (except for cerebellar pathways)

Myelination within the brain stem appears to advance later than in the spinal cord, with only the medial longitudinal fasciculus myelinated early. A few other tracts contain some myelin visible by microscopy at midgestation. Those characterized by a rapid course of myelination, such as the medial and lateral lemniscus and the spinal trigeminal tract, are rather well-myelinated at birth, whereas others starting myelination before the end of the second trimester of gestation present active myelination during third trimester, but do not display a similar level of myelination at birth. During the last weeks before birth, myelination is more evident in the corticospinal tract than at the level of the spinal cord (Fig. 48). Finally, myelin is present in all mesencephalic and rhombencephalic pathways at birth except for the medial and lateral crus pedunculi of the mesencephalon (Kinney et al., 1988).

Cerebellum and its peduncles

The cerebello-petal and cerebello-fugal pathways begin the myelination process during fetal life, but the time of onset has

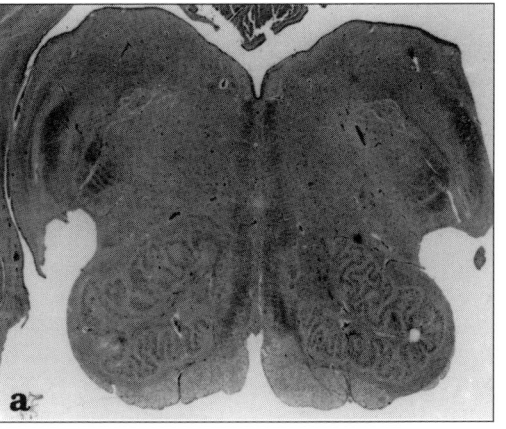
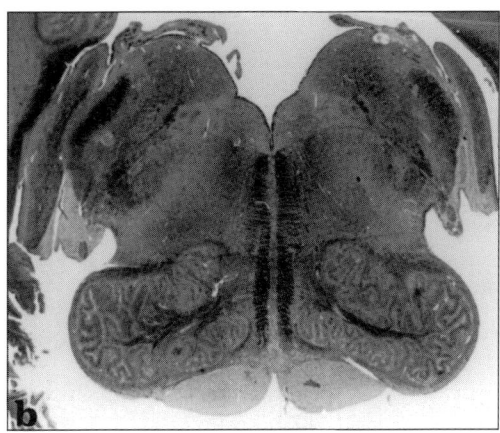

Fig. 48. Myelination of medulla.

(a) at 30 weeks of development; (b) at birth;
Kluver-Barrera.

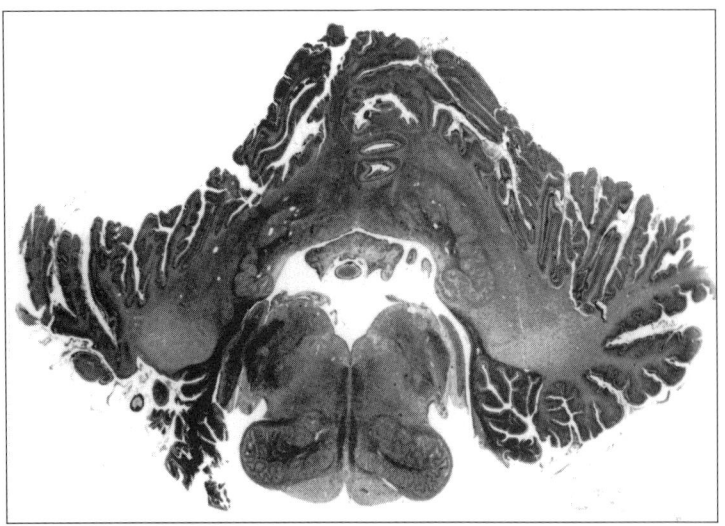

nation in the middle cerebellar peduncle later, around birth. The cerebellar white matter presents an evident difference in time of myelination in archi- and neocerebellar components (Fig. 49). Myelination in the cerebellar vermis (parasagital portion of the cerebellum) begins before birth, during the third trimester of gestation, and in the cerebellar hemispheres, two months later at birth (Gilles et al., 1983; Larroche, 1977; Brody et al., 1987). In both parts, the process is protracted, and in the cerebellar hemispheres, it extends past 1 year postnatally (Kinney et al., 1987).

Cerebral hemispheres

Myelination within the cerebral hemispheres embraces many structures. The observations of Brody et al. (1987) and Kinney et al. (1988) confirmed most previous opinions on the general rules of this process and added some new ones. The most important observation appears to be that myelination in telencephalic structures progresses from the central sulcus outward to the poles and that myelination in posterior sites precedes that in anterior and fronto-temporal sites (Fig. 50).

Fig. 49 (above). Myelination of archi- and neocerebellar components at birth. Kluver-Barrera.

Fig. 50 (below). Myelination of frontal lobe (U-fibers unmyelinated) at 1 year of age; Kluver-Barrera.

been variably reported. The cerebellar inferior and superior peduncles begin myelination at the beginning of the third trimester of gestation and the middle peduncle (ponto-cerebellar) some weeks later but still before birth. The course of myelination is prolonged after birth, as was estimated by Gilles et al. (1983) and Sarnat (1992c). Yakovlev and Lecours (1967) are in agreement with Brody and coworkers (1987) in estimating the beginning of myeli-

Only the occipital pole acquires myelin somewhat earlier than the posterior-parietal white matter. Thus the posterior part of the CC (corpus and splenium) becomes myelinated before its rostral parts, which are connected with late myelinizing frontal pathways. The exception to this general rule about the direction of myelination is represented by U-fibers, which myelinate later and in their own order. The differences in the time of U-fiber myelination reflect the earlier and shorter myelination time of the primary projection system as compared with associative connections. The most detailed studies on myelination of the cerebral hemispheres performed on 62 selected white matter sites were done by Brody et al. (1987) and Kinney and coworkers (1988); the reader is referred to those reports for data concerning time and topography of

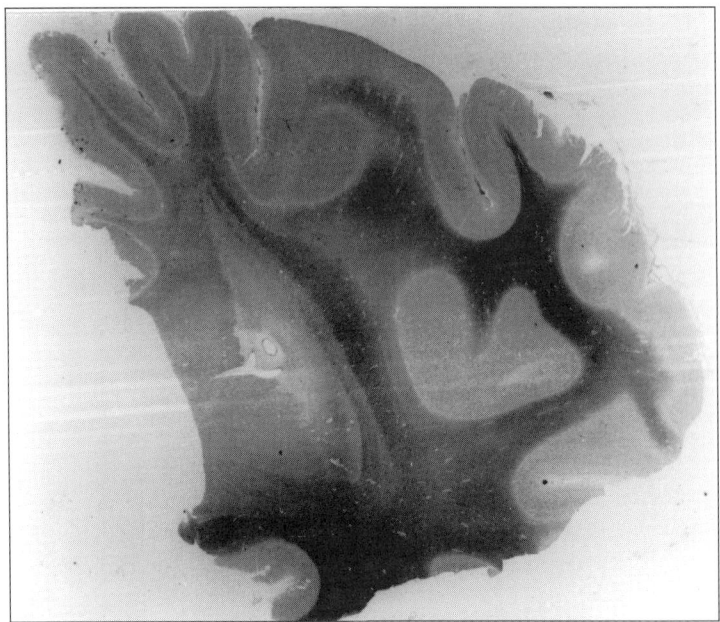

Table 3. Myelination (estimated in light microscopy)

Pyramidal system

White matter deep to precentral gyrus			± 3.5 m → 2 y
Internal capsule – lateral limb midthalamic level			
	(1) lateral half		at birth ± 1 y
	(2) medial half		at birth ± 1 y 2.5 m
Cortico-spinal tract		midbrain	± 1 m → 1 y
		pons	± 7 m → 11 m
		spinal thoracic	± 8 m → >2 y
		cervical	± 10 m → >2 y
		lumbar	± 1 m → >2 y

Optic system

Optic chiasm		± 3 m → 4.5 m
Optic tract		± birth → 11 m
Optic radiation		1.5 m proximal → 11 m
		distal → 7 m
Calcarine cortex (subcortical)		6 m → >2 y

Commissures

Corpus callosum	rostrum	± 8 m → >2 y
	corpus	± 5.5 m → >2 y
	splemium	± 3.5 m → ± 1 y 8 m
Anterior commissure	anterior	± 4.5 m → >2 y
	inner	± 11 m → >2 y
External capsule		± 6.5 m → >2 y
Internal capsule		± 1 y 8 m → >2 y

Hemispheric lobes

Occipital	pole	± 6 m → 1 y 5.5 m
	pole subcortical	± 1 y 2 m → >2 y
Parietal	posterior	± 6 m → 1 y 10 m
	posterior subcortical	± 9.5 m → ± 2 y
	central	± 2 m → >2 y
Temporal	central	± 2 m → >2 y
	pole	± 1 y 2 m → >2 y
	at lat. genicul. level	± 11 m → ± 1 y 9 m
	subcortical	± 1 y 7.5 m → >2 y
Frontal	posterior	± 3 m → >2 y
	pole	± 6 m → >2 y
	pole subcortical	± 1 y 6 m → >2 y

myelination in individual structures/or areas of the cerebral hemispheres (Table 3).

Within basal ganglia, the globus pallidus with some myelinated fibers seen at birth has been examined most often. On the basis of morphological evaluation, it has been determined that myelination starts here around 37 WG and is completed during the second postnatal year. The MBP examination indicates an earlier onset of this process, at 25 weeks (Hasegawa et al., 1992). Those authors proposed a similar time of myelination onset for the thalamus, and at 37 weeks for the striatum. The internal capsule appears to begin myelination in the posterior part at 25 WG, and in the anterior part, at 37 weeks. In histologic staining, myelin is visible at birth in the posterior and after birth in the anterior part of the capsula interna, and myelination continues even after the second postnatal year (Kinney et al., 1988).

Optic pathways reveal the beginning of the myelination process during the third trimester of gestation in the optic chiasm and optic tract; in the latter, Gilles et al. (1983) have estimated even some weeks earlier. The optical radiation is estimated to begin myelination around birth (Gilles et al., 1983; Kinney et al., 1988; Sarnat, 1992c), and MBP analysis reveals only 2 weeks earlier, around 37 WG (Hasegawa et al., 1992). The optic tract may complete myelination between 6 months and one year postnatally. In the optic chiasm, the process appears to be protracted beyond 1 year postnatally. Within the optic radiation, myelination was variably estimated as completed at 6 months (Sarnat, 1992c), and up to 2 years postnatally (Kinney et al., 1988). The subcortical associative fibers in the calcarine cortex become myelinated between the third month and 1–2 years after birth.

The temporal lobe white matter begins myelination around birth within the hippocampal formation. Six tracts seen in this area acquire myelin consecutively. Histological analysis indicates that myelination is completed during the third postnatal year (Dąmbska & Laure-Kamionowska, 1990), although measurement of the area of myelin staining suggests that myelin content increases until adulthood, as observed particularly in the subicular region and presubiculum (Benes et al., 1994). The subcortical association fibers within the temporal pole begin the myelination process around 6 months after birth, within the posterior parietal cortex between the fifth and sixth months, and within the frontal pole even later. The maturation of myelin sheaths within those areas was not complete even at the end of the observation period of two postnatal years (Kinney et al., 1988).

Corpus callosum

Within the main interhemispheric commissure, the myelination process begins within its body at the second postnatal month, within the splenium at the third month, and within the rostrum at the fourth month. The process continues for 1–2 years (Kinney et al., 1988) and some authors have estimated up to 10 years (Sarnat, 1992c).

We would like to express our conviction that despite the doubts about when normal myelination of particular tracts is definitely accomplished, this general overview of the myelination process within the CNS may be helpful in comparisons with results of MRI, which has proven to be a good tool for *in-vivo* estimation of CNS myelination in infants (Hasegawa et al., 1992; Staudt et al., 1993; Hittmair et al., 1994; Huppi et al., 1998).

Vascularization of the CNS

The CNS receives its blood supply from extrinsic precursors. From the very early stages of development, after the closure of the neural tube (fourth week of development), the future nervous system is encircled by epiparenchymal vascular plexus

(Kuban & Gilles, 1985). According to Duckett (1971), this is the first step in the external phase of the formation of the cerebral blood vessel system. During subsequent development, the vessels of the base of the future brain can be identified. Around the fifth week of developmental age, the majority of vessels supplying the blood for the CNS can be distinguished, and after the end of sixth week, the arterial circle (circle of Willis) is complete (Streeter, 1915, 1918; Allsopp & Gamble, 1979). Those young vessels give rise to the same distinct channels over the surface of the CNS, but above all, participate in the formation of the epiparenchymal plexus, which extends between the pia and the arachnoid. This plexus is the principal source of channels perforating the brain structures; therefore, at this stage, it is difficult to distinguish definite vascular branches as vascularizing particular brain structures. Just when perforating channels invade the nervous tissue, the phase of internal vascularization begins. This process increases with time. During the fifth to sixth week, only a few young vessels perforate the newly forming rhombencephalic derivatives, the mesencephalon and the basal part of the diencephalon. One week later, they are evidently more numerous. With time, branches are observed from the basilar, anterior cerebellar and posterior and posterior communicating arteries entering the brain stem, and those of the choroid and posterior communicating arteries that participate in the vascularization of the diencephalon (Allsopp & Gamble, 1979). All those perforating vessels retain the structure of capillaries. The correlation between the internal development of the brain stem and the diencephalic structures and the formation of their vascular system is clearly visible.

Within the telencephalon, only the basal part receives perforating vessels, mainly from the meningeal plexus before the end of the sixth week of development. Later, the vessels entering the caudate nucleus clearly originate from the anterior, Heubner, middle and choroidal arteries (De Reuck, 1971). The striatal vessels from the middle cerebral artery supply blood to the germinal matrix, putamen, thalamus, and a part of the internal capsule, i.e. the structures originating from both the telencephalon and diencephalon. Those of the amygdaloid nucleus were considered as deriving from the middle cerebral and choroid anterior arteries (Nelson et al., 1991). Recent studies of Goetzen and Sztamska (1996) demonstrated that the amygdaloid nucleus is vascularized by anterior choroidal arteries only.

The pallial portion of the brain hemispheres is avascular at this time. The first perforating channels from the epiparenchymal plexus enter the hemispheric pallium during the seventh to eigth week of development, just when neuronal migration to the cortical plate begins. The long endothelial channels extending ventriculopetaly from the convexity are very visible during the next weeks (Fig. 51). They reach the ventricular area around the 12th week of development and ramify there (De Reuck, 1971; Bar, 1980; Kuban & Gilles, 1985). The notion that some of these channels may terminate as centrifugal ones forming the hypovascular end zones with other ventriculopetal vessels (De Reuck, 1971; Takashima & Tanaka 1978) has not been confirmed by most recent studies (Kuban & Gilles, 1985; Nelson et al., 1991; Nakamura et al., 1994).

The further vascularization of the cerebral pallium progresses along with its growth by increasing the number of penetrating vessels. The observations in animal models of pallial vascular system development (Bar, 1980) are consistent with those in humans (Kuban & Gilles, 1985; Markovic & Marinkovic, 1991). It has long been observed that vascularization follows the structural organization of the cortical stripe. In the six-layered neocortex, each layer has its proper net of vessels. The cerebellar cortex, which is perforated very early by endothelial channels, acquires its

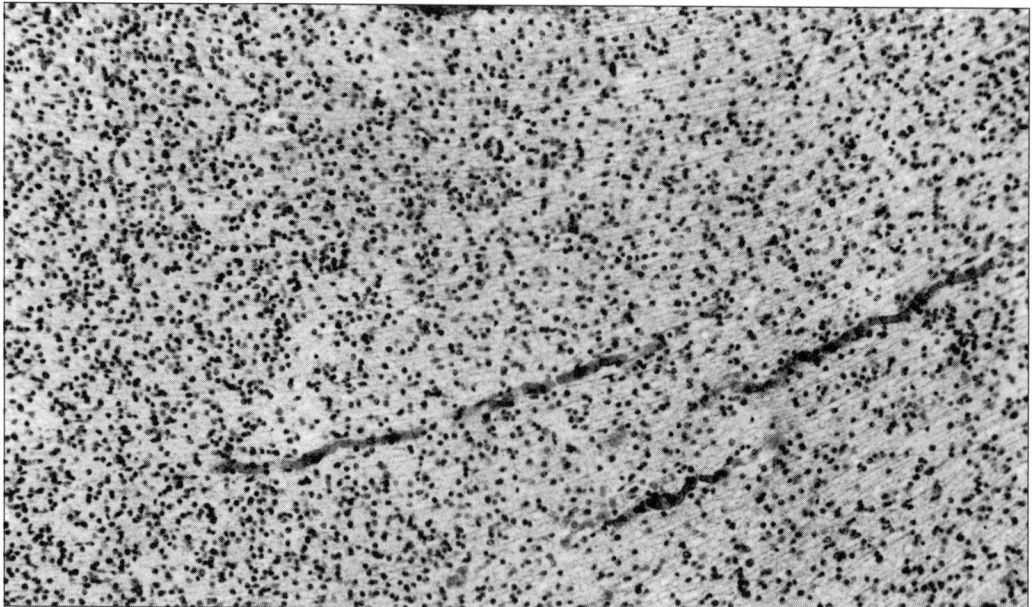

Fig. 51. Endothelial channels penetrating the subcortical white matter. Cresyl violet, × 100.

vascular system along the development of this structure (De Reuck, 1972). Within the cortex, the density and diameter of the vessels increase at about 26 weeks of development, reaching a peak at 36 weeks (Mito et al., 1991), but development of the cortical capillaries continues after birth (Norman & O'Kusky, 1986).

Vessel development in the subcortical white matter is similar to the process within the cortex (Mito et al., 1991). Hypovascularization of the subcortical area, which was proposed by Takashima and coworkers (1978), denied by Kuban and Gilles (1985), but was recently seen by Kdzia (1995), remains an unresolved question.

Recent studies have shown that angiogenesis can be regulated during brain development, particularly its intensive growth stimulated by the vascular endothelial growth factor (VEGF). Localized in epithelial cells and myocytes, VEGF exerts its paracrine activity to modulate the endothelium of the vessels (Shifren et al., 1994).

The maturation of the vascular walls within the meningeal plexus and cerebral hemispheres occurs rather late. This presents a problem for early differentiation of the veins and arteries. Veins have been thought to develop later than arteries (Padget, 1948, 1956, 1957). Recent investigations using postmortem angiography permitted differentiation of the superficial and deep venous drainage of the hemispheres during development; the deep veins were found to drain the blood into the subependymal veins and further to the internal cerebral vein and the basal vein of Rosenthal (Nakamura et al., 1994).

The walls of the cerebral vessels mature in correlation with the developmental age of the vascularized structures (Fig. 52). In the brain hemispheres, near the middle stages of pregnancy, the leptomeningeal vessels and those entering from their side to the lateral striatum have been characterized as a thin endothelium-lined walls that develop an evident media. The majority of the extrastriatal vessels of various diameters (10–100 µm) retain such endothelium-lined vascular walls until the end of gestation (Kuban & Gilles 1985), maturing together with the vascularized tissue.

Development of blood–brain barrier (BBB)

The morphological maturation of the vascular walls plays a role in the development of the blood–brain barrier (BBB). The penetrating vessels present an intrusion of the mesodermal elements into the ectodermal nervous tissue. The characteristics of the CNS, i.e. lack of lymphatic channels; the production, circulation and 'sink action' of the CSF (see Chapter 8); the peculiarities of the nervous tissue metabolism; and the special features of vascular permeability contribute to the formation of a BBB. The BBB represents the contact between the mesoderm and ectoderm, i.e. between the blood and the nerve tissue. It should be remembered that not only the BBB, but also the BBB and the CSF-brain-barrier comprise the vasculature of the CNS (Dzi gielewska et al., 1988). This special barrier protects the nervous tissue from substances brought by the blood to ensure a selective transport and the necessary modification of substances deriving from blood or nervous tissue (Risau & Wolburg, 1990).

The vascular channels that invade the developing nervous system gradually become tightly encircled by astrocytic processes. The vascular channels and astrocytic processes are currently defined as the two basic elements for the development of the BBB, despite the complex cellular system representing the barrier. The pericytes and perivascular microglia appear to be involved in BBB functions, but their precise role is not clear. The most important role in addition to that of the endothelial cells was attributed to astrocytes, which are separated from the endothelial cells only by a basal lamina. The astrocytes may transfer inductive signals from brain tissue. The interaction of endothelial cells with astrocytes may regulate the function of the BBB, which starts early in fetal life, and is definitively mature probably after birth (Goldstein et al., 1988). Some recent data raise doubt about the necessity of the intimate contact between the neural tissue and the vessel wall for BBB expression; thus, the role of astrocytes requires further evaluation (Stewart & Hayakawa, 1994). The microvessels in the early developing brain acquire a complex structure at the level of the tight junctions between endothelial cells. They constitute the principal morphological and functional basis for the BBB (Risau & Wolberg, 1990).

The formation and maturation of the BBB have been examined from both the morphological and functional points of view in various animal species and in humans. Results of those studies provides an overview of the events occurring during the gradual maturation of the BBB.

Ultrastructural studies of the mouse cerebral cortex revealed the morphological features of the BBB after the start of its vascularization (Bauer et al., 1992, 1993).

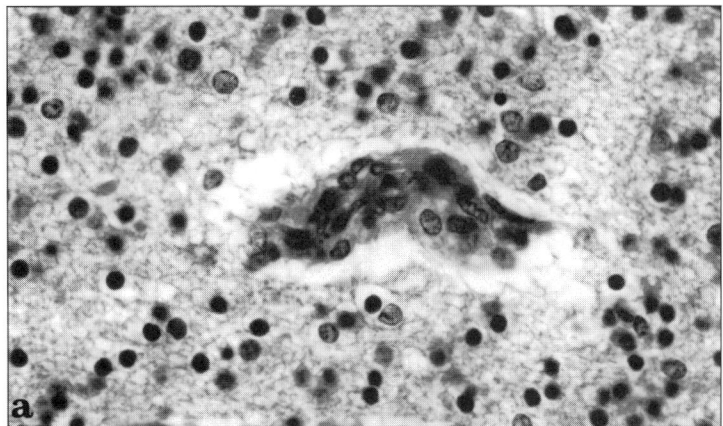
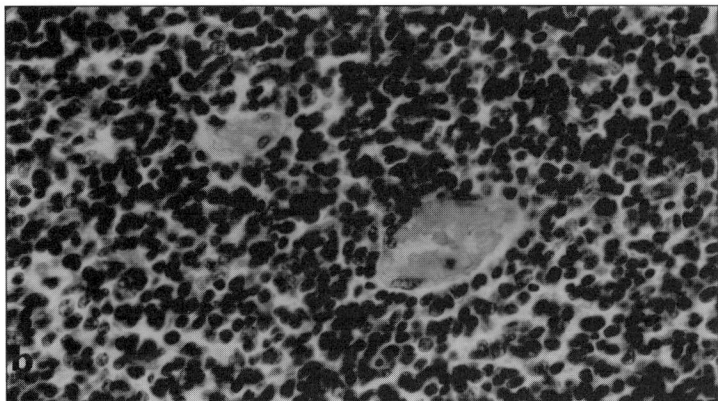

Fig. 52. Maturation of vascular walls at 28 WG.

(a) in striatum, × 400; (b) within periventricular matrix zone, × 400.

The presence of tight junctions between the cerebral endothelial cells and the choroid plexus epithelial cells was observed along with differentiation of these cells very early in other species (Saunders & Mollgard, 1984). After further maturation of the BBB, endothelial cell fenestration allowing for increased permeability were observed; the numbers of fenestrated vessels declines in midgestation period (Stewart & Hayakawa, 1994). Another sign of BBB maturation, i.e. the gradual thickening of the basement membrane, was observed in rats after birth (Bradbury, 1979). Analysis of anionic domains in the developing BBB confirmed the gradual maturation of this barrier. The time of the appearance of anionic sites on both endothelial fronts during BBB maturation confirmed that this process in mice continues beyond the day of birth (Vorbrodt et al., 1986a, 1990; Lossinsky et al., 1986).

In humans, junctions between endothelial cells were reported at 10–13 WG (Bradbury, 1979). In general, BBB maturation in humans appears to depend on CNS structural maturation. It is now known that the BBB in the spinal cord forms earlier than in the telencephalon, consistent with previous observations (Farkas-Bargeton & Arsenio-Nunes, 1970), and that not only the morphology, but also the enzymatic equipment of the vessel walls progress during maturation in parallel with the vascularized structures. The subependymal zone containing germinal cells illustrates the parallel immaturity of this structure and vascular channels without well developed tight junctions or glial processes around the vessels (Sotrel & Lorenco, 1989). This developing subependymal zone may not serve as a barrier (Sarnat, 1992c). It was suggested that BBB closure occurs at some earlier time before the rapid maturation of given cerebral structures. Bradbury (1979) proposed that the rapid maturation of the BBB within the cerebral cortex in humans occurs by 12–16 WG. Thus, a search of the literature demonstrates that BBB maturation varies from one mammalian species to another. In humans, sheep and other animals, BBB maturation occurs *in utero* (Bradbury, 1979), whereas in rodents, maturation of this barrier appears to occur *de novo* (Vorbrodt et al., 1986b; Lossinsky et al., 1986).

The physiological observations confirm the gradual maturation of the BBB, but also raise some new questions about the correlation between its morphological basis and function. In humans, the immaturity of the barrier during fetal life was confirmed by some observations. The highest levels of protein and albumen content in the CSF were detected at 20 WG; they probably decrease thereafter because of barrier thickening (Bradbury, 1979). Protein concentration in the CSF falls from 100 µg at birth to 15–20 µg in the adult, suggesting that further maturation of the BBB occurs after birth. According to some experimental data obtained in animals, the maturation of the BBB occurs not only gradually, but also at different rates for various substances. Analysis of CSF and blood levels of magnesium, chloride, potassium and calcium ions in fetal brains revealed that the concentration of these ions changes with time at different rates until adulthood. It also appears that the restriction in permeability becomes established later than the development of tight junctions present earlier in the growing vessels. The contribution of the intracellular vesiculo-tubular system, the capillary basement membrane, and astroglial processes in regulating permeability must also be considered. It is possible that in early ontogeny, the route from blood to the brain may recapitulate phylogeny, i.e. transcellular, not only intercellular. Clearly, much remains unknown about BBB development, particularly in humans, despite the continuous progress in this field of study.

Meninges – skull bones

O'Rahilly and Müller (1986) have called the origin of meninges 'shrouded in mystery'.

To date, the origin of the cells involved in the formation of meninges is to some degree controversial. Since the beginning of the century, all meningeal layers were considered to be of mesenchymal derivation (reviewed in O'Rahilly & Müller, 1986). Nevertheless, Oberling (1922) postulated the participation of neuroepithelial cells in the origin of meninges, which was supported by observations in meningeal tumors (Dąmbska, 1964). Harvey and other authors (1926, 1933) proposed the involvement of neural crest cells in the formation of meninges. The morphological characteristics of meninges were also debated, and the question was raised whether pia matter and arachnoidea constitute one or two separate sheaths (Oberling, 1922). The observations by O'Rahilly and Müller (1986), covering brain development between 18–57 days (stages 8–23), provided insight into the process of meninges formation and are summarized below.

At days 22–24 (stages 10, 11), the prechordal plate produces mesenchyme and the neural crest provides the material for formation of the pia matter. The meningeal sheath is seen first around the caudal part of the medulla and somewhat later at the mesencephalic level. During this time, vascularization of the brain occurs, first forming the vascular net on its surface, then penetrating the nerve tissue. The cell layer between nerve tissue and epiparenchymal vascular network can be recognized as the developing pia matter. Subsequently, the entire telencephalon becomes surrounded by loose mesenchyme, which is recognizable at around day 33 (stage 15) as the primary meninx. Its ingrowth in the direction of the further tentorium cerebelli is also seen a few days later at day 44 (stage 18). The primary meninges undergo cavitation forming the meshwork where fluid penetrates between the nerve tissue and skeletogenous layer. This meshwork constitutes the forming subarachnoid space. At 46 days (stage 19), the falx cerebri starts to appear. During the last days of observations by O'Rahilly and Müller (52–57 = stages 21–23), the chondrocranium is visible and the more internal dural layer is differentiated. The division between pia and the pachymeninx becomes marked by the variably condensing meshwork between them, which is seen even in the areas of the cerebral hemispheres that develop relatively later. At the end of the embryonic period, the dural limiting layer is visible to the midbrain, the tissue of the subarachnoid space is evident, connections between the skeletogenous layer and the pachymeningeal tissue are also well defined, and most of the cisternae are present. The tentorium represents a separation between subtentorial and infratentorial subarachnoid areas. The meninges at the level of the spinal cord follow a similar course of development. The first indication of the pia matter is detectable at around day 33 (stage 15). The dura encircles the spinal canal at 8 weeks (stage 23); only formation of the arachnoid is prolonged, completed around birth.

Together, these observations lead to the conclusion that mesodermal cells from various sources, including the prechordal plate, periaxial mesoderm and mesectoderm derived from neural crest, provide the material for formation of the meninges, although the participation of some cells from the neural tube has not been definitively excluded.

From a structural point of view, the development of the meninges results in formation of the following consecutive layers (O'Rahilly & Müller, 1986): (1) pia matter adjacent to nerve tissue, (2) subarachnoid space, including arachnoid cells, (3) arachnoid barrier layer, (4) dural border layer, and (5) dura matter. Layers 1–3 constitute the leptomeninx, whereas layers 4–5 constitute the pachymeninx. The border layers between lepto- and pachymeninx (3–4) form the interface layer, i.e. the arachnoid membrane.

Skull and vertebral column bones

The skeletal system deriving from the mesodermal germ layer start to form during the third week of development. Its parts enveloping and protecting the CNS include the vertebral column and the skull.

Formation of the vertebral column starts within the sclerotome, a medial portion of somite which give rise to connective tissue and cartilage. The sclerotomic tissue differentiate according to segmentation order and starting at the cervical level, progresses rostrally and caudally. Intervertebral discs, neural arches and transverse processes appear successively, the arches being completed at the thoracic and upper lumbar levels at the 64th day (French, 1983) of development. Chondrification of centers gives rise to cartilagineous vertebra formed without segmental arrangement from elements of adjoining somites (French, 1983); their ossification occurs in the course of the long-lasting maturation process.

The cranium is composed from viscerocranium and neurocranium deriving from the craniofacial mesenchyme. The viscerocranium comprises the facial skeleton, including jaw skeleton. Among the mesodermal population, which is the source of mesenchymal cells, the neural crest mesenchyme participate, giving material particularly to facial bones (Noden, 1988). The neurocranium includes two parts: the cartilaginous (basal) and the membranous (the vault of the skull). The most cephalic somites are involved in the formation of the cartilaginous neurocranium whose elements develop successively, changing into cartilages (Lemire, 1986). This process starts between days 40 and 44 in the basiocciput and the body of the sphenoid (French, 1983). Finally the process of endochondral ossification occurs. The large bones of the membraneous cranial vault derive by direct ossification of mesenchymal tissue in the course of so-called membraneous ossification. Membraneous bones are joined by squamal sutures. Their closure occurs successively until the 12th year of life, but complete bony fusion is even more prolonged (Jacobson, 1991; Enlow, 1986).

The parameters for evaluation of CNS development

The review of CNS development visualizes how much the maturation rates of particular brain structures differs. Therefore, for evaluation of developmental age of the brain from the second trimester of gestation until the neonatal period, we propose, according to our experience, to compare macroscopic evaluation of the development of cortical gyrification and microscopic evaluation of the amount of matrix cells around the anterior horn of lateral ventricle, the level of maturation of cerebral cortex and neocerebellar cortex, the maturation of brain stem motor nuclei, and myelination of medulla oblongata and frontal lobe for postnatal age. Taking into account that the CNS is relatively spared of developmental disturbances during fetal life, the comparison of brain, lung and placental developmental age may help in estimation of possible (or probable) pathology of pregnancy.

References to Part One

Aboitiz, F. (1988): Epigenesis and the evolution of the human brain. *Med. Hypotheses* **25**, 55–59.

Allsopp, G. & Gamble, H.J. (1979): Light and electron microscopic observations on the development of the blood vascular system of the human brain. *J. Anat.* **128**, 461–477.

Angevine, J.B., Jr. & Sidman, R.L. (1961): Autoradiographic study of cell migration during histogenesis of cerebral cortex in the mouse. *Nature* **192**, 766–768.

Angevine, J.B., Jr. (1965): Time of neuron origin in the hippocampal region. An autoradiographic study in the mouse. *Exp. Neurol.* (suppl.) **2**, 1–70.

Angevine, J.B., Jr. (1970): Critical cellular events in the shaping of neural centers. In: *The Neurosciences Second Study Program*, ed. F.O. Schmitt, pp. 62–72. New York: University of Rockefeller, Press.

Angevine, J.B., Jr. (1975): Development of the hippocampal region. In: *Hippocampus* eds. R.L. Isaacson & K.H. Pribram, vol. I, pp. 61–94. New York, London: Plenum Press.

Armstrong, E., Schleicher, A., Omran, H., Curtis, M. & Zilles, K. (1995): The ontogeny of human gyrification. *Cereb. Cortex* **5**, 56–63.

Asou, H., Murakami, K., Toda, M. & Uyemura, K. (1995): Development of oligodendrocyte and myelination in the central nervous system. *Keio J. Med.* **44**, 47–52.

Bar, T. (1980): The vascular system of the cerebral cortex. *Adv. Anat. Embryol. Cell. Biol.* **59**, IBVI, 1–62.

Barinaga, M. (1996): Guiding neurons to the cortex [news]. *Science* **274**, 1100–1101.

Baron, M. & Gallego, A. (1973): The relation of the microglia with the pericytes in the cat cerebral cortex. *Z. Zellforsch. Mikrosk. Anat.* **128**, 42–57.

Bauer, H.C., Steiner, M. & Bauer, H. (1992): Embryonic development of the microvasculature in the mouse: new insight into the structural mechanism of early angiogenesis. *EXS* **61**, 64–68.

Bauer, H.C., Bauer, H., Lametschwandtner, A., Amberger, A., Ruiz. P. & Steiner, M (1993): Neovascularization and the appearance of morphological characteristics of the blood–brain barrier in the embryonic mouse central nervous system. *Brain Res.* **75**, 269–278.

Becker, L.E., Armstrong, D.L., Chan, F. & Wood, M.M. (1984): Dendritic development in human occipital cortical neurons. *Brain Res.* **13**, 117–124.

Benes, F.M., Turtle, M., Khan, Y. & Farol, P. (1994): Myelination of a key relay zone in the hippocampal formation occurs in the human brain during childhood, adolescence, and adulthood. *Arch. Gen. Psychiatry* **51**, 477–484.

Berry, M. (1986): Neurogenesis and gliogenesis in the human brain. *Food Chem. Toxicol.* **24**, 79–89.

Bodhireddy, S.R., Lyman, W.D., Rashbaum, W.K. & Weidenheim, K.M. (1994): Immunohistochemical detection of myelin basic protein is a sensitive marker of myelination in second trimester human fetal spinal cord. *J. Neuropathol. Exp. Neurol.* **53**, 144–149.

The Boulder Committee (1970): Embryonic vertebrate central nervous system: revised terminology. *Anat. Rec.* **166**, 257–261.

Bourgeois, J.P. (1994): Synaptogenesis in the neocortex of primates. *Brain Pathol.* **4**, 296.

Bowen, I.D. (1993): Apoptosis or programmed cell death? *Cell. Biol. Int.* **17**, 365–380.

Boya, J. (1975): Contribution to the ultrastructural study of microglia in the cerebral cortex. *Acta Anat.* **92**, 364–375.

Bradbury, M. (1979): The concept of a blood–brain barrier. Chichester, Brisbano, Toronto: John Wiley & Sons.

Brody, B.A., Kinney, H.C., Kloman, A.S. & Gilles, F.H. (1987): Sequence of central nervous system myelination in human infancy. I. An autopsy study of myelination. *J. Neuropathol. Exp. Neurol.* **46**, 283–301.

Brown, J.W. (1983): Early prenatal development of the human precommissural septum. *J. Comp. Neurol.* **215**, 331–350.

Brun, A. (1965): The subpial granular layer of the foetal cerebral cortex in man. Its ontogeny and significance in congenital cortical malformations. *Acta Pathol. Microbiol. Scand. Suppl.* **179** 3–98.

Budka, H., Costanzi, G., Cristina, S., Lechi, A., Parravicini, C., Trabattoni, R. & Vago, L. (1987): Brain pathology induced by infection with the human immunodeficiency virus (HIV). A histological, immunocytochemical, and electron microscopical study of 100 autopsy cases. *Acta Neuropathol.* **75**, 185–198.

Caley, D.W. & Maxwell, D.S. (1968): An electron microscopic study of the neuroglia during postnatal development of the rat cerebrum. *J. Comp. Neurol.* **133**, 45–70.

Cameron, R.S. & Rakic, P. (1994): Identification of membrane proteins that comprise the plasmalemma junction between migrating neurons and radial glial cells. *J. Neurosci.* **14**, 3139–3155.

Candy, J.M., Perry, E.K., Perry, R.H., Bloxham, C.A., Thompson, J., Johnson, M., Oakley, A.E. & Edwardson, J.A. (1985): Evidence for the early prenatal development of cortical cholinergic afferents from the nucleus of Meynert in the human foetus. *Neurosci. Lett.* **61**, 91–95.

Caviness, V.S., Jr., Kennedy, D.N., Bates, J.F. & Makris, N. (1996): The developing human brain. A morphometric profile. In: *Developmental neuroimaging*, eds. R.W. Thatcher, G.R. Lyon, J. Rumsey & N. Krasnegov, pp. 3–14. San Diego: Academic Press.

Chi, J.G. & Dooling, E.C. (1976): Gyral development of the human brain. *Arch. Neurol.* **33**, 387 (Abstract).

Chi, J.G., Dooling, E.C. & Gilles, F.H. (1977): Gyral development of the human brain. *Ann. Neurol.* **1**, 86–93.

Choi, B.H. (1981): Hematogenous cells in the central nervous system of developing human embryos and fetuses. *J. Comp. Neurol.* **196**, 683–694.

Choi, B.H. (1981): Radial glia of developing human fetal spinal cord: Golgi, immunohistochemical and electron microscopic study. *Brain Res. Dev. Brain Res.* **227**, 249–267.

Choi, B.H. (1986): Glial fibrillary acidic protein in radial glia of early human fetal cerebrum: a light and electron microscopic immunoperoxidase study. *J. Neuropathol. Exp. Neurol.* **45**, 408–418.

Choi, B.H. (1988): Developmental events during the early stages of cerebral cortical neurogenesis in man. A correlative light, electron microscopic, immunohistochemical and Golgi study. *Acta Neuropathol. (Berl.)* **75**, 441–447.

Choi, B.H. & Kim, R.C. (1984): Expression of glial fibrillary acidic protein in immature oligodendroglia. *Science* **223**, 407–409.

Choi, B.H. & Kim, R.C. (1985): Expression of glial fibrillary acidic protein by immature oligodendroglia and its implications. *J. Immunol.* **8**, 215–235.

Choi, B.H., Kim, R.C. & Peckham, N.H. (1987): Ultrastructural and immunohistochemical studies of radial glia and astroglia in the developing mouse forebrain. *J. Neuropathol. Exp. Neurol.* 1987, 46, 352 (Abstract).

Chugani, D.C., Kedersha, N.L. & Rome, L.H. (1991): Vault immunofluorescence in the brain: new insights regarding the origin of microglia. *J. Neurosci.* **11**, 256–268.

Cowan, W.M., Fawcett, J.W., O'Leary, D.D.M. & Stanfield, B.B. (1984): Regressive events in neurogenesis. *Science* **225**, 1258–1265.

Crosby, E.C., Humphrey, T. & Lauer, E.W. (1962): Correlative anatomy of the nervous system. New York: MacMillan.

Dąmbska, M. (1964): Histoire naturelle et classification des meningiomatoses à propos de cinq observations anatomiques. *Neuropath. Pol.* **2**, 55–82.

Dąmbska, M. & Maślińska, D. (1982): Development of neuronal junctions in different phylogenetic regions of rabbit's cerebral cortex. *Zwierz ta Laboratoryjne* **19**, 131–137.

Dąmbska, M., Wiśniewski, K.E. & Sher, J.H. (1986): Marginal glioneuronal heterotopia in nine cases with and without cortical abnormalities. *J. Child Neurol.* **1**, 149–157.

Dąmbska, M. & Laure-Kamionowska, M. (1990): Myelination as a parameter of normal and retarded brain maturation. *Brain Dev.* **12**, 214–220.

Davson, H. (1967): Physiology of the cerebrospinal fluid. London: Churchill.

De Reuck, J. (1971): The human periventricular arterial blood supply and the anatomy of cerebral infarctions. *Eur. Neurol.* **5**, 321–334.

De Reuck, J. (1972): The cortico-subcortical arterial angio-architecture in the human brain. *Acta Neurol. Belg.* **72**, 323–329.

del Rio-Hortega, P. (1919): Eltercer elemento de los centros nervosos. 1. La microglia estado normal. *Bol. Soc. Espan. Biol.* **9**, 68–83.

Dickson, J.G., Kesselring, J., Walsh, F.S. & Davison, A.N. (1985): Cellular distribution of 04 antigen and galactocerebroside in primary cultures of human foetal spinal cord. *Acta Neuropathol.* **68**, 340–344.

Duckett, S. (1971): The establishment of internal vascularization in the human telencephalon. *Acta Anat. (Basel)* **80**, 107–113.

Dzi gielewska, K.M., Hinds, L.A., Mollgard, K., Reynolds, M.L. & Saunders, N.R. (1988): Blood–brain, blood-cerebrospinal fluid and cerebrospinal fluid-brain barriers in a marsupial (Macropus eugenii) during development. *J. Physiol. (Lond.)* **403**, 367–388.

Eckenhoff, M.F. & Rakic, P. (1991): A quantitative analysis of synaptogenesis in the molecular layer of the dentate gyrus in the rhesus monkey. *Brain Res. Dev. Brain Res.* **64**, 129–135.

Enlow, D.H. (1986): Normal craniofacial growth. In: *Craniosynostosis: diagnosis, evaluation, and management*, ed. M.M. Cohen, pp. 131–156. New York: Raven Press.

Evrard, P., de Saint Gorges, P., Gadisseaux, J.F. et al. (1989): Abnormal development and destructive processes of the human brain during the second half of gestation. In: *Developmental neurobiology*, eds. P. Evrard, A. Minkowski, Nestlé Nutrition Workshops Series, Vevey, Switzerland, vol. 12, pp. 21–41. New York: Raven Press.

Farbman, A.I. (1990): Olfactory neurogenesis: genetic or environmental controls? *Trends Neurosci.* **13**, 362–365.

Farkas-Bargeton, E. & Thieffry, S. (1967): Maturation histoenzymologique de la substance blanche et des parois vasculaires du cerveau de l'enfant. *C.R. Acad. Sci. Hebd. Seances Acad. Sci. D.* **264**, 669–672.

Farkas-Bargeton, E. & Arsenio-Nunes, M.L. (1970): Maturation de l'equipment enzymatique des parois vasculaires du système nerveux. *Acta Neuropathol. (Berl)* **15**, 251–271.

Farkas-Bargeton, E., Diebler, M.F., Rosenberg, B. & Wehrle, R. (1984): Histochemical changes of the developing human cerebral neocortex. Studies on two enzymes of energy metabolism in three cortical layers. *Neuropediatrics* **15**, 82–91.

Feremutsch, K. (1962): Die embryonale Fundamental gliederuno der Hirnrinde. *Z. Anat. Entwickelungsgesch.* **123**, 264–270.

Ferri, R.T. & Levitt, P. (1993): Cerebral cortical progenitors are fated to produce region-specific neuronal populations. *Cereb. Cortex* **3**, 187–198.

Filimonov, I.N. (1947): A rational subdivision of the cerebral cortex. *Arch. Neurol. Psychiatr.* **58**, 296–311.

Filimonov, I.N. (1965): Paleocortex, archicortex and neocortex. Amygdala nucleus and claustrum. In: *Development of the child's brain*, ed. S.A. Sarkisov, pp. 218–239. Leningrad: Meditsina.

Fine, R.E. & Rubin, J.B. (1988): Specific trophic factor-receptor interactions. Key selective elements in brain development and 'regeneration'. *J. Am. Geriatr. Soc.* **36**, 457–466.

Fishell, G., Mason, C.A. & Hatten, M.E. (1993): Dispersion of neural progenitors within the germinal zones of the forebrain. *Nature* **362**, 636–638. [published erratum appears in *Nature* (1993), **363**, 286].

Flechsig, P. (1920): Anatomie des menschlichen Gehirns und Rückenmarks auf myelogenetischer Grunlage, vol. I, pp. 7–44. Leipzig: Thieme.

Flower, M.J. (1985): Neuromaturation of the human fetus. *J. Med. Philos.* **10**, 237–251.

Forger, N.G. & Breedlove, S.M. (1987): Motoneuronal death during human fetal development. *J. Comp. Neurol.* **264**, 118–122.

French, B.N. (1983): The embryology of spinal dysraphism. *Clin. Neurosurg.* **30**, 295–340.

Friede, R.L. (1961): A histochemical study of DPN-diaphorase in human white matter with some notes on myelination. *J. Neurochem.* **8**, 17–30.

Friede, R.L. (1989) *Developmental neuropathology*, 2nd rev. and expanded. Berlin: Springer Verlag.

Friede, R.L. & Samorajski, T. (1968): Myelin formation in the sciatic nerve of the rat. A quantitative electron microscopic, histochemical and autoradiographic study. *J. Neuropathol. Exp. Neurol.* **27**, 546–570.

Fujita, S. & Kitamura, T. (1976): Origin of brain macrophages and the nature of the microglia. In: *Progress in neuropathology*, ed. H.M. Zimmerman, 3, pp. 1–50. New York: Grune & Stratton.

Fujita, S. (1992): Molecular mechanisms of neuroblast differentiation. In: *Molecular basis of neuronal connectivity*, eds. M. Satake, K. Obata, H. Hatanaka, E. Miyamoto, T. Okuyama, pp. 1–4. Japan: Hohko-da Niigata.

Gadisseaux, J.F. & Evrard, P. (1985): Glial-neuronal relationship in the developing central nervous system. A histochemical-electron-microscopic study of radial glial cell particulate glycogen in normal and reeler mice and human fetus. *Dev. Neurosci.* **7**, 12–32.

Gadisseaux, J.F., Goffinet, A.M., Lyon, G. & Evrard, P. (1992): The human transient subpial granular layer: an optical, immunohistochemical, and ultrastructural analysis. *J. Comp. Neurol.* **324**, 94–114.

Galas-Zgorzalewicz, B., Neuhoff, V., Zimmer, H.G. & Dąmbska, M. (1986): Myelin associated glycoprotein of the developing rabbit optic nerve. Separation by micro-polyacrylamide gel electrophoresis and identification by concavalin A binding. *Lectins Biol. Biochem. Clin. Biochem.* **5**, 593–598.

Gallstone, G.W., Robertson, P. & Betz, A.L. (1988): Update on the role of the blood–brain barrier in damage to immature brain. *Pediatrics* **81**, 732–734.

Garcia-Segura, L.M. & Rakic, P (1985): Differential distribution of intermembranous particles in the plasmalemma of the migrating cerebellar granule cells. *Brain Res.* **23**, 145–149.

Gardner, W.J. (1973): The dysraphic states from syringomyelia to anencephaly. Amsterdam: Excerpta Medica.

Garey, L.J. & de Courten, C. (1983): Structural development of the lateral geniculate nucleus and visual cortex in monkey and man. *Behav. Brain Res.* 10, 3–13.

Gershon, M.D. (1993): Development of the neural crest. *J. Neurobiol.* **24**, 141–145.

Gehrmann, J., Gold, R., Linington, C., Lannes-Vieira, J., Wekerle, H. & Kreutzberg, G.W. (1993): Microglial involvement in experimental autoimmune inflammation of the central and peripheral nervous system. *Glia* **7**, 50–59.

Ghosh, A. & Shatz, C.J. (1993): A role for subplate neurons in the patterning of connections from thalamus to neocortex. *Development* **117**, 1031–1047.

Gilles, F.H., Shankle, W. & Dooling, E.C. (1983): Myelinated tracts: growth patterns. In: *The developing human brain: growth and epidemiologic neuropathology*, eds. F.H. Gilles, A. Leviton & E.C. Dooling, pp. 117–183. Boston: Wright.

Giulian, D. & Baker, T.J. (1986): Characterization of ameboid microglia isolated from developing mammalian brain. *J. Neurosci.* 6, 2163–2178.

Goetzen, B. & Sztamska, E. (1996): Comparative study of arterial vascularization of the amygdaloid body in man and sheep. *Folia Neuropathol.* **34**, 143–148.

Golden, J.A. & Chernoff, G.F. (1995): Multiple sites of anterior neural tube closure in humans: evidence from anterior neural tube defects (anencephaly). *Pediatrics* **95**, 506–510.

Goldman-Rakic, P.S. (1987): Development of cortical circuitry and cognitive function. *Child. Dev.* **58**, 601–622.

Goldstein, G.W., Robertson, P. & Betz, A.L. (1988): Update on the role of the blood–brain barrier in damage to immature brain. *Pediatrics* **81**, 732–734.

Goodlett, C.R., Hamre, K.M. & West, J.R. (1990): Regional differences in the timing of dendritic outgrowth of Purkinje cells in the vermal cerebellum demonstrated by the MAP^2 immunocytochemistry. *Brain Res.* **53**, 131–134.

Gould, S.J. & Howard, S. (1987): An immunohistochemical study of the germinal layer in the late gestation human fetal brain. *Neuropathol. Appl. Neurobiol.* **13**, 421–437.

Govender, S., Charles, R.W. & Haffejee, M.R. (1989): Level of termination of the spinal cord during normal and abnormal fetal development. *S. Afr. Med. J.* **75**, 484–487.

Graeber, M.B. & Streit, W.J. (1990): Microglia: immune network in the CNS. *Brain Pathol.* **1**, 2–5.

Gross, G.W. & Goldberg, B.B. (1995): Neurosonography of the fetal neonatal and infant brain and spine. In: *Pediatric neuropathology*, ed. Serge Duckett, pp. 830–881. Baltimore: Williams & Wilkins.

Gruner, J.E. (1970): The maturation of human cerebral cortex in electron microscopy study of post-mortem punctures in premature infants. *Biol. Neonate* **16**, 243–255.

Guillery, R.W. & Killackey, H.P. (1987): Neurobiology. Disappearing developing cells [news]. *Nature* **325**, 578–579.

Hager, H. (1975): EM findings on the source of reactive microglia on the mammalian brain. *Acta Neuropathol. Suppl. (Berl)*, **6**, 279–283.

Hallonet, M.E., Teillet, M.A. & Le Duarin, N.M. (1990): A new approach to the development of the cerebellum provided by the quail-chick marker system. *Development* **108**, 19–31.

Hao, C., Richardson, A. & Fedoroff, S. (1991): Macrophage-like cells originate from neuroepithelium in culture: characterization and properties of the macrophage-like cells. *Int. J. Dev. Neurosci.* **9**, 1–14.

Harvey, S.C. & Burr, H.S. (1926): The development of the meninges. *Arch. Neurol. Psychiatr.* **15**, 545–567.

Harvey, S.C., Burr, H.S. & Van Campenhout, E. (1933): Development of the meninges. Further experiments. *Arch. Neurol. Psychiatr.* **29**, 683–690.

Hasegawa, M., Houdou, S., Mito, S., Takashima, S., Asanuma, K. & Ohno, T. (1992): Development of myelination in the human fetal and infant cerebrum: a myelin basic protein immunohistochemical study. *Brain Dev.* **14**, 1–6.

Hawass, N.D., el-Badawi, M.G., Fatani, J.A., Meshari, A.A., Abbas, F.S., Edrees, Y.B. Jabbar, F.A. & Banna, M. (1987): Myelographic study of the spinal cord ascent during fetal development. *A.J.N.R.* **8**, 691–695.

Herrup, K. & Silver, J. (1994): Cortical development and topographic maps: patterns of cell dispersion in developing cerebral cortex. *Curr. Opin. Neurobiol.* **4**, 108–111.

Hevner, R.F. & Kinney, H.C. (1996): Reciprocal entorhinal-hippocampal connections established by human fetal midgestation. *J. Comp. Neurol.* **372**, 384–394.

Hewitt, K. (1959): The mammalian caudate nucleus. *J. Anat.* **93**, 169–176.

Hewitt, W. (1958): The development of the human caudate and amygdaloid nuclei. *J. Anat.* **92**, 377–382.

Hickey, W.F. & Kimura, H. (1988): Perivascular microglial cells of the CNS are bone marrow-derived and present antigen *in vivo*. *Science* **239**, 290–292.

His, W. (1889): Uber die Entwicklung des Riechganglions und uber diejenige des Verlangevtenmarks. *Verl. Anat. Ges. Anat. Anal. (Erg Herz)* **4**, 63–66.

Hittmair, K., Wimberger, D., Rand, T., Prayer, L., Bernert, G., Kramer, J. & Imhof, H. (1994): MR assessment of brain maturation: comparison of sequence. *AJNR* **15**, 425–433.

Humphrey, T. (1967): The development of the human tuberculum olfactorium during the first three months of embryonic life. *J. Hirnforsch.* **9**, 437–469.

Humphrey, T. (1967a): The development of the human hippocampal fissure. *J. Anat.* **101**, 655–676.

Huppi, P.S., Warfield, S., Kikinis, R., Barnes, P.D., Zientara, G.P., Jolesz, F.A., Tsuji, M.K. & Volpe, J.J. (1998): Quantitative magnetic resonance imaging of brain development in premature and mature newborns. *Ann. Neurol.* **43**, 224–235.

Huttenlocher, P.R. (1984): Synapse elimination and plasticity in developing human cerebral cortex. *Am. J. Ment. Defic.* **88**, 488–496.

Imamoto, K. (1981): Origin of microglia: cell transformation from blood monocytes into macrophagic ameboid cells and microglia. In: *Glial and neuronal cell biology*, Eleventh International Congress of Anatomy, Part A, Editors-in-chief, E. Acosta Vidrio & S. Fedoroff, pp. 125–139. New York: Liss.

Jacobson, M. (1991): *Developmental neurobiology*, 3rd edn. New York: Plenum Press.

Jacobson, M. & Rutishauser, U. (1986): Induction of neural cell adhesion molecule (NCAM) in Xenopus embryos. *Dev. Biol.* **116**, 524–531.

Jotereau, F.V. & Le Douarin, N.M. (1978): The development relationship between osteocytes and osteoclasts: a study using the quail-chick nuclear marker in endochondral ossification. *Dev. Biol.* **63**, 253–265.

Jurevics, H. & Morell, P. (1995): Cholesterol for synthesis of myelin is made locally, not imported into brain. *J. Neurochem.* **64**, 895–901.

Kadhim, H.J., Gadisseux, J.F. & Evrard, P. (1988): Topographical and cytological evolution of the glial phase during prenatal development of the human brain: histochemical and electron microscopic study. *J. Neuropathol. Exp. Neurol.* **47**, 166–188.

Kahle, W. (1956): Zur Entwicklung des menschlichen Zwischenhirns. Studien uber die Matrixphasen und die orliche Reifungsunterschiede im embryonalen menschlichen Gehirn. *Dtsch. Z. Nervenheilk.* **175**, 259–318.

Kahle, W. (1969): *Die Entwicklung der menschlichen Grosshirnhemispäre.* Springer-Verlag, Berlin, Schriftenr. Neurol. 1, 1–116.

Kamada, H., Kawai, Y., Sato, S., Fujiwara, H., Ara, S., Ogasawara, T., Hotta, T., Nakamura, J., Saruta, T. & Suematsu, K. (1984): [The immunohistochemical study of developing human spinal cord – the localization of vimentin, GFAP in radial glial cell.] *No to Shinkei (Japanese)* **36**, 229–235.

K dzia, A. (1995): Evaluation of human telencephalon microangioarchitecture in fetal period. *Folia Neuropathol.* **33**, 181–186.

Kershman, J. (1939): Genesis of microglia in the human brain. *Arch. Neurol. Psychiatr.* **41**, 24–50.

Kinney, H.C., Brody, A.B., Kloman, A.S. & Gilles, F.H. (1988): Sequence of central nervous system myelin ation in human infancy. II. Patterns of myelination in autopsied infants. *J. Neuropathol. Exp. Neurol.* **47**, 217–234.

Kinney, H.C., Karthigasan, J., Borenshteyn, N.I., Flax, J.D. & Kirschner, D.A. (1994): Myelination in the developing human brain: biochemical correlates. *Neurochem. Res.* **19**, 983–996.

Kishi, K., Peng, J.Y., Kakuta, S., Murakami, K., Kuroda, M., Yokota, S., Hayakawa, S., Kuge, T. & Asayama, T. (1990): Migration of bipolar subependymal cells, precursor of the granule cells of the rat olfactory bulb, with reference to the arrangement of the radial glial fibers. *Arch. Histol. Cytol.* **53**, 219–226.

Kitamura, T., Miyake, T. & Fujita, S. (1984): Genesis of resting microglia in the gray matter of mouse hippocampus. *J. Comp. Neurol.* **226**, 421–433.

Klose, M. & Bentley, D. (1989): Transient pioneer neurons are essential for formation of an embryonic peripheral nerve. *Science* **245**, 982–984.

Knobler, R.L. (1995): Demyelinating and dysmyelinating diseases. In: *Pediatric neuropathology*, ed. Serge Duckett, pp. 293–301. Baltimore: Williams & Wilkins.

Koester, S.E. & O'Leary, D.D. (1993): Connectional distinction between callosal and subcortically projecting cortical neurons is determined prior to axon extension. *Dev. Biol.* **160**, 1–14.

Konigsmark, B.W. & Sidman, R.L. (1963): Origin of brain macrophages in the mouse. *J. Neuropathol. Exp. Neurol.* **22**, 643–676.

Kostovic, I. & Rakic, P. (1984): Development of prestriate visual projections in the monkey and human fetal cerebrum revealed by transient cholinesterase staining. *J. Neurosci.* **4**, 25–42.

Kostovic, I. (1986): Prenatal development of nucleus basalis complex and related fiber systems in man: a histochemical study. *Neuroscience* **17**, 1047–1077.

Kostovic, I., Skavic, J. & Strinovic, C. (1988): Acetylcholinesterase in the human frontal associative cortex during the period of cognitive development: early laminar shifts and late innervation of pyramidal neurons. *Neurosci. Lett.* **90**, 107–112.

Kostovic, I., Lukinovic, N., Judas, M., Bogdanovic, N., Mrzljak, L., Zecevic, N. & Kubat, M. (1989): Structural basis of the developmental plasticity in the human cerebral cortex: the role of the transient subplate zone. *Metab. Brain Dis.* **4**, 17–23.

Krmpotic-Nemanic, J., Kostovic, I., Kelovic, Z., Nemanic, D. & Mrzljak, L. (1983): Development of the human fetal auditory cortex: growth of afferent fibers. *Acta Anat.* (Basel) **116**, 69–73.

Krmpotic-Nemanic, J., Kostovic, I., Bogdanovic, N., Fucic, A. & Judas, M. (1988): Cytoarchitectonic parameters of developmental capacity of the human associative auditory cortex during postnatal life. *Acta Otolaryngol. (Stockh).* **105**, 463–466.

Kronquist, K.E., Crandall, B.F., Macklin, W.B.& Campagnoni, A.T. (1987): Expression of myelin proteins in the developing human spinal cord: cloning and sequencing of human proteolipid protein cDNA. *J. Neurosci. Res.* **18**, 395–401.

Kuban, K.C.K. & Gilles, F.H. (1985): Human telencephalic angiogenesis. *Ann. Neurol.* **17**, 539–548.

Kuchna, I. (1994): Quantitative studies of human newborns' hippocampal pyramidal cells after perinatal hypoxia. *Folia Neuropathol.* **32**, 9–16.

Landau, E. (1923): Anatomie des Grosshirns, Formanalytische Untersuchungen E. Bircher, Bern.

Langman, J. (1963): *Medical embryology: human development – normal and abnormal*, pp. 260–261. Baltimore: Williams and Wilkins.

Larroche, J.C. & Bandey, J. (1961): Cavum septi lucidi, cavum Vergae, cavum veli interpositi: les cavites de la ligne mediane. Etude anatomique et pneumoencephalographique dans la periodeneonate. *Biol. Neonate* **3**, 193–236.

Larroche, J.C. (1977): Developmental pathology of the neonate. Amsterdam: Excerpta Medica.

Larroche, J.C. (1981): The marginal layer in the neocortex of a 7 week-old human embryo. A light and electron microscopic study. *Anat. Embryol. (Berl)* **162**, 301–312.

Larroche, J.C., Privat, A. & Jardin, L. (1981): Some fine structures of the human fetal brain. In: *Physiological and biochemical, basis for perinatal medicine*, Levine Conference, Paris, eds. M. Monset-Couchard, A. Minkowski & Z. Samuel, pp. 350–358. Basel: Karger.

Larsell, O. (1947): The development of the cerebellum in man in relation to the comparative anatomy. *J. Comp. Neurol.* **87**, 85–127.

LeBrun, D.P., Warnke, R.A. & Cleary, M.L. (1993): Expression of bcl-2 in fetal tissues suggests a role in morphogenesis. *Am. J. Pathol.* **142**, 743–753.

Lehmann, S., Kuchler, S., Theveniau, M., Vincendon, G. & Zanetta, J.P. (1990): An endogenous lectin and one of its neuronal glycoprotein ligands are involved in contact guidance of neuron migration. *Proc. Natl. Acad. Sci. USA* **87**, 6455–6459.

Lemire, R.J. (1986): Embryology of the skull. In: *Craniosynostasis: diagnosis, evaluation and management*, ed. M.M. Cohen Jr., pp. 105–129. New York: Raven Press.

Levi-Montalcini, R. & Angeletti, P.U. (1968): Nerve growth factor. *Physiol. Rev.* **48**, 534–569.

Ling, E.A. (1978): Brain macrophages in rats following intravenous labeling of mononuclear leucocytes with colloidal carbon. *J. Anat.* **125**, 101–106.

Ling, E.A. & Wong, W.C. (1993): The origin and nature of ramified and amaeboid microglia: a historical review and current concepts. *Glia* **7**, 9–18.

Linnemann, D. & Bock, E. (1989): Cell adhesion molecules in neural development. *Dev. Neurosci.* **11**, 149–173.

Lossinsky, A.S., Vorbrodt, A.W. & Wiśniewski, H.M. (1986): Characterization of endothelial cell transport in the developing mouse blood–brain barrier. *Dev. Neurosci.* **8**, 61–75.

Macchi, G. (1951): The ontogenic development of the olfactory telencephalon in man. *J. Comp. Neurol.* **95**, 245–305.

Marcusson, J.O., Morgan, D.G., Winblad, B. & Finch, C.E. (1984): Serotonin-2 binding sites in human frontal cerebral cortex and hippocampus. Selective loss of S-2A sites with age. *Brain Res. Dev. Brain Res.* **311**, 51–56.

Marin-Padilla, M. (1983): Structural organization of the human cerebral cortex prior to the appearance of the cortical plate. *Anat. Embryol. (Berl.)* **168**, 21–40.

Marin-Padilla, M. (1988): Early ontogenesis of the human cerebral cortex. In: *Cerebral cortex*, eds. A. Peters & E.G. Jones, vol. 7, pp. 1–34. New York: Plenum Press.

Marin-Padilla, M. (1995): Prenatal development of human cerebral cortex: an overview. *Int. Pediatr.* **10** (suppl.), 6–15.

Markovic, L. & Marinkovic, R. (1991): [Microvascularization of the human cerebral cortex during development.] Published in Serbo-Croatian. *Roman. Med. Pregl.* **44**, 447–450.

Maślińska, D. & Muzylak, M. (1995): Apoptosis, programmed cell death in the central nervous system. *Folia Neuropath.* **33**, 69–76.

Martinez, J. & Friede, R.L. (1970): Changes in the nerve cell bodies during the myelination of their axons. *J. Comp. Neurol.* **138**, 329–338.

Matthews, M.A. (1974): Microglia and reactive 'M' cells of degenerating central nervous system: does similar morphology and function imply a common origin? *Cell Tissue Res.* **148**, 477–491.

McConnell, S.K. (1992): The control of neuronal identity in the developing cerebral cortex. *Curr. Opin. Neurobiol.* **2**, 23–27.

Meyer, G. & Gonzalez-Hernandez, T. (1993): Developmental changes in layer I of the human neocortex during prenatal life: a DiI-tracing and AChE and NADPH-d histochemistry study. *J. Comp. Neurol.* **338**, 317–336.

Michel, A.E. & Garey, L.J. (1984): The development of dendritic spines in the human visual cortex. *Hum. Neurobiol.* **3**, 223–227.

Miller, R.H., Zhang, H. & Fok-Seang, J. (1994): Glial cell heterogeneity in the mammalian spinal cord. *Perspect. Dev. Neurobiol.* **2**, 225–231.

Milligan, C.E., Cunningham, T.J. & Levitt, P. (1991): Differential immunochemical markers reveal the normal distribution of brain macrophages and microglia in developing rat brain. *J. Comp. Neurol.* **314**, 125–135.

Milokhin, A.A. (1983): Early synaptogenesis in the spinal cord of human embryos. *Acta Biol. Hung.* **34**, 231–245.

Milokhin, A.A. & Iakushova, A.M. (1988): [Synapses of the human brain in early prenatal ontogeny.] Published in Russian. *Biull. Eksp. Biol. Med.* **105**, 357–359.

Mito, T., Konomi, H., Houdou, S. & Takashima, S. (1991): Immunohistochemical study of the vasculature in the developing brain. *Pediatr. Neurol.* **7**, 18–22.

Mollgard, K. & Jacobsen, M. (1984): Immunohistochemical identification of some plasma proteins in human embryonic and fetal forebrain with particular reference to the development of the neocortex. *Brain Res.* **13**, 49–63.

Morys, J., Narkiewicz, O. & Wiśniewski, H.M. (1993): Neuronal loss in the human claustrum following ulegyria. *Brain Res. Dev. Brain Res.* **616**, 176–180.

Mrzljak, L., Uylings, H.B.M., Kostovic, I. & Van Eden, C.G. (1988): Prenatal development of neurons in the human prefrontal cortex: I. A qualitative Golgi study. *J. Comp. Neurol.* **271**, 355–386.

Müller, F. & O'Rahilly, R. (1983): The first appearance of the major divisions of the human brain at stage 9. *Anat. Embryol. (Berl.)* **168**, 419–432.

Müller, F. & O'Rahilly, R. (1985): The first appearance of the neural tube and optic primordium in the human embryo at stage 10. *Anat. Embryol. (Berl.)* **172**, 157–169.

Müller, F. & O'Rahilly, R. (1986): The development of the human brain and the closure of the rostral neuropore at stage 11. *Anat. Embryol. (Berl.)* **175**, 205–222.

Müller, F. & O'Rahilly, R. (1987): The development of the human brain, the closure of the caudal neuropore, and the beginning of secondary neurulation at stage 12. *Anat. Embryol. (Berl.)* **176**, 413–430.

Müller, F. & O'Rahilly, R. (1988a): The development of the human brain from a closed neural tube at stage 13. *Anat. Embryol. (Berl.)* **177**, 203–224.

Müller, F. & O'Rahilly, R. (1988b): The first appearance of the future cerebral hemispheres in the human embryo at stage 14. *Anat. Embryol. (Berl.)* **177**, 495–511.

Müller, F. & O'Rahilly, R. (1988c): The development of the human brain, including the longitudinal zoning in the diencephalon at stage 15. *Anat. Embryol. (Berl.)* **179**, 55–71.

Müller, F. & O'Rahilly, R. (1989a): The human brain at stage 16, including the initial evagination of the neurohypophysis. *Anat. Embryol. (Berl.)* **179**, 551–569.

Müller, F. & O'Rahilly, R. (1989b): The human brain at stage 17, including the appearance of the future olfactory bulb and the first amygdaloid nuclei. *Anat. Embryol. (Berl.)* **180**, 353–369.

Müller, F. & O'Rahilly, R. (1990a): The human brain from at stages 18–20 including the choroid plexuses and the amygdaloid and septal nuclei. *Anat. Embryol. (Berl.)* **182**, 285–306.

Müller, F. & O'Rahilly, R. (1990b): The human brain at stages 21–23, with particular reference to the cerebral cortical plate and to the development of the cerebellum. *Anat. Embryol. (Berl.)* **182**, 375–400.

Murabe, Y. & Sano, Y. (1982): Morphological studies on neuroglia. VI. Postnatal development of microglial cells. *Cell Tissue Res.* **225**, 469–485.

Nakamura, Y., Okudera, T. & Hashimoto, T. (1994): Vascular architecture in white matter of neonates: its relationship to periventricular leukomalacia. *J. Neuropathol. Exp. Neurol.* **53**, 582–589.

Nelson, M.D. Jr., Gonzalez-Gomez, I. & Gilles, F.H. (1991): Dyke Award. The search for human telencephalic ventriculofugal arteries. *Am. J. Neuroradiol.* **12**, 215–222.

Nikolic, I. & Kostovic, I. (1986): Development of the lateral amygdaloid nucleus in the human fetus: transient presence of discrete cytoarchitectonic units. *Anat. Embryol. (Berl.)* **174**, 355–360.

Noble, M., Fok-Seang, J., Wolswijk, G. & Wren, D. (1990): Development and regeneration in the central nervous system. *Philos Trans. R. Soc. (Lond.) Biol. Sci.* **327**, 127–143.

Noden, D.M. (1988): Interaction and fates of avian craniofacial mesenchyme. *Development* **103** (suppl.), 121–140.

Noetzel, H. (1966): Autoradiographische Untersuchungen zur Entwicklung und Differenzierung der Glia. In: *Proceedings of the 5th International Congress of Neuropathology*; 1965, Zurich, eds. F. Luthy & A. Bischoff, pp. 802–806. Amsterdam: Excerpta Medica (International Congress series, no. 100).

Norman, M.G. & O'Kusky, J.R. (1986): The growth and development of microvasculature in human cerebral cortex. *J. Neuropathol. Exp. Neurol.* **45**, 222–232.

Norman, M.G., Mc Gillivray, B.C., Kalousek, D.K., Hill, A. & Paskitt, K.J. (1995): Congenital malformations of the brain: pathologic, embryologic, clinical, radiologic, and genetic aspects. New York: Oxford University Press.

Northcutt, R.G. & Kaas, J.H. (1995): The emergence and evolution of mammalian neocortex. *Trends Neurosci.* **18**, 373–379.

Nowakowski, R.S., Hayes, N.L. & Egger, M.D. (1992): Competitive interactions during dendritic growth: a simple stochastic growth algorithm. *Brain Res.* **576**, 152–156.

Oberling, C. (1922): Les tumeurs des meninges. *Bull. Assoc. Fr. Etud. Cancer* **11**, 365–394.

Ogawa, M. (1992): Sequential generation of neurons and glial cells from isolated cerebral cortical cells in culture. In: *Molecular basis of neuronal connectivity*, eds. M. Satake, K. Obata, H. Hatanaka, E. Miyamoto & T. Okuyama, pp. 5–7. Japan: Kohko-do Niigata.

Okamoto, H. & Mitani, S. (1992): Inductive differentiation of neural lineages reconstituted and analyzed in a microculture system derived from Xenopus early gastrula cells. In: *Molecular basis of neuronal connectivity*, eds. M. Sataka, K. Obata, H. Hatanaka, E. Miyamoto & T. Okuyama, pp. 8–10. Japan: Kohko-do Niigata.

Oksche, A. (1968): Die pranatale und vergleichende Entwicklungsgeschichte der Neuroglia. *Acta Neuropathol. (Berl.)* (suppl. IV), 4–19.

O'Rahilly, R. (1965): The optic vestibulocochlear and terminal vomeronasal neural crest in staged human embryos. In: *The structure of the eye: II symposium*, ed. J.W. Rohen, pp. 557–564. Stuttgart: Schattauer.

O'Rahilly, R. & Müller, F. (1981): The first appearance of the human nervous system at stage 8. *Anat. Embryol. (Berl.)* **163,** 1–13.

O'Rahilly, R. & Müller, F. (1985): The origin of the ectodermal ring in staged human embryos of the first 5 weeks. *Acta Anat. (Basel)* **122,** 145–157.

O'Rahilly, R. & Müller, F. (1986): The meninges in human development. *J. Neuropathol. Exp. Neurpathol.* **45,** 588–608.

O'Rahilly, R., Müller, F., Hutchins, G.M. & Moore, G.W. (1987): Computer ranking of the sequence of appearance of 73 features of the brain and related structures in the staged human embryos during the sixth week of development. *Am. J. Anat.* **180,** 69–86.

O'Rahilly, R. & Gardner, E. (1979): The initial development of the human brain. *Acta Anat. (Basel)* **104,** 123–133.

O'Rahilly, R. & Müller, F. (1987): Developmental stages in human embryos including a revision of Streeter's 'Horizons' and a survey of the Carnegie collection, Pub. 637. Washington DC: Carnegie Institute of Washington.

O'Rahilly, R. & Müller, F. (1994): Neurulation in the normal human embryo. Ciba Found Symp.,vol. 181, pp. 70–82, discussion 82–89.

O'Rourke, N.A., Dailey, M.E., Smith, S.J. & McConnell, S.K. (1992): Diverse migratory pathways in the developing cerebral cortex. *Science* **258,** 299–302.

Ostertag, B. (1956): Missbildungen. Grundzuge der Entwicklung und Fehlentwicklung. Die Formbestimmenden Faktoren. In: *Handbuch der speziellen pathologischen anatomie und histologie*, Bd. 13 + 4, eds. F. Henke, O. Lubarsch, R. R ssle & W. Scholz, pp. 283–362. Berlin: Springer-Verlag.

Otani, H. & Tanaka, O. (1988): Development of the choroid plexus anlage and supraependymal structures in the fourth ventricular roof plate of human embryos: scanning electron microscopic observations. *Am. J. Anat.* **181,** 53–66.

Ozawa, H., Nishida, A., Mito, T. & Takashima, S. (1994): Development of ferritin-containing cells in the pons and cerebellum of the human brain. *Brain Dev.* **16,** 92–95.

Padget, D.H. (1957): The development of the cranial venous system in man from the viewpoint of comparative anatomy. *Contrib. Embryol.* **36,** 79–140.

Padget, D.H. (1948): The development of the cranial arteries in the human embryo. *Contrib. Embryol.* **32,** 205–261.

Padget, D.H. (1956): The cranial venous system in man in reference to development, adult configuration, and relation to the arteries. *Am. J. Anat.* **98,** 307–355.

Papalopulu, N. & Kintner, C.R. (1994): Molecular genetics in neurulation. *Ciba Foundation Symp.* **181,** 90–99; discussion 99–102.

Pardanaud, L., Yassine, F. & Dieterlen-Lievre, F. (1989): Relationship between vasculogenesis, angiogenesis and hemopoiesis during avian ontogeny. *Development* **105,** 473–485.

Pardanaud, L. & Dieterlen-Lievre, F. (1993): Emergence of endothelial and hemopoietic cells in the avian embryo. *Anat. Embryol. (Berl.)* **187,** 107–114.

Parkinson, D. & Del Bigio, M.R. (1996): Posterior 'septum' of human spinal cord: normal developmental variations, composition, and terminology. *Anat. Rec.* **244,** 572–578.

Paxinos, G. (1990): *The human nervous system*. San Diego: Academic Press.

Perry, E.K., Smith, C.J., Atack, J.R., Candy, J.M., Johnson, M. & Perry, R.H. (1986): Neocortical cholinergic enzyme and receptor activities in the human fetal brain. *J. Neurochem.* **47,** 1262–1269.

Perry, V.H. & Gordon, S. (1988): Macrophages and microglia in the nervous system. *Trends Neurosci.* **11,** 273–277.

Price, J., Williams. B. & Grove, E. (1992): The generation of cellular diversity in the cerebral cortex. *Brain Pathol.* **2,** 23–29.

Privat, A. (1975): Postnatal gliogenesis in the mammalian brain. *Int. Rev. Cytol.* **40,** 281–323.

Purves, D. & Lichtman, J.W. (1985): *Principles of neural development.* Sinauer Associates, Sunderland, Mass.

Rabinowicz, T. (1964): The cerebral cortex of the premature infant of the eigth month. *Prog. Brain Res.* **4,** 39–86.

Rabinowicz, T., Courten Myers, G.M., Petetot, J.M., XI, G. & de los Reyes, E. (1996): Human cortex development estimates of neuronal numbers indicate major loss late during gestation. *J. Neuropathol. Exp. Neurol.* **55,** 320–328.

Rafałowska, J. & Krajewski, S. (1991): Do astroglial cells participate in the process of human spinal cord myelination. *Neuropathol. Pol.* **29,** 41–47.

Raff, M.C. (1989): Glial cell diversification in the rat optic nerve. *Science* **243,** 1450–1455.

Raff. M.C., Miller, R.H. & Noble, M. (1983): A glial progenitor cell that develops in vitro into an astrocyte or an oligodendrocyte depending on culture medium. *Nature* **303,** 390–396.

Raff, M.C., Barres, B.A., Burne, J.F., Coles, H.S., Ishizaki, Y. & Jacobson, M.D. (1993): Programmed cell death and the control of cell survival: lessons from the nervous system. *Science* **262,** 695–700.

Rakic, P. & Yakovlev, P.I. (1968): Development of the corpus callosum and cavum septi in man. *J. Comp. Neurol.* **132,** 45–72.

Rakic, P. (1982): Early developmental events: cell lineages, acquisition of neuronal positions, and areal and laminar development. *Neurosci. Res. Program. Bull.* **20,** 439–451.

Rakic, P. (1985): Limits of neurogenesis in primates. *Science* 227, 1054–1056.

Rakic, P. (1995): The development of the frontal lobe. A view from the rear of the brain. *Adv. Neurol.* **66,** 1–6; discussion 6–8.

Reske–Nielsen, E., Oster, S. & Reintoft, I. (1987): Astrocytes in the perinatal central nervous system. From 5th to 28th week of gestation. An immunohistochemical study on paraffin–embedded material. *Acta Pathol. Microbiol. Immunol. Scand.* [A], **95,** 339–346.

Risau, W. & Wolburg, H. (1990): Development of the blood–brain barrier. *Trends Neurosci.* **13,** 174–178.

Rizvi, T.A., Wadhwa, S., Mehra, R.D. & Bijlani, V. (1986): Ultrastructure of marginal zone during prenatal development of human spinal cord. *Exp. Brain Res.* **64,** 483–490.

Roback, H.N. & Scherer, H.J. (1935): Uber die feinere Morphologie des fruhkindlichen Gehirns unter besonderer Berucksichtigung der Gliaentwicklung. *Virchows. Archiv. Pathol. Anat. Physiol.* **294,** 365–413.

Roessmann, U. & Gambetti, P. (986): Astrocytes in the developing human brain. An immunohistochemical study. *Acta Neuropathol. (Berl.)* **70,** 308–313.

Rorke, L.B. & Riggs, H.E. (1969): Myelination of the brain in the newborn. Philadelphia: Lippincott.

Rorke, L.B. (1994): A perspective: the role of disordered genetic control of neurogenesis in the pathogenesis of migration disorders. *J. Neuropathol. Exp. Neurol.* **53,** 105–117.

Rose, M. (1926): Uber das histogenetische Princip der Einteilung der Grosshirnrinde. *J. Psychol. Neurol.* **32,** 97–160.

Samorajski, T. & Friede, R.L. (1968): A quantitative electron microscopic study of myelination in the pyramidal tract of rat. *J. Comp. Neurol.* **134,** 323–338.

Sariola, H., Ekblom, P., Lehtonen, E. & Saxen, L. (1983): Differentiation and vascularization of the metanephric kidney on the chorioallantoi membrane. *Dev. Biol.* **96,** 427–435.

Sariola, H., Peault, B., Le Douarin, N., Buck, C., Dieterlen-Lievre, F. & Saxen, L. (1984): Extracellular matrix and capillary ingrowth in interspecies chimeric kidneys. *Cell Differ.* **15,** 43–51.

Sarnat, H.B. (1991): Cerebral dysplasias as expressions of altered maturational processes. *Can. J. Neurol. Sci.* **18,** 196–204.

Sarnat, H.B. (1992a): Role of human fetal ependyma. *Pediatr. Neurol.* **8,** 163–178.

Sarnat, H.B. (1992b): Regional differentiation of the human fetal ependyma: immunocytochemical markers. *J. Neuropathol. Exp. Neurol.* **51,** 58–75.

Sarnat, H.B. (1992c): *Cerebral dysgenesis: embryology and clinical expression*. New York: Oxford University Press.

Sarnat, H.B. (1992): Disturbances of neuroblast migrations after 20 weeks in the human fetus and neonate. In: *Fetal and perinatal neurology*, eds. Y. Fukuyama, Y. Suzuki, S. Kamoshita & P. Casaer, pp. 108–117. Basel: Karger.

Sasaki, A., Hirato, J., Naka ato, Y. & Ishida, Y. (1988): Immunohistochemical study of the early human fetal brain. *Acta Neuropathol. (Berl.)* **76,** 128–134.

Saunders, N.R. & Mollgard, K. (1984): Development of the blood–brain barrier. *J. Dev. Physiol.* **6,** 45–57.

Schmechel, D.E. & Rakic, P. (1979a): A Golgi study of radial glial cells in developing monkey telencephalon: morphogenesis and transformation into astrocytes. *Anat. Embryol. (Berl.)*, **156,** 115–152.

Schmechel, D.E. & Rakic, P. (1979b): Arrested proliferation of radial glial cells during midgestation in rhesus monkey (Letter). *Nature* **277,** 303–305.

Schelper, R.L. & Adrian, E.K., Jr. (1986): Monocytes become macrophages; they do not become microglia: a light and electron microscopic autoradiographic study using 125–iododeoxyuridine. *J. Neuropathol. Exp. Neurol.* **45,** 1–19.

Seifert, R., Zhao, B. & Christ, B. (1992): Cytokinetic studies on the aortic endothelium and limb bud vascularization in avian embryos. *Anat. Embryol. (Berl.)*, **186,** 601–610.

Shaw, C.M. & Alvord, E.C. Jr. (1969): Cava septi pellucidi et vergae: their normal and pathological states. *Brain* **92,** 213–224.

Shifren, J.L., Doldi, N., Ferrara, N., Mesiano, S. & Jaffe, R.B. (1994): In the human fetus vascular endothelial growth factor is expressed in epithelial cells and myocytes, but not vascular endothelium: implication for mode of action. *J. Clin. Endocrinol. Metab.* **79,** 316–322.

Sidman, R.L. & Rakic, P. (1973): Neuronal migration, with special reference to developing human brain: a review. *Brain Res. Dev. Brain Res.* **62,** 1–35.

Sidman, R.L. & Rakic, P. (1982): Development of the human central nervous system. In: *Histology and histopathology of the nervous system*, Vol. 1, eds. W. Haymaker & R.D. Adams, pp. 3–145. Springfield, Illinois: Thomas.

Smart, I.H. (1972): Proliferative characteristics of the ependymal layer during the early development of the spinal cord in the mouse. *J. Anat.* **111,** 365–380.

Smith, J.C. & Slack, J.M.W. (1983): Dorsalization and neural induction: properties the organizer in xenopus laevis. *J. Embryol. Exp. Morphol.* **78,** 299–317.

Snow, D.M., Steindler, D.A. & Silver, J. (1990): Molecular and cellular characterization of the glial roof plate of the spinal cord and optic tectum: a possible role for a proteoglycan in development of an axon barrier. *Dev. Biol.* **138,** 359–376.

Sotrel, A. & Lorenzo, A.V. (1989): Ultrastructure of the blood vessels in the ganglionic eminence of premature rabbits with spontaneous germinal matrix hemorrhages. *J. Neuropathol. Exp. Neurol.* **48,** 462–482.

Spatz, H. (1924): Zur Ontogenese des Striatum und des Pallidum. *Dtsch. Z. Nervenheik.* **81,** 185–188.

Spatz, H. (1925): Uber die Entwicklungsgeschichte der basalen Ganglien des menschlichen Grosshirns. *Anat. Anz.* **60**, 54–58.

Stagaard, M. & Mollgard, K. (1989): The developing neuroepithelium in human embryonic and fetal brain studied with vimentin-immunocytochemistry. *Anat. Embryol. (Berl.)* **180**, 17–28.

Staudt, M., Schropp, C., Staudt, F., Obeletter, H., Bise, K. & Breit, A. (1993): Myelination of the brain in MRI: a staging system. *Pediatr. Radiol.* **23**, 169–176.

Stewart, P.A. & Wiley, M.J. (1981): Developing nervous tissue induces formation of blood–brain characteristics in invading endothelial cells: a study using quail-chick transplantation chimeras. *Dev. Biol.* **84**, 183–192.

Stewart, P.A. & Hayakawa, K. (1994): Early ultrastructural changes in blood–brain barrier vessels of the rat embryo. *Brain Res.* **78**, 25–34.

Streeter, G.L. (1915): The development of the venous sinuses of the dura matter in human embryo. *J. Anat.* 1915, **18**, 145–178.

Streeter, G.L. (1918): The developmental alterations in the vascular system of the brain of the human embryo. *Contrib. Embryol.* 1918, **8 (24)**, 7–38 & plates 1–5.

Streeter, G.L. (1927): Archetypes and symbolism. *Science* **65**, 405–412.

Streit, W.J., Graeber, M.B. & Kreutzberg, G.W. (1988a): Functional plasticity of microglia: a review. *Glia* **1**, 301–307.

Streit, W.J., Graeber, M.B. & Kreutzberg, G.W. (1989): Expression of a antigen on perivascular and microglial cells after sublethal and lethal motor neuron injury. *Exp. Neurol.* 1989, **105**, 115–126.

Streit, W.G. & Kincaid-Colton, C.A. (1995): The brain's immune system. *Sci. Am.* 1995, **273**, 54–55, 58–61.

Sturrock, R.R. (1981): A quantitative and morphological study of vascularization of the developing mouse spinal cord. *J. Anat.* **132**, 203–221.

Sturrock, R.R. (1982): A quantitative study of vascularization of the prenatal rabbit spinal cord. *J. Anat.* **135**, 89–96.

Takashima, S., Armstrong, D.L. & Becker, L.E. (1978): Subcortical leukomalacia. Relationship to development of the cerebral sulcus and its vascular supply. *Arch. Neurol.* **35**, 470–472.

Takashima, S. & Tanaka, K. (1978): Development of cerebrovascular architecture and its relationship to periventricular leukomalacia. *Arch. Neurol.* **35**, 11–16.

Takashima, S. & Becker, L.E. (1983): Developmental changes of glial fibrillary acidic protein in cerebral white matter. *Arch. Neurol.* **40**, 14–18.

Takashima, S., Becker, L.E., Nishimura, M. & Tanaka, J. (1984): Developmental changes of glial fibrillary acidic protein and myelin basic protein in perinatal leukomalacia: relationship to a predisposing factor. *Brain Dev.* **6**, 444–450.

Takashima, S. & Becker, L.E. (1986): Prenatal and postnatal maturation of medullary 'respiratory centers'. *Brain Res.* **26**, 173–177.

Tan, S.S. & Breen, S. (1993): Radial mosaicism and tangential cell dispersion both contribute to mouse neocortical development (Letter). *Nature* **362**, 638–640.

Tanaka, O., Yoshioka, T. & Shinohara, H. (1988): Secretory activity in the floor plate neuroepithelium of the developing human spinal cord: morphological evidence. *Anat. Rec.* **222**, 185–190.

Tanaka, S., Mito, T. & Takashima, S. (1995): Progress of myelination in the human fetal spinal nerve roots, spinal cord and brain stem with myelin basic protein histochemistry. *Early Hum. Dev.* **41**, 49–59.

Tapscott, S.J., Bennett, G.S., Toyama, Y., Kleinbart, F. & Holtzer H. (1981): Intermediate filament proteins in the developing chick spinal cord. *Dev. Biol.* **86**, 40–54.

Van Allen, M.J., Kalousek, D.K., Chernoff, G.F., Juriloff, D., Harris, M., McGillivray, B.C., Yong, S.L., Langlois, S., MacLeod, P.M., Chitayat, D. et al. (1993): Evidence for multi-site closure of the neural tube in humans. *Am. J. Med. Genet.* **47,** 723–743.

Van der Knaap, M.S., van Wezel-Meijler, G., Barth, P.G., Barkhof, F., Ader, H.J. & Valk, J. (1996): Normal gyration and sulcation in preterm and term neonates: appearance on MR images. *Radiology* **200,** 389–396.

Van Essen, D.C. (1997): A tension-based theory of morphogenesis and compact wiring in the central nervous system. *Nature* **385** 313–318.

Van Straaten, H.W.N. & Hekking, J.W.N. (1991): Development of floor plate neurons and axonal outgrowth pattern in the early spinal cord of the notochord-deficient chick embryo. *Anat. Embryol. (Berl.)* **184,** 55–63.

Vaughn, J.E. & Peters, A. (1968): A third neuroglial cell type. An electron microscopic study. *J. Comp. Neurol.* **133,** 269–288.

Vladimirov, S.V.& Altukhova, V.I. (1983): Maturation of the human hypothalamo-hypophyseal neurosecretory system in prenatal ontogeny. A light-optical and electron-microscope study. *Sov. J. Dev. Biol.* 14, 322–328. Translated from *Ontogenez,* **14,** 510–517.

Vogt, O. & Vogt, C. (1919): Algemeine Ergebnisse unserer Hirnforschung. *J. Psychol. Neurol.* **25,** 279–461.

Vorbrodt, A.W., Lossinsky, A.S., Dobrogowska, D.H. & Wiśniewski, H.M. (1986a): Distribution of anionic sites and glycoconjugates on the endothelial surfaces of the developing blood–brain barrier. *Brain Res. Dev. Brain Res.* **29,** 69–79.

Vorbrodt, A.W., Lossinsky, A.S. & Wiśniewski, H.M. (1986b): Localization of alkaline phosphatase activity in endothelia of developing and mature blood–brain barrier. *Dev. Neurosci.* **8,** 1–13.

Vorbrodt, A.W., Lossinsky, A.S., Dobrogowska, D.H. & Wiśniewski, H.M. (1990): Sequential appearance of anionic domains in the developing blood–brain barrier. *Brain Res. Dev. Brain Res.* **52,** 31–37.

Wagner, M., Thaller, C., Jessell, T. & Eichele, G. (1990): Polarizing activity and retinoid synthesis in the floor plate of the neural tube. *Nature* **345,** 819–822.

Weidenheim, K.M., Kress, Y., Epshteyn, I., Rashbaum, W.K. & Lymann, W.D. (1992): Early myelination in the human fetal lumbosacral spinal cord: characterization by light and electron microscopy. *J. Neuropathol. Exp. Neurol.* **51,** 142–149.

Weiss, S., Reynolds, B.A., Vescovi, A.L., Morshead, C., Craig, C.G. & van der Kooy, D. (1996): Is there a neural stem cell in the mammalian forebrain? *Trends Neurosci.* **19,** 387–393.

Wilkinson, M., Hume, R., Strange, R. & Bell, J.E. (1990): Glial and neuronal differentiation in the human fetal brain 9–23 weeks of gestation. *Neuropathol. Appl. Neurobiol.* **16,** 193–204.

Wiśniewski, H.M., W giel, J., Wang, K.C., Kujawa, M. & Lach, B. (1989): Ultrastructural studies of the cells forming amyloid fibers in classical plaques. *Can. J. Neurol. Sci.* **16,** 535–542.

Wiśniewski, B., Kida, K.E., Kuchna, E.,Wierzba-Bobrowicz, I. & Dąmbska, M. (1997): Regulators of neuronal survival (Bcl-2, Bax, c-Jun) in prenatal and postnatal human frontal and temporal lobes in normal and Down syndrome brain. In: *Normal and abnormal development of cortex,* R*esearch perspectives in the neurosciences,* eds. A.M. Galaburda & Y. Christen, pp. 179–195. New York: Springer-Verlag.

Wozniak, W., O'Rahilly, R. & Olszewiski, B. (1980): The fine structure of the spinal cord in human embryos and early fetuses. *J. Hirnforsch.* **21,** 101–124.

Yakovlev, P.J. & Lecours, A.R. (1967): The myelogenetic cycles of regional maturation of the brain. In: *Regional development of the brain in early life,* ed. A. Minkowski, pp. 3–70. Oxford: Blackwell.

Zheng, D.R., Guan, Y.L., Luo, Z.B. & Yew, D.T. (1989): Scanning electron microscopy of the development layer I of the human visual cortex (area 17). *Dev. Neurosci.* **11,** 1–10.

Zilles, K., Werners, R., Busching, U. & Schleicher, A. (1986): Ontogenesis of the laminar structure in areas 17 and 18 of the human visual cortex. A quantitative study. *Anat. Embryol. (Berl.)*, **174**, 339–353.

Part Two

Abnormal Brain and Spinal Cord Development

Chapter 4

Etiologic Factors of Abnormal CNS Development

Genetic factors

Morphologically abnormal CNS development may start with very early occurring disturbances of cell differentiation, then faulty migration of neuroectodermal cells and formation of dysplastic structures. Abnormal or evidently delayed further maturation also belongs to the group with disturbed CNS development. All these groups will be the subject of our presentation and will be classified according to their morphological picture. Nevertheless, the question of their etiology has to be reviewed. The genetic factors are the first to be analyzed as causes of CNS maldevelopment.

At present, it is estimated that many disorders affecting the world's population have a major or minor genetic component (Harding & Copp, 1997). In North America, this group is estimated to include 40 per cent of patients in pediatric clinics and 12 per cent of those admitted to general hospitals (Nora & Fraser, 1994). The frequency among these cases of disorders affecting CNS development is difficult to establish. They include not only the direct sequelae of genetic abnormalities, but also the interaction of genes with environmental factors, which, for instance appear to occur particularly often in dysraphic anomalies. Disturbances of the developmental processes within the CNS may also occur secondarily to genetically determined syndromes or diseases impairing normal development of the nervous system. The disorders of genetic origin may occur at each stage of CNS formation and maturation, all these processes most likely being genetically controlled. For instance, we could assume by comparing cortical development in humans with that in lower animal forms that the background of all its steps, such as neuronal proliferation, migration with neuronal-glial interaction, programmed cell death, and final neuronal position, should be controlled by appropriate genes involved in neurogenesis (Rorke, 1994).

The genetic causes affecting CNS development include (a) chromosomal aberration and (b) single-gene mutation.

(a). Among chromosomal abnormalities various types of chromosomal aberration occur. Those with an abnormal number of chromosomes (aneuploids) include trisomy, monosomy and polyploidy. The abnormal chromosomal structure is seen as a deletion of a part of the chromosome, duplication of an additional segment, translocation, inversion or mosaicism. Among chromosomal abnormalities is the fragile site of the X chromosome (Norman et al., 1995) causing the common syndrome, fragile X syndrome. Chromosomal abnormalities occurring in humans are in large part lethal. According to Jacobs and Hassold (1987), the chromosomal abnormalities are found in 50 per cent of spontaneous abortions. In contrast, in more than 66 per cent of neuropathologically examined cases with chromosomal abnormalities, no CNS changes were found (Gullotta et al., 1981). In term newborns only 5 per cent of malformations were recognized as due to chromosomal aberrations; those resulting from gene mutation reached 15 per cent and to known teratogens, 3–5 per cent. Seventy-five per cent were of unknown origin (Shepard, 1986). Chromosomal aberrations are as likely to lead to major or minor malformations as to moderate disturbances of CNS development. The first type of change is often observed in trisomy 13 and 18, and the last is dominant in trisomy 21 and in fragile X syndrome. Therefore, we choose the syndromes due to these chromosomal aberrations for a more detailed description from the neuropathological point of view. The observed changes will be summarized and discussed in Chapter 7.

(b). The majority of syndromes caused by a single gene mutation are transmitted in an autosomal dominant fashion; less common are autosomal recessive conditions, and even rarer, X-linked disorders. Inheritance of such syndromes affecting the CNS occurs in particular families; therefore, study of the pedigree of affected individuals helps determine in which fashion the pathologic syndrome is inherited and to what degree gene penetrance and expressivity are evident. We must take into account that if the penetrance is reduced, some individuals bearing the gene may not present with clinical changes and that when expressivity is not total, individuals may be less affected than other family members. The syndrome may also appear as a new mutation. Among syndromes involving CNS development, microcephaly may occur as a result of autosomal dominant or recessive inheritance, and holoprosencephaly was sometimes also reported as transmitted in a recessive way (Anderson, 1995). In the group of diseases named phakomatoses (Ph), gene changes play a fundamental role. They will be described in Chapter 5.

Exogenous factors

Many factors are known or only suspected to be teratogens. Shepard (1992) published a list of such agents. Until now, many more teratogens are known for animals, and around 30 as producing developmental anomalies in humans. Among them, x-rays, antimitotic, and some other drugs (including those used in medical treatment), fetal asphyxia, ischemia, infectious diseases, and many other environmental factors are listed. The exogenous agents may act in various ways and impair normal development at various stages, inducing mutations, disturbances of mitotic activity, abnormal metabolism because of lack of substances or enzymatic inhibition, among other changes. When development is disturbed as a sequel of early-occurring clastic lesions, embryopathies (disruptions) arise. All extrinsic factors disturbing CNS development and further maturation could be treated jointly as a group of teratogens according to Shepard (1986). The final result of each teratogenic influence is strictly related to the time of its activity and of dosage of injurious agent.

Ionizing radiation may, depending on such circumstances, lead to fetal death or result in major or minor lesions (Altman et al., 1968; Ferrer et al., 1984; Miller, 1990).

Drugs have a poorly known influence. Lesions on fetal brains were observed in experimental animals after administration of antimitotic drugs during pregnancy (Dąmbska et al., 1979a; Dąmbska & Maślińska, 1981). According to an experimental study, phenobarbital may exert an unfavorable influence on brain development (Dąmbska et al., 1979b; Chmielik, 1996). The sequelae of antiepileptic drug administration interact with the threat of a mother's epileptic attacks, which may induce hypoxic lesions in the fetus, which were observed in animals (Dąmbska et al., 1984a). Although those changes have to be compared carefully with possible ones in humans, it is known that anticonvulsant drugs may induce lesions in the brain of fetuses of mothers with epilepsy (Holmes, 1994). Phenytoin may provoke microcephaly and other rather mild anomalies (Buchler et al., 1990), and valproic acid is known to increase the risk of spina bifida, whereas carbamazepine imposes only a small risk (Lammer et al., 1987; Rosa, 1991; Nau, 1994).

Among other chemicals, alcohol has for a long time been suspected to cause fetal damage, and fetal alcohol syndrome (FAS) has been studied (Jones et al., 1973). In such newborns, microcephaly, some major anomalies such as agenesis of the corpus callosum (CC), meningocele and syringomyelia, and minor changes including glio-neuronal meningeal heterotopies were reported (Pfeiffer et al., 1979; Wiśniewski et al., 1983). Nevertheless, little is known about the direct and indirect actions of alcohol on the developing brain (Norman et al., 1995).

Infectious diseases in a mother could lead to fetal infection across the placenta or during delivery. Other broad influences are also possible. Viruses (cytomegalovirus [CMV], rubella, herpes, and human immunodeficiency virus [HIV]), bacteria (often listeria monocytogenes), and parasites (particularly, toxoplasma gondi) have to be taken into account. Early-transmitted infections often provoke pregnancy loss. They may also damage the fetal CNS at various stages of development. Therefore, infection may be responsible for early-arising malformation (Byrne et al., 1987), but they are rare. The later-arising anomalies consecutive to fetal infections, such as polymicrogyria combined with periventricular lesions, are seen more often (Bignami & Appicciutoli, 1964; Dąmbska et al., 1983a).

Among intrauterine infections, HIV exerts a particular role due to its neurotrophic properties. In addition to possible HIV encephalitis, impairment of CNS growth and maturation are observed (Kozłowski, 1995; Kozłowski et al., 1997).

Some maternal diseases may also be found in the group of factors damaging the fetal brain. For instance, severe diabetes in the mother may cause not only some malformations (Holmes, 1994), but also according to our own observation, retardation of brain maturation in newborns too tall and too heavy for conceptional age.

The list of exogenous factors damaging the CNS during development could change, but even if the number of affected individuals diminishes thanks to better prevention of exposure to these factors, the list of threats will grow larger with increasing environmental pollution.

Correlations between time and type of developing brain damage

Organogenesis, consecutive development, and final maturation of the CNS in humans constitute a very long process. It starts from the appearance of the neural plate at 16–18 days after conception, and biochemically and ultrastructurally detectable developmental events continue after the second decade of life. The morphological characteristics of normal and abnormal brain development are perceptible on routine light microscopic examination until the second or third year of life. We will restrict our presentation to this stage of CNS maturation.

The review of CNS development (Part One) demonstrated the different rates of formation and maturation of CNS structures. When the intensively differentiating structures are most susceptible to damage, leading to their erroneous development, reparative processes correlate with maturity of the damaged tissue. Differences in reactions to damage of different CNS structures are evident.

The teratogenic time for the spinal cord is very early, before the end of the first month of gestation; some midline malformations even due to an earlier defect may appear at the second and third month, and cortical anomalies may start around the end of this month. Long-lasting neuronal migration and organization of the cerebral cortex result in a prolonged period even beyond the moment of birth, when cortical anomalies may arise. Their picture and severity depend on the time of appearance.

The particularities of the uneven timing of the development of CNS structures must be taken into account when analyzing for malformation and secondary lesions of the CNS. When an injurious agent induces general damage to the developing brain, the changes in different structures depend on their maturity. An insult at the third to fifth gestational month can cause necrotic lesions in the brain stem and spinal cord and evident malformations of the hemispheric cortex. Malformations of the cortical mantle differ in type according to the degree of maturation of the particular part at the time the lesion develops. For instance, the agyric frontal lobes and pachygyric hippocampal formation may help establish the time of damage. The different character of changes may also be the result of their causal interdependence. Necrotic changes within hemispheric white matter may be responsible for cortical anomalies – we will describe them as late, secondary changes.

Very early-arising malformations may also influence the abnormal topographical conditions for further brain development, inducing the chain of consecutive developmental abnormalities.

The final maturation of gray matter structures and myelination of CNS pathways also occur at different rates in various areas. Therefore, their susceptibility for damage proportional to metabolic patterns may differ at various steps of the maturation process. This leads to the age-dependent topography of perinatal lesions. Asphyxia in preterm newborns (mainly between 24 and 32 WG) leads to periventricular hemorrhages within germinal nests; later-occurring insults result in white matter infarcts and cortical necrotic lesions. All such necrotic lesions influence the last phase of the maturation process, resulting in a complicated picture of lesions as the morphological background of cerebral palsy syndromes in infants.

In our presentation, we will take into account the results of this complicated pathomechanism of abnormalities occurring during the lengthy CNS development.

Chapter 5

The Phakomatoses – the Ecto-mesodermal Syndromes

The phakomatoses (Ph) constitute a group of diseases encompassing many entities. Their clinical, morphological, and genetic criteria have been elaborated step by step since van Hoeve introduced this systematic diagnosis in 1923. The name for these diseases is derived from the Greek term *phakos*, which means spot or figure; these diseases are characterized by spots. The phakomatoses present such changes in the skin and tumor-like formations in the CNS and in other organs. Neuronal and mesodermal elements are involved in such pathologic formations. Because many may involve neural crest derivatives, even the term neurocristopathies has been used to refer to such neuromesodermal syndromes (Reznik & Pierard, 1995). The focal changes present the traits of disturbances of cell differentiation, and those cytological abnormalities differentiate them from other dysplasias (Francois, 1972; Sarnat, 1992). Therefore, to discuss normal and pathologic brain development, we must first take into account this group of diseases. The failures of development or formation of anomalies are secondary. The relation between early cellular anomalies and the blastomatic changes that often appear later in Ph are still a subject of discussion (Bolande, 1984; Norman *et al.*, 1995). The blastomatous tendency in Ph has already been emphasized by van Bogaert (1949), and the transitional position of lesions seen in these syndromes between dysplasia and neoplasia is also actually evoked. Malformations, secondary to defective cytological differentiation and often presenting disturbances in cell migration, are observed particularly within the CNS. They are the final of the four cardinal, morphological features of Ph according to Francois (1972), small spots, tumor-like hyperplastic formations, tumors, and other congenital malformations.

It was found that Ph are genetically determined, with autosomal-dominant inheritance, but with various levels of gene penetration. In sporadic cases, gene mutations are suspected. The diseases show a great phenotypic variability, but observation of changes existing at various steps of development suggests that disturbances within paracrine growth factors (peptides, cytokines, and nerve growth factors, etc.) play an important role in their pathomechanism. It has even been proposed that the term paracrinopathies (Kousseff, 1990). The list of Ph designated as disembryoplasias with blastomatous tendency (van Bogaert, 1949, 1961), familiar hamartoblastoses (Zülch, 1958), and, finally, the ecto-mesodermal syndromes (Norman et al., 1995) differ in consecutive classifications. Some neuropathologists have even concealed them as a separate group of disorders. Avoiding such an extreme point of view, we could see four entities nearly generally accepted as representative for phakomatoses: tuberous sclerosis (TS), neurofibromatosis (NF), (recently divided into two separate entities), and Hippel–Lindau and Sturge–Weber syndromes. Recently, Norman et al. (1995) suggested that Sturge–Weber syndrome be reclassified as a vascular malformation, but Reznik and Pierard (1995) consider it together with Hippel–Lindau syndrome as representative of vascular phakomatoses, usually involving the CNS structures. We decided to present both of them in their traditional position.

We would like to present these syndromes and some others involving the nervous system as demonstrating the continuous course of developmental disturbances from erroneous cellular differentiation to structural anomalies, even joined with blastomatous metaplasia.

Tuberous sclerosis (Bourneville disease)

Tuberous sclerosis is a genetically heterogenous disease. The genes responsible for its autosomal dominant inheritance were found in chromosomes 9, 11, 14 and 16, and their exact localization is still being studied (Sampson et al., 1992; Anonymous, 1993; Reznik & Pierard, 1995). The frequency of TS is estimated, with a great divergence of opinions, to be from 1:10,000–1:170,000 births (Gomez, 1988). Some authors found it to be even 1:6,000 (Editorial Progress in TS, 1990).

The disease is characterized by tumors of various sizes, numbering from only a few to many millimeters in diameter and localized in the CNS. Small spots also appear within time in the skin, as angiofibromas named Pringle nevus or amelanotic skin spots, and perineural fibroma known as Kenan's knobs. Tumors of various sites, verified as hematoma, fibroma, and lipoma are also found in the skin and internal organs. Rarely is cardiac rhabdomyoma seen.

Clinical manifestations depend on topography and the degree of changes. They may appear and increase in number during infancy. Melanotic skin spots are seen very early, and Pringle nevus on the face is observed later, even in children 8–9 years of age. Neurological abnormalities consist of mental retardation in around 50 per cent of cases and epileptic seizures in 90 per cent. CNS tumors can be detected by computed tomography (CT) or magnetic resonance image (MRI) techniques, which are helpful for clinical diagnosis of changes within the CNS (Halimi et al., 1989; Truhan & Filipek, 1993). Growth of tumors may impede the normal circulation of the CSF; therefore, secondary hydrocephalus may arise in TS.

Neuropathologically, CNS tumefactions are localized most often within the white matter, many times subpendymally or in the cortex, and are seen macroscopically on the external face of cerebral convolutions. They include a group of abnormal cells that are often very elongated, testifying of their disturbed differentiation and migration. The cells can be recognized often as astrocytes and sometimes as nerve cells; several others could not be verified at all (Fig. 53). Chou and Chou (1989) performed an immunohistochemical study and found that a great number of abnormal cells were characterized by a positive reaction for GFAP (glial fibrillary acidic proteins), but many of them reveal heterogenous reactions. They considered them as heterogenous from the point of view of neuronal differ-

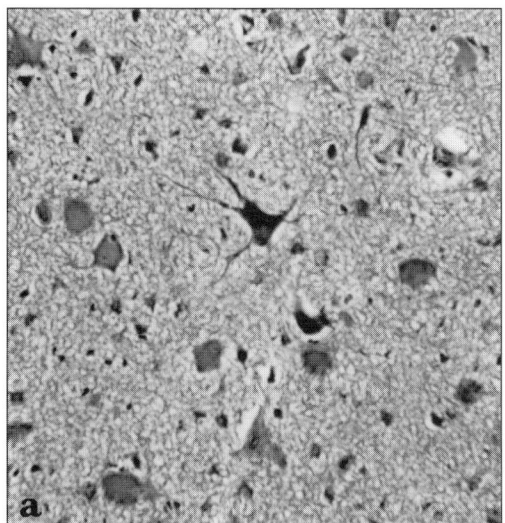
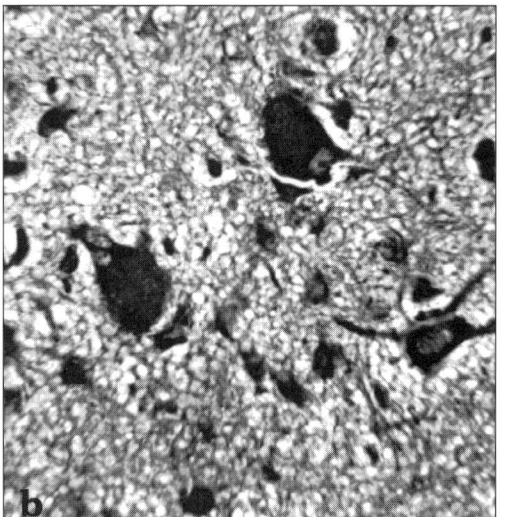

Fig. 53. Large, poorly differentiated neurocytes and glial cells in tuberous sclerosis. Cresyl violet;

(a) × 120; (b) × 400.

entiation. Calcification of nodules occurs rather often. The abnormal cells are not only seen in nodules, but are also disseminated in different brain structures (Roach et al., 1992).

The tumor often appearing in TS is a giant cell astrocytoma localized in the subpendymal area (Fig. 54).

Neurofibromatosis

Neurofibromatosis (NF) has been recognized during recent years as including two separate entities: neurofibromatosis type 1 (NF1) and type 2 (NF2). This classification was introduced at the National Institutes of Health Consensus Developmental Conference (Anonymous, 1988). It was concluded that both entities are due primarily to affected cell growth of neuronal tissue, but resulting from different genes. As a particular feature of the examined entities, it was found that in NF1, the majority of intracranial neoplastic tumors appearing in addition to peripheral ones develop from the primary components of the CNS (astroglial cells and neurons), and in NF2 the coverings are involved in a intracranial neoplastic process (Schwann and meningeal cells) (Aoki et al., 1989).

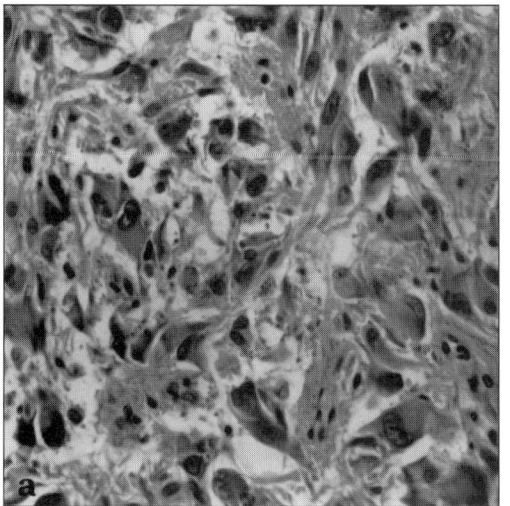
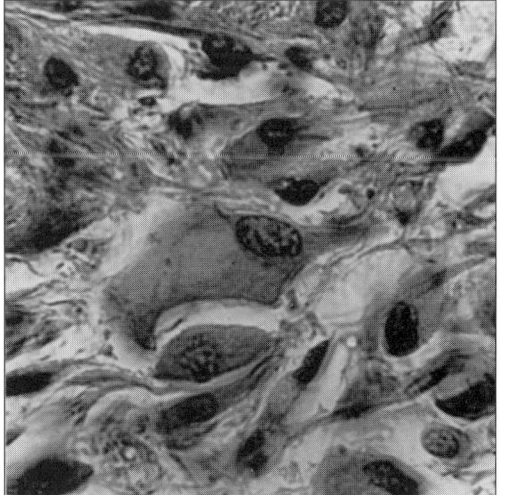

Fig. 54. Giant cell astrocytoma in a case of tuberous sclerosis. HE;

(a) × 200; (b) × 400.

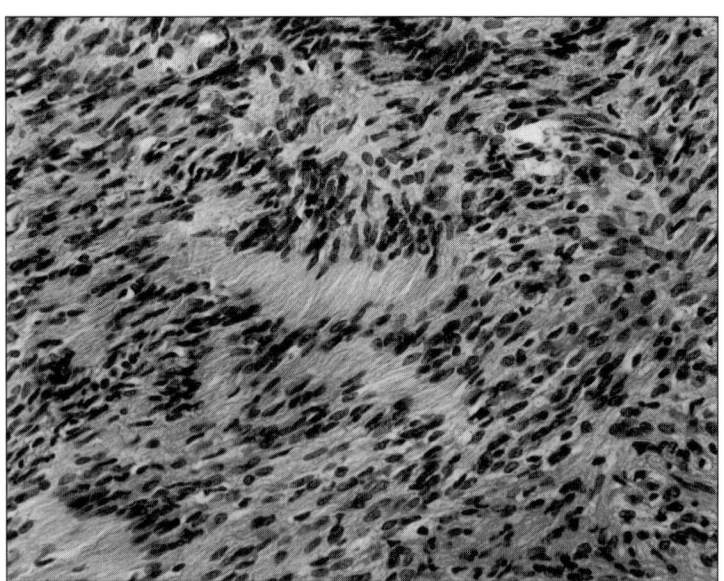

Fig. 55. Schwannoma in neurofibromatosis type II. HE, × 160.

NF 1 = von Recklinghausen disease (the peripheral form)

This disease is relatively common, being observed in 1:2,000–1:4,000 births. Its autosomal dominant inheritance is due to a gene located on chromosome 17 (Barker et al., 1987; Wallace et al., 1990; Marchuk, 1991). The structure and function of gene products – among others, neurofibromin, which may play the role of a tumor suppressor – are under investigation (Guttmann & Collins, 1992; Gregory et al., 1992). Gene expression in NF1 is variable. Therefore, the intensity of changes differs from one case to another (Braffman & Naidich, 1994a). The disease is characterized by the appearance of tumors, from small to large, on the peripheral and intracranial nerves. They grow between nerve fibers, forming complex convolutions. They are recognized as neurofibromas (known also as lemmocytomas). Secondarily, café au lait spots are disseminated in the skin, occurring mostly in infancy. The presence of six spots 1.5 cm in diameter justifies the diagnosis of NF, when they coexist with one of the other characteristic traits, which include small benign hamartomas within the iris (Lisch tumors), freckling of the axillary or inguinal region, skeletal malformations, and optic glioma (Anonymous, 1988).

Clinically, the course of the disease is usually slowly progressive, presenting symptoms secondary to localization of pathologic changes. In more severe cases, epileptic seizures and mental retardation have been observed. From the pathological point of view, the tumors (neurofibromas) of the peripheral nerves include in their structure fibroblasts, Schwann cells, and collagen fibers. In up to 10 per cent of cases, they reveal the tendency to become malignant. In the CNS, glioma of optic nerves occur rather often, in 30–80 per cent of cases (NIH CDC, 1988). Other changes, corresponding probably to some undetermined foci, seen on MRI with increased signal T2 (Aoki et al., 1989), consist of neuropathologically described small, subependymal gliofibrillary tumors (Rubinstein, 1986), and some vascular anomalies (Woody et al., 1992). Among rare, but more severe CNS anomalies, coexisting with NF1, hemimegalencephaly was reported (Cusmai et al., 1990). Syringomyelia also was observed, for which Ostertag (1957) underlined the blastomatic tendency, suggesting its nosological position between malformations and Ph.

NF2 B the central form

This disease reached its independent position definitively when the gene responsible for its appearance was detected on chromosome 22 (Rouleau et al., 1987; Trofatter et al., 1993). Previously known as a central form of neurofibromatosis, NF2 is rather rare, appearing in 1:50,000 births (Anonymous, 1988). The bilateral acoustic Schwannomas are most characteristic of NF2 (Fig.55).

Together with multiple CNS meningiomas, they may induce clinical manifestations of the disease. The hearing loss and balance disturbances occur rather late and often progress more or less slowly. Only CT or

MRI examination help detect NF2 relatively early. Tumors of cranial and spinal nerves, and intramedullary tumors are also seen in this disease.

von Hippel–Lindau disease

Except for sporadic cases, hemangioblastoma cerebelli and retinae depend on a gene located on chromosome 3 (Seizinger et al., 1988). The disease consists of development of angioblastic tumors in the cerebellum and retina, and sometimes also in the brain stem, spinal cord and meninges. Pheochromocytoma, carcinoma, and cystic tumors are seen within internal organs, particularly the kidneys and pancreas (Seizinger et al., 1988; Braffman & Naidich, 1994b). Syringomyelia and bony cysts complete the list of changes seen in von-Hippel–Lindau disease. A cerebellar tumor is often recognized clinically in an adult presenting cerebellar symptoms and/or symptoms of a tumor of the posterior fossa. Neuroimaging techniques are essential for its diagnosis.

Pathologically, angioblastic tumors within the CNS have a cystic appearance, containing yellowish fluid. The tumor itself is attached to the cystic wall and contains angioblasts, cushioning many cysts. The only treatment is surgical.

Sturge–Weber disease – angiomatosis cerebrofacialis

The genetic defect for this disease has still not been found, and it often appears as sporadic and only sometimes as familiar. The disease is characterized by angioma of the face, often topographically related to the innervation of trigeminal nerves. Glaucoma can be also seen. Considering this disease a primary anomaly of blood vessels (Norman & Schoene, 1977), some authors have classified it among the vascular malformations. Angiomatic changes including

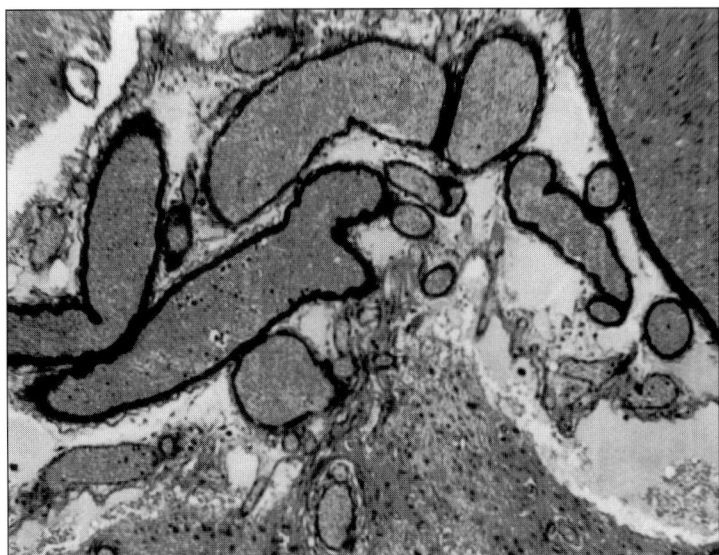

Fig. 56. Angiomatic changes of meningeal vessels. van Gieson, × 60.

large, thin-walled veins are seen also within meninges in the subarachnoidal space, most often on the parieto-occipital level (Fig. 56). The thin walls of veins are often composed only by endothelium and a collagen layer (Alexander & Norman, 1960). The progressive calcification of vessels occurs, leading to pressure on underlying cortical convolutions and their secondary atrophy. Such changes increase with time, which are clearly visible on repeated radiographic examination (Braffman & Naidich, 1994b). The focal cortical malformations that may also be seen, coinciding with angiomatic changes, testify to early formation of vascular anomalies. The progressive lesion of the brain hemisphere underlying angiomatic changes induces epilepsy, mental retardation, and other syndromes depending on the topography of the changes. Sometimes intractable seizures lead to the decision for hemispherectomy, which should be considered during the first six months of life (Ogunmekan et al., 1989).

The list of other Ph reaches 10–20 syndromes (Francois, 1972; Haberland, 1987; Norman et al., 1995; Reznik & Pierard, 1995). We choose four of them representing different types and pathomechanisms of such disturbances.

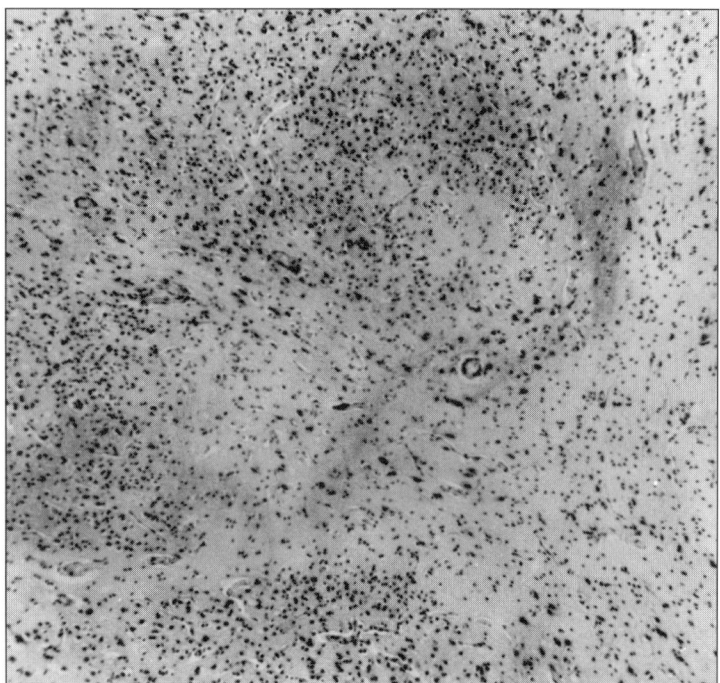

Fig. 57. Disturbed cortical organization in a case of hemimegalencephaly. Cresyl violet, × 100.

The Jadassohn linear nevus

This syndrome occurs very rarely. Its genetic characteristics have not been found, but its morphological features allow classification of this syndrome in the group of Ph (Zaremba et al., 1978; Kousseff, 1992). The disease is characterized by skin nevi localized on the midline of the body, angiomata of the retina, and malformations within the CNS and internal organs. In the CNS, disseminated tumors may be similar to those observed in tuberous sclerosis. Hemimegalencephaly was also observed to be associated with this syndrome.

Clinically, in the Jadassohn nevus, even without this last association, epilepsy, mental retardation, and other symptoms may appear secondary to CNS changes.

Hemimegalencephaly

Hemimegalencephaly is found more often with Jadassohn linear nevus than with other neurocutaneous syndromes (Sarnat, 1992). This unusual anomaly bears the morphological traits of phakomatoses. In hemimegalencephaly, only one cerebral hemisphere is enlarged. It includes the anomalies of neuronal migration and deeply disturbed cortical organization without normal layering (Fig. 57). The nerve and glial cells rather disseminated in the abnormal cortex present features of disturbed differentiation. Among them, giant cells are observed (Dąmbska et al., 1984b; Barth, 1987; Manz et al., 1979).

Clinically, head, face and entire body asymmetry may or may not be seen. The neurological syndromes also are not constant. Most characteristic are epileptic seizures and mental retardation (Pavone et al., 1991; Trounce et al., 1991). Even hemispherectomy is taken into account for intractable seizures (Vigevano et al., 1989; Mischel et al., 1995). Neuroimaging techniques are very useful for the accurate diagnosis of heminegalencephaly.

Neurocutaneous melanosis

Neurocutaneous melanosis, named by van Bogaert (1949), is a very rare syndrome presenting as pigmented nevi on the skin, the CNS, and meninges. They are sometimes very large, in the form of the so-called bathing trunk nevus. The nevi include cells containing melanin droplets, without the tendency to malignancy (Faillace et al., 1984). This entity is usually symptomless, except for the large melanotic spots in meninges that may disturb the circulation of the CSF, leading to hydrocephaly. Melanomas coexist rather sporadically (Russell & Rubinstein, 1989).

Lhermitte–Duclos disease-dysplastic gangliocytoma of the cerebellum

We decided to mention this disease because of its nosological position, illustrating the difficulties in classification and existence of transitional forms of some entities. This was described by Lhermitte and Duclos (1920) and then by Hallervorden (1959) and was considered more a malformation than a neoplasm (Leech et al., 1977). It appears sporadically and more often in males. The syndrome most often consists of enlargement of one cerebellar hemisphere in which the abnormal structures of the cortex are seen. Below the molecular layer, instead of normal Purkinje cells, the large cells are accumulated in the outer part of granular layer. Myelinated fibers arise from the population of abnormal cells. These cells arise verisimiliter mostly from the granular cells (Beuche et al., 1983; Hair et al., 1992). Mineral deposits can be seen within the changes. Recently, it was suggested that this disease is identical to Cowden disease, which is a multiple hamartomas syndrome with autosomal dominant inheritance (Albrecht et al., 1992; Reznik & Pierard, 1995; Norman et al., 1995). In Cowden disease, multiple hamartomas and tumors of the face, anus, breast and ovaries are seen. An association with a syndrome presenting characteristics of Lhermitte–Duclos disease was observed, suggesting the diagnosis of Lhermitte–Duclos–Cowden syndrome (Padberg et al., 1991). Lhermitte–Duclos disease was until now known as autosomal dominant inheritance. The gene for Cowden disease was recently localized to chromosome 10q 22–23 (Nelen et al., 1996).

Lhermitte–Duclos disease was found in a newborn (Roesmann & Wongmongkolrit, 1984), but the clinical symptoms occur most often during the second decade of life, presenting brain stem dysfunction, headache, and other features of increased intracranial pressure. Even sudden death was reported, but its duration was observed from few months to several years.

Chapter 6

Malformations of the CNS

The majority of abnormalities that arise within the CNS in the course of developmental processes before birth deserve the name of malformations. The terms dysplasia, dysgenesis or malformation are synonymous. Particular types of developmental disturbances such as ectopia or heterotopia (displacement of nerve tissue), aplasia or hypoplasia (primary deficiency of tissue development), or hamartoma (focally disorganized arrangement of tissue) also belong to this group of changes (Sarnat, 1992). Among the disturbances mentioned last, most localized in the hypothalamic region, present as 'tumor-like' (Willis, 1958) malformations; therefore, they will not be included in our review of developmental abnormalities.

The etiopathomechanism of CNS malformations is, for many reasons, very difficult to establish (see Chapter 4). A large group of malformations can be considered as multifactorial or from unknown etiology. The morphological picture of primary and secondary malformations is often identical. Taking into account the complex or undetermined etiology of so many cases, we are obliged to adopt the traditional classification of malformations according to their morphology. Analysis of each particular case of CNS malformation, in correlation with the history of its development, may help to reconstruct the mechanism of formation of the observed changes.

Neural tube defects – the dysraphic syndromes

Malformations related to the defects of the neural tube, known also as dysraphic disorders, belong to the most common dysgeneses of the CNS. Campbell *et al.* (1986) estimate that they occur in one to eight cases per 1,000 live births. Bremer (1927), who introduced the term dysraphic syndrome according to the suggestion of Henneberg and Bielschowsky, proposed that they embrace a very large spectrum of early-arising abnormalities, not only of the nervous system, but also involving the ribs, feet, hands and other organs. According to the precise meaning of dysraphic syndrome, this term should be reserved only for malformations deriving from primary or secondary impairment of closure of the neural tube. Nevertheless, the more recently accepted enlargement of this group named by the more general term 'neural tube defects' allows inclusion of the developmental abnormalities that arise even before the formation of the neural plate and also after the closure of the neural tube (French, 1983; O'Rahilly & Müller, 1994). Thus, it embraces the neural tube defects, combined with anomalies of surrounding mesodermal tissues.

The earliest tube defects have to be related to the time of the induction of the neuroectoderm by the chordamesoderm, which occurs during the third week of embryonal development. The split, that is, the partial duplication (Bentley & Smith, 1960), of the notochord or other mechanisms, like abnormal separation of tissue layers, may cause several malformations: neurenteric cysts, combined anterior and posterior spina bifida, and diastematomyelia with septum, belonging to the so-called occult spinal dysraphism (James & Lassman, 1981; French, 1983).

The pathomechanism of malformations arising during the primary and secondary neurulations is still controversial, and several theories have been advanced (Warkany, 1977). The concept of developmental arrest leading to failure of closure is known from von Recklinghausen (1886). The mesodermal deficiency assumed by Marin-Padilla and Marin-Padilla (1981) may be of importance in this process. The hypothesis of overgrowth of neural folds suggests that it may disturb the fusion of the neural tube (French, 1983). Several experimental studies provide support for the opinion that lack of closure of the neural tube is the cause of many malformations (Smith & Huntington, 1981; Takeuchi & Takeuchi, 1985). The opposite hydrodynamic theory, supported mostly by Gardner (1973), proposed the reopening of the just-closed neural tube disrupted by overpressure of primary cerebrospinal fluid (CSF). This theory being criticized (French, 1983), mechanisms other than CSF pressure have been proposed. Among these is the lack of correlation between the growth of mesodermal and neuro-ectodermal elements as leading to neural tube defects. All of the proposed pathomechanisms of dysraphic disorders were discussed also in relation to Chiari malformation, which belongs to the group of neural tube defects (Padget, 1972; Marin-Padilla & Marin-Padilla, 1981; French, 1983).

Finally, it appears that all the theories (Dias & Walker, 1992; David, 1993) on the pathomechanism of neural tube defects do not totally exclude each other, and we can only conclude, according to Friede (1989), that changes, known as dysraphic, present the disturbances of neuroectodermal and mesodermal structures that are susceptible to damaging factors in a given time of development. Indeed, studies concerning the pathomechanisms of the neural tube disorders are tightly associated with the search for the timing of their appearance. The analysis of particular cases in this field was very helpful (Dekaban & Bartelmez, 1964; Müller & O'Rahilly, 1984). After a comprehensive review, Campbell et al. (1986) divided the neural tube defects into those occurring in an open neural tube and others arising when primary neurulation is accomplished, and the neural tube is closed. Summarizing the existing data, Lemire (1987) attributed the occurrence of such malformations to consecutive developmental stages. His studies were supplemented recently by the experience of O'Rahilly and Müller (1994). The postulated timing of the morphological appearance of neural tube defects is presented in Table 4. The data available in the papers of five authors were collected. Day 26 is underlined as the time when it can be concluded the neural tube is closed. To resolve the problem of the pathomechanism of neural tube defects, we should mention that Campbell et al. (1986), after a review of experimental studies on animals, supported the suggestion presented above, obtained from examination of human material, and concluded that neural tube defects may be produced by many different pathomechanisms.

The etiology of neural tube malformations was also studied in multidisciplinary ways. In humans, not a single teratogen was found to produce malformations belonging to this group (Copp et al., 1990). Folic acid deficiency (Wald, 1994) and maternal diabetes

6 Malformations of the CNS

Table 4. Postulated timing of neural tube and related defects formation

	Norman 1996	O'Rahilly & Müller 1994	Lemire 1987	Campbell et al. 1986	French 1983
Diastematomyelia	18 d				16–17 d
Spina bifida antero-posterior					16–17 d
Cystae neuroentericae					16–17 d
Craniorachischisis			18–20 d	< 26 d	
Anencephaly	22–26 d		23–24 d	< 26 d	
Meningomyelocele		22–24 d	20–24 d	< 26 d	
Chiari malformation	2.5–3.5 WG				28 d
Encephalocele	3–7–8 WG			< 26 d	
Meningocele			6–8 WG		
Spina bifida occulta			5–> WG		

Legend: Closure of neural tube

(Myrianthopoulos & Melnik, 1987; Holmes, 1994) are suspected to induce neural tube defects, and valproic acid may also play an injurious role (Nau, 1994). An increased number of cases of spina bifida were noted after an epidemic of rubella. Some geographical regions (e.g. Great Britain) are known to have greater incidence of such malformations than other countries. Seasonal differences in their appearance were also observed. Among genetic factors, only a generally increased susceptibility seems to be important. The malformations were observed to appear more often in some families. Also, in some groups, a prevalence of females exists. Chromosomal abnormalities (more often trisomy 13 and 18) were observed with rather small incidence.

The discovery in experimental studies of some specific genes and gene products expressed during neurulation opens new possibilities of identifying precisely the manner by which neural tube anomalies form. They look like the result of the interaction between genetic predisposition and environmental factors (Copp et al., 1990; Copp, 1994).

Ultrasound examination is very useful for prenatal diagnosis of neural tube defects. Examination of amniotic or fetal-protein level is also very sensitive, but it is important to remember that false-positive results were observed in approximately 50 per cent of cases (Main & Mennuti, 1986). The last observation suggests that treatment with folic acid may play a role in prevention of neural tube defects (Oakley et al., 1994).

We will present a review of neural tube defects and related anomalies following the topographical sequence (Ingraham, 1944; Gross & Hoff, 1959a; Berry & Patterson, 1991) from brain to spinal cord changes.

Dysraphic cerebral changes

Craniorachischisis is the most severe anomaly in this group of malformations. In embryos or fetuses the great majority aborted very early, and the neural tube is entirely open, with the absence of brain and in great part the spinal cord also, presenting the total amyelia. In other cases, only the disorganized stripe of nervous tissue may be found, instead of a spinal cord with angiomata-like proliferation of vessels. The anomaly makes survival impossible. It seems unbelievable, but it has been proved by a few observations (Lemire et al., 1978) that some fetuses with anencephaly and total dysraphism were seen at 8 months' developmental age.

Anencephaly has been mentioned during the last two centuries using various terms (Dekaban, 1964; Lemire et al., 1978; Lemire, 1987) expressing the severity of dysraphic lesions or the phase of development of this abnormality. It always occurs with the absence of cranial vault bones (acrania), and the base of the skull reveals anomalies within the anterior and median fossa (Fields et al., 1978). The level at which the bones of the spinal column are involved in malformations suggests differentiation into two types of anencephaly: (1) holoacrania – with a maldeveloped foramen magnum and more or less advanced rachischisis, sometimes in continuity with an open cranium, sometimes only at the lumbar level (lumbar myelocele), or finally without rachischisis; and (2) meroacrania – when anencephaly occurs with a normal foramen magnum. This type appears to be the most common (Lemire, 1987; Chaurasia, 1984).

The eyes of anencephalic fetuses are usually rather well-developed, but the optic nerves beyond the orbits are absent. On the open base of the skull, a relatively small mass of disorganized nervous tissue is attached, containing glial elements, ependymal nests, and some immature nerve cells, which usually do not form any recognizable structures. Only some fragments of abnormal, most often cerebellar, elements may be seen in several cases. The abnormal tissue is highly vascularized by vessels presenting embryonal features, being probably both persistent primitive vessels and developed abnormally in response to destruction of nerve tissue (Norman et al., 1995). The entire abnormal structure is known as the area cerebro-vasculosa. It may be surrounded by meningeal tissue and finally is covered by squamous epithelium (Bell & Green, 1982). The cerebellum and the anterior part of the brain stem are more or less lacking in the majority of cases; only in a few of them are the subtentorial structures relatively spared. In such cases, dysplasia of corticospinal tracts and some abnormalities of neuronal arrangement are seen.

Anencephalic fetuses with a more or less well-developed brain stem, usually born as premature during the last trimester of pregnancy, can rarely survive 2–3 days (Dąmbska & Kansy, 1963; Baird & Sadownick, 1984). Anencephaly with a well-developed spinal canal usually has an underdeveloped spinal cord, with a lack of all brain-deriving pathways.

Anencephaly usually occurs with malformations of many organs, and it is hard to differentiate to which degree the malformations may be considered as secondary to CNS underdevelopment or as coexisting with them. Such malformations are seen in facial bones, limbs, heart, lungs, the gastrointestinal tract, or endocrine glands (Cooney & Thurlbeck, 1985; Van Allen & Myrhe, 1985; Lemire, 1987). The diagnosis of anencephaly can be made during intrauterine life by ultrasound. It often occurs with polyhydramnios.

Exencephaly, the term used by Sarnat (1992) interchangeably with encephaloceles, could also be considered a variant of anencephaly (Norman et al., 1995), as it is an earlier stage of the same malformation (Wood & Smith, 1984). The nervous tissue, found in a greater amount than within an anencephalic, area cerebro-vasculosa on the base of the skull, deprived of the cranial vault, may include several abnormal and immature, but to some degree, organized compounds. It should be admitted that necrotic changes, occurring within this tissue, deprived of protection against surrounding injurious factors may finally result in the already known picture of anencephaly. The incidence of anencephaly is estimated as 0.5–2.0 per 1,000 births, and this anomaly comprises nearly one-third of the malformations seen among all abnormal newborns (Coffey & Jessop, 1957; Lemire et al., 1972), when such cases were not diagnosed prenatally and pregnancies interrupted.

Iniencephaly is a complex malformation in which the basic features are (1) occipital bone defect, (2) cervical dysraphic changes, and (3) retro-flexia of the whole spine (Nishimura & Okamoto, 1976; Lemire et al., 1972). The iniencephaly may be 'closed' when the occipital bone is not 'open', but if so it is rather hypoplastic (Scherrer et al., 1992). Anomalies of the nervous system may present many types, from lesions similar to those in anencephaly to less-advanced dysgeneses of the brain, protruding within the encephalocele through cranial defect (Aleksic et al., 1983; Scherrer et al., 1992).

Encephaloceles consist of a developmental cranial defect, embracing herniations of the brain tissues. When herniation contains only meninges, we recognize meningocele, and a midline cranial defect without any herniation is termed cranium bifidum. The meningoceles are less common than the meningo-encephaloceles. Only in some statistics do they rise to nearly similar frequency (Guthkelch, 1970). Not involving the brain tissue, they present a much better clinical prognosis. In encephaloceles, the midline bone defect and protruding tissues are usually covered by normal skin, and concomitant cranial anomalies other than the midline defect are usually seen. The encephaloceles may be localized at various levels.

The most common form in Europe and North America appears to be the occipital encephaloceles (Ingraham & Swam, 1943; Matson, 1969; Sarnat, 1992). They consist of skeletal and neural cleft formation, including, in varying degrees, bones from the occipital squame to the vertebral arches, with secondary defects and other apparently unrelated changes (Karch & Urich, 1972). Two types of anomalies are seen. In the first type, the cranial defect is localized in the occipital bones; the second type involves foramen magnum, and the first cervical arch is not closed. Depending on the type of cranial defect, encephaloceles may embrace the brain stem, cerebellum, and one or both cerebral hemispheres. Often, one occipital pole is trapped into the sac with or without cerebellar elements. The adhesion of the occipital pole to the wall of the protruding cyst leads to various asymmetrical abnormalities during further development of brain hemispheres (Karch & Urich, 1972). They may involve subcortical gray structures, change the shape of lateral ventricles, and even induce abnormalities of the cortical ribbon, as was evident in our case presented in Fig. 58. The coexistence of occipital encephaloceles with other anomalies, such as midline malformations, is also seen.

Hydrocephalus is one of the possible complications of both occipital meningoceles and, more frequently, of encephaloceles (Lorber, 1967; Guthkelch, 1970). Secondary anomalies of the brain stem, olives, and cortico-spinal tract decussation are also seen. Anomalies within meningeal vessels, presenting fetal features, are common (see Chapter 6, on Changes related to vascular, skull bone and menungeal anomalies (p. 146).

Anterior encephaloceles (or sincipital) are not frequent, but are seen more often in Asians than in Caucasians (Sarnat, 1992). They can protrude through the fronto-ethmoidal junction (Suwanwele & Suwanwele, 1972) and present various types: the nasofrontal type is seen between the orbits and contains the brain tissue; the nasoethnoidal type appears between the nasal bones and nasal cartilages (David & Proudman, 1989), and protrusion of encephaloceles into the orbit is very rare.

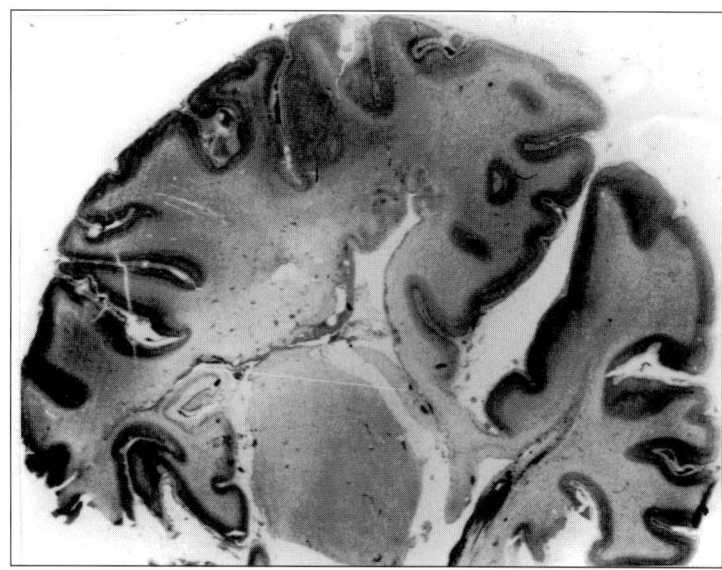

Fig. 58. Asymmetry of cerebral hemispheres in a case with occipital encephaloceles. Cresyl violet, × 3.

Midline encephaloceles between the parietal bones and on the fontanel are rather rare. The basal encephaloceles are the least common type (Modesti et al., 1977). It is supposed that impairment of closure of the anterior neuropore may play a role in their pathomechanism, which would be exceptional among the encephaloceles, arising in the closed neural tube. The coexistence often seen with midline malformations supports this theory. The protrusion of encephaloceles may be transphenoidal (Wiese et al., 1972), sphenoethmoidal, or transenthmoidal (Pollock et al., 1968). According to Naidich et al. (1983), it is possible to differentiate the superior type, affecting the nose and eventually the orbits, and the inferior type, involving the lip and occurring with hypertelorism.

Encephaloceles may be observed sporadically beyond the midline on the parietal level (McLaurin, 1987). The problem of frequent coincidence of encephaloceles with other malformations or their occurrence in some known syndromes warrants their mention here. Encephalocele was described in Meckel–Gruber syndrome as invariably lethal, presenting as cranial and CNS malformations, which may or may not include, occipital encephalocele, rachischisis, microcephaly, eye anomalies, malformation of other organs, and cystic dysplasia of the kidney (Blankenberg et al., 1987; Ahdab-Bamada & Claassen, 1990). It was found also in Joubert syndrome (p. 135) and Walker–Warburg syndrome (p. 128). We would like to mention fronto-nasal dysplasia with fronto-nasal encephalocele, hypertelorsim, and abnormal nose. The autosomal-dominant inheritance of this syndrome was observed (DeMyer, 1967; Gorlin et al., 1971). Apert syndrome, with cranial dysostosis and polydactyly (Waterson et al., 1985), dyssegmental dwarfism (Gruhn et al., 1978), and some other syndromes were also observed as coinciding with encephaloceles. The clinical syndromes and the course of encephaloceles depend on their localization and degree of lesions. Radiologic and neuroimaging diagnosis is helpful for surgical treatment of such cases.

Chiari (Arnold–Chiari) malformation

This malformation of the brain stem and cerebellum was described by Cleland (1883), Chiari (1891, 1896), and Arnold (1894) from various points of view. Finally, it was accepted, following Chiari's suggestion, three types of Arnold–Chiari malformations should be recognized. The originally proposed type IV, consisting of cerebellar hypoplasia, was the first type withdrawn from this set of anomalies. Type III was most recently proposed to be diagnosed as encephalocervical meningocele, and type I as downward displacement of the cerebellar tonsils (Norman et al., 1995). Because this last suggestion has generally not been accepted and discussed by many authors, we decided to present type I as controversial, from the classification point of view (Sarnat, 1992).

Chiari type I consists only of herniation of cerebellar tonsils. Friede (1989) stressed that when Chiari described such changes, the tonsillar herniation due to increased intracranial pressure was not known. At present, we can discuss such a syndrome only without supratentorial changes leading to increased intracranial pressure. Harding (1992) insists against abandoning the term Chiari type I malformation for cerebellar herniation of tonsils, which may be atrophic. Friede (1989) suggests that the problem consists rather of the degree of changes that allow differentiation between the chronic herniation of cerebellar tonsils, which may not be so rare (Friede & Roessmann, 1976), and Chiari malformation, which in addition presents some anomalies particularly of the bones at the cranio-spinal junction. However, the borderline between both syndromes seems to be indistinct. Norman et al. (1995) considers them as synonymous and proposes the recognition of the cerebellar developmental anomaly as being the sequel of the primary hypoplastic fossa and leading to herniation of cerebellar tonsils. Such herniation was seen with anomalies of the posterior fossa such as platybasia or basal impression (Spillane et al., 1957; Nyland & Krogness, 1978; Schady et al., 1987). This anomaly, often asymptomatic, may sometimes cause pain, and brain stem and cerebellar symptoms (Paul et al., 1983). It may also lead to hydrocephaly, not improving even after shunt treatment (Hoffman & Tucker, 1976). The coincidence of tonsillar herniation, posterior fossa deformities, and syringomyelia was often observed (Williams & Fahy, 1983; Paul et al., 1983; Mohr et al., 1977; Schady et al., 1987) in various combinations in this not finally classified type of malformation. Treatment is surgical, including decompression of the posterior fossa.

Chiari II malformation is generally recognized as the most typical for this dysgenesis of the nervous system, which has been studied extensively by many authors (Peach, 1965; Variend & Emery, 1974; Bell et al., 1980; Gilbert et al., 1986; Bamberger-Bozo, 1987). The earliest arising anomalies that define the Chiari II malformation according to the definition of Norman et al. (1995) are 'the neural tube defect and the brain stem-cerebellum/posterior fossa malformation'. Its basic symptoms are elongation of inferior vermis and the brain stem and their displacement into the cervical spinal canal (Fig. 59).

The bone anomalies are typical for this malformation. The posterior fossa is shallow, the torcular is in low position, and the foramen magnum is enlarged (Kruyff & Jeffs, 1966). Craniolacuniae of the cerebral vault are demonstrated very often in radiological examination (Tajima et al., 1977). The spinal anomalies may involve the posterior arch of the atlas (Blaauw, 1971). The severity of dysraphic changes differs in particular cases. Meningocoeles and, more often, myelocoeles coincide in large part with cases of Chiari II malformation and also other anomalies of the spinal cord-like hydromyelia or diastematomyelia (Emery & MacKenzie, 1973; Emery & Lendon, 1973). Crowding of the posterior fossa leads to compression of the fourth ventricle, to focal dysplasia, or to necrotic changes within the cerebellar structures displaced into the foramen magnum, vermis, uvula, nodulus and pyramis (Russell & Donald, 1935; Daniel & Strich, 1958). The brain stem pushed caudally may even bend over the cervical spinal cord. The anomalies in the topography of brain stem structures are seen as sequels of such basic abnormalities. Abnormal positioning of cranial nerves and spinal roots is also evident. Hydrocephalus usually occurs with more or less advanced stenosis of the aqueduct (Emery, 1974; MacFarlane & Maloney, 1957) and is the cause of cortical abnormalities in the cerebral hemispheres. Among them, secondary lesions and polymicrogyria were observed (McLendon et al., 1985; Gilbert et al., 1986).

The clinical syndrome induced by such abnormalities of subtentorial structures include (a) symptoms of intracranial pressure, (b) palsies of cranial nerves, (c)

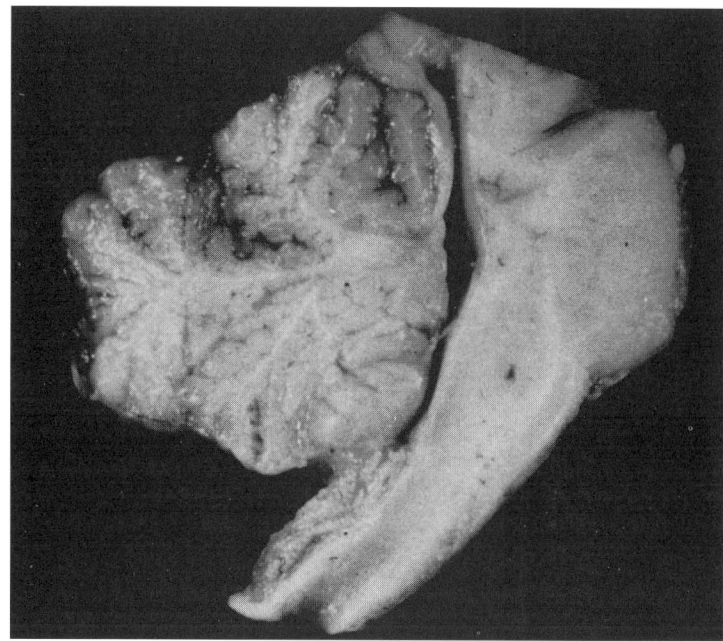

Fig. 59. Downward displacement of cerebellar structures in Chiari II malformation.

syndromes from the brain stem and spinal cord, which are compressed, and (d) cerebellar symptoms. The diagnosis of Chiari II malformation may start prenatally by ultrasound; then, CT and MRI complete the evaluation of the character and the severity of changes (Naidich et al., 1980a,b,c, 1983). They constitute a basic examination for advice on surgical treatment.

The pathomechanism of Chiari II malformation has been discussed many times. The mesodermal defect is considered by Marin-Padilla and Marin-Padilla (1981) a primary failure. Osaka et al. (1978) suggested that the spinal neural tube defect is an initial event, and Norman et al. (1995) agree with this speculation. The next event may be disproportion of growth of the small posterior fossa and its contents, the brain stem, and cerebellum. Experimental studies support the opinion that nervous system abnormalities may occur secondary to skeletal defects, and observation of human cases appears to confirm that small posterior fossa play a role in formation of brain stem and cerebellar deformities (Bell et al., 1980).

When Sarnat (1992), Norman et al. (1995), and some other authors restricted the analysis of previous Arnold–Chiari malformations to presentation of Chiari type II, considering it essential for this dysgenesis, the problem of the eponym of those unquestionable complex developmental abnormalities arose. The terms Arnold–Chiari, or only Chiari, malformations are both used at present, until a common agreement for one term is reached.

Dysraphic and related anomalies of the spinal cord

Spinal dysraphism includes a range of malformations from mild to severe. We will present the most characteristic types, which were described and discussed many years ago (Ingraham et al., 1943; French, 1983).

Spina bifida is a less severe type of anomaly, presenting a lack of fusion of the posterior lamina of the spinal canal. The meninges and spinal cord are not involved; only minor abnormalities within the spinal cord roots, or filum terminale, may appear. Nevertheless, such types of bone anomalies present a potential canal for herniation of meninges and the spinal cord. Spina bifida, like other dysraphic malformations, appears most often at the lumbar level, but may be observed at any other one. A very rare malformation is anterior spina bifida, consisting of separation of the two halves of vertebrae, and it belongs to the earliest defects, as mentioned previously.

Meningocele presents the herniation of dura and arachnoid meninges through the lack of a spinal canal junction (Fig. 60). The spinal cord remains in the canal, but it may present some developmental anomalies. The thin skin layer over the meningocele is often covered by hairs; vascular nevus or lipomas are also seen. Similar changes are sometimes also found at the level of spina bifida without meningocele, and they may serve as an indication for radiologic detection of a clinically silent malformation. Meningocele may be clinically asymptomatic, when the malformation did not severely involve the spinal cord. In such cases, surgical treatment gives good results.

In some instances, the enlarged central canal in this anomaly forms a kind of pouch, entering into the meningocele and forming the meningocystocele (Steinbok & Cochrane, 1991). *Meningomyelocele* is a more severe malformation in which the herniated sack contains the spinal cord elements together with the meninges. In 80 per cent of cases, it is localized at the lumbo-sacral level (Larroche, 1977), but it is also common at the cervical and cervico-thoracic levels because, unfortunately, this type of malformation is more common than meningocele. Meningomyelocele is often covered by thin skin. In other cases, the herniated tissue containing the spinal cord elements connected with the open spinal canal (i.e. not covered by skin) forms an abundantly vascularized area medullovasculosa, which is usually epithelized *in utero* or after birth. The spinal cord above and sometimes below the meningomyelocele may be normal, but most often presents different types of developmental anomalies (Fig. 61). The clinical symptoms and the results of surgical treatment depend upon the type and degree of spinal cord malformation.

Hydromyelia belongs to the anomalies often found in cases with various forms of spinal dysraphism. It presents as a large central canal persisting from early developmental stages and may be seen at different levels of the spinal cord. The large canal is clothed in part by ependymal cells and subependymal glia.

Syringomyelia, although sometimes omitted in descriptions of spinal-cord anomalies, must be mentioned as requiring differential diagnosis between developmental abnormality and secondarily acquired lesion. It consists of the formation of cavities in the spinal cord most often dorsally to the central canal, involving dorsal horns, sometimes dorsal columns, and even other parts of the spinal cord (Fig. 62). The cavities could be the sequelae of lesions in the mature spinal cord deserving the diagnosis of pseudo-syringomyelia. The mesodermal elements are abundant within their walls, and sometimes even remnants of necrotic changes are seen. Nevertheless, the cavities could also derive during development, when the dorsal raphe of the spinal cord is forming (4–10 WG). Such cavities are clothed by fibrillary glia, with a few mesodermal elements, in contrast to the

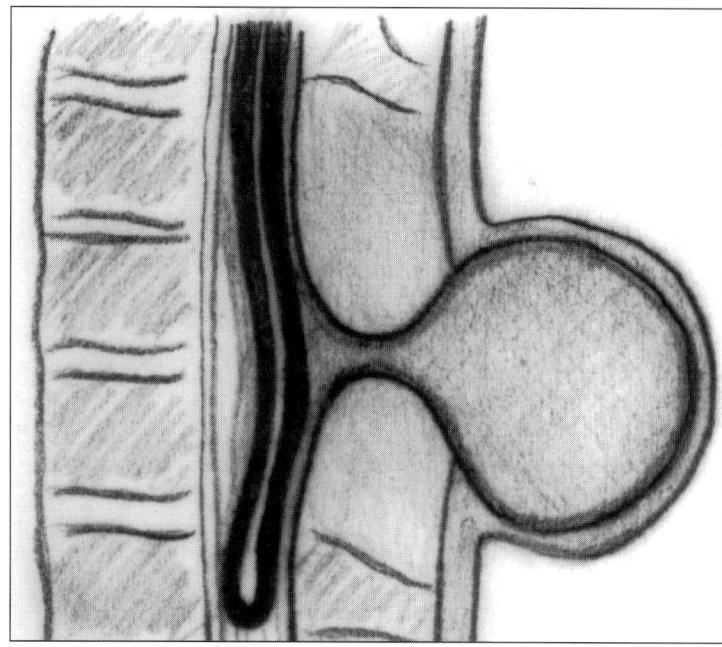

Fig. 60 (above). Meningocele – topography of changes.

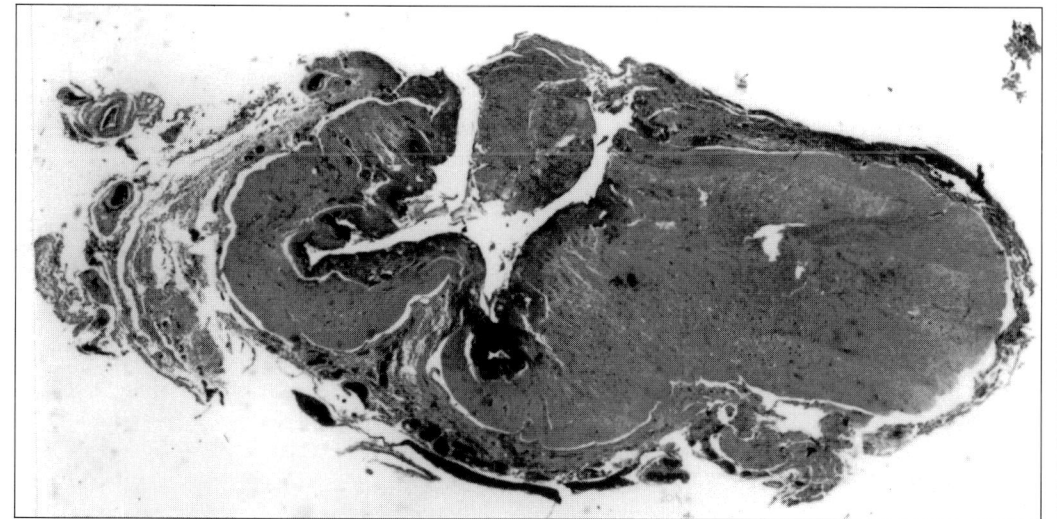

Fig. 61 (left). Dysraphic changes within the spinal cord above lumbar meningomyelocele. Cresyl violet, × 8.

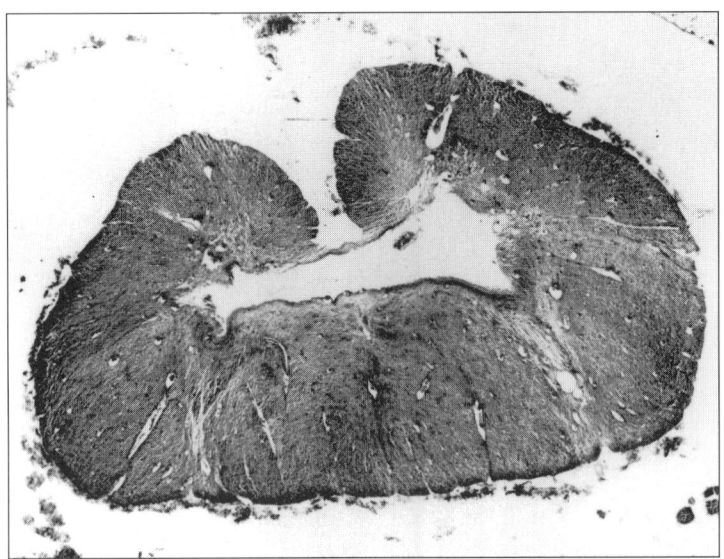

Fig. 62 (above). Syringomyelitic cavity in the spinal cord. HE, × 8.

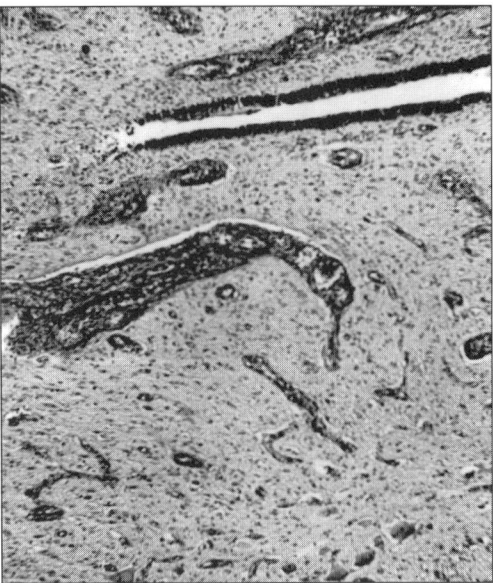

Fig. 63 (right). Vascular abnormalities in the spinal cord with dysraphic changes. van Gieson, × 100.

modification of the clinical course of syringomyelia. The vascular anomalies (Fig. 63), with secondary changes observed sometimes at the level of cavities, may play a similar role (Dąmbska et al., 1970). The cavities may occupy each level of the spinal cord and may also be found in the medulla oblongata, resulting in the clinicopathological syndrome of syringobulbia.

The typical picture of syringomyelia includes the split sensation disturbances, indicating the level of spinal cord cavities, central and/or peripheral motor deficiency, and other signs depending on topography of changes. The clinical symptoms may appear in adulthood, with deterioration during the following years. The surgical treatment of cavernous malformations of the spinal cord may improve the neurological function of patients (McCormick et al., 1988).

There also exist anomalies that are very probably not associated with primary neurulation, but as stated at the beginning of this chapter, arise earlier, during the third week of development. Sarnat (1992) and Pang et al. (1992) consider these anomalies the result of partial duplication (split) of the notochord.

Diastematomyelia, the most representative malformation within this group, consists of division of the spinal cord into two separate hemicords located in two individual or in one dural sac and turned toward each other at a 90° angle. The hemicords are separated by connective tissue and sometimes by bony septum. Lipomas may also be observed at this level. Diastematomyelia is a sister anomaly of diplomyelia, each forming various degrees of spinal cord duplication arising at the beginning of embryonic life, but when the cells are already distributed in germ layers.

cavities resulting from destructive processes.

Ostertag (1956) concluded that syringomyelia is a malformation including the same traits of blastomatic tendency, because glial proliferation in the central part of the spinal cord can extend above and below the spinal cavities. The proliferative or regressive changes within this glial tissue may contribute to modification in shape and dimension of cavities, which results in

Diplomyelia presents as two separate spinal cords (Fig. 64) located alongside each other, or occasionally one behind the other. Such malformation is most often seen at the lumbar level, but also at the cervical level. It is

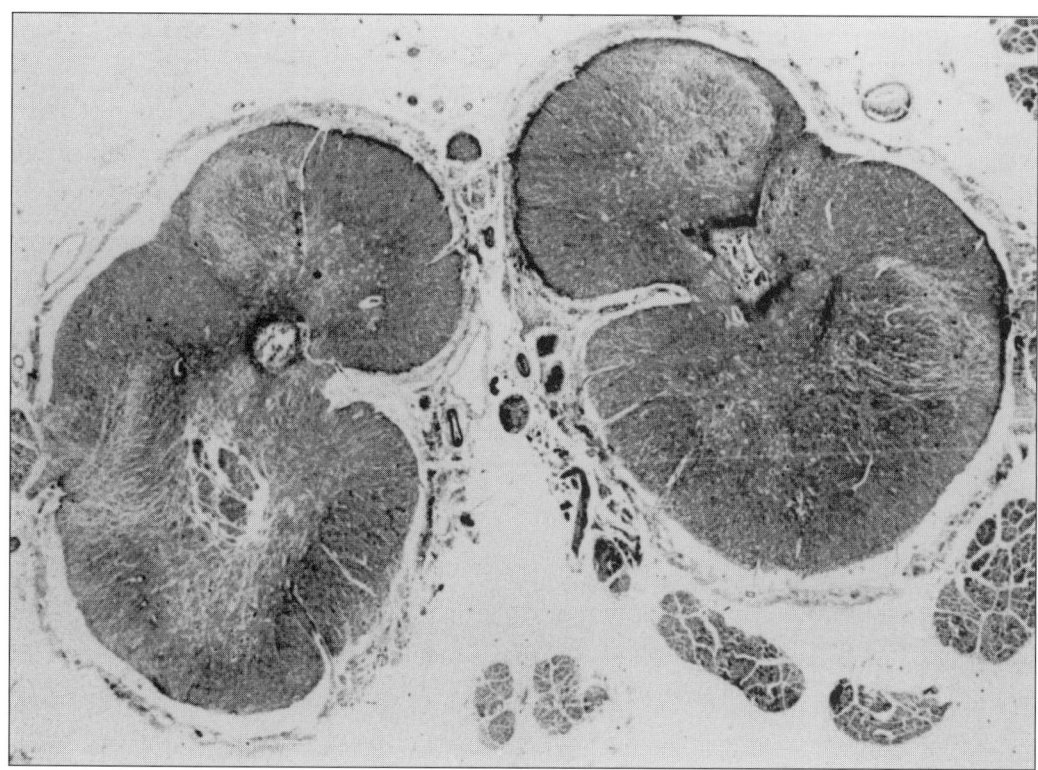

Fig. 64. Diplomyelia with two separate spinal cords at the lumbar level. HE, × 8.

often associated with spina bifida (also anterior, meningo- or meningo-myelocele), sometimes with other vertebral abnormalities. The endodermal tissue entering between the two parts of the duplicated spinal cord may form neurenteric cysts (see below). Some clinical symptoms of diplomyelia and diastematomyelia may appear in children, and an accurate diagnosis can be made with MRI examination (Kuharik et al., 1985–86). Nevertheless, such abnormalities may often fail to be diagnosed during life, because of the paucity of clinical deficit and may appear as an autopsy finding.

Abnormalities associated with duplication of the spinal cord may appear in very complicated forms. In a case we observed, with spinal cord duplication on the cervical level in one of the cords, the central canal was divided into two, and even a third hypoplastic cord appeared (Fig. 65). The duplication of the spinal central canal is the slightest form of spinal cord duplication. Malformations of the diastomyelitic type have been observed in association with dysembrogenetic tumors.

Fig. 65. Duplication of the spinal cord at the cervical level. HE, × 8.

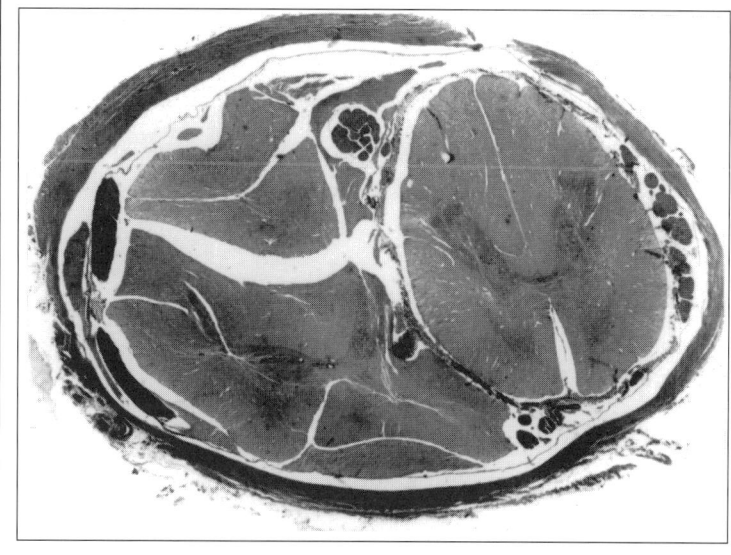

Other anomalies belonging to the same group

Neuroenteric cysts are very rare anomalies; no more than 30 cases were described until Fernandes et al.'s (1991) publication. They are intradural, localized intramedullary or extramedullary, often between the cervical and thoracic levels, but they were described also at the level of the brain stem (Lach et al., 1989) and supratentorially (Dom et al., 1990). The walls of such cysts may include cells proper to various neighboring organs (Ho & Tiel, 1989; Lach et al., 1989). Malformations of vertebrae and intrathoracic cysts may coexist with them.

Combined *anterior and posterior spina bifida* is also an extremely rare finding: the majority of cases are found in stillborn infants. Posterior spina bifida communicates in such cases with longitudinal division of vertebral bodies. Such cases also present severe complex malformations in other organs.

The spinal dermal sinus consists in small ducts most often in midline at the lumbosacral level, which may only reach the subcutaneous area, but sometimes are attached even to the spinal cord. Spinal dermal sinus may coincide with spina bifida occulta. Dermoid sinuses may be prolonged by tracts connected with dermoid cysts, extradural or even situated within the fourth ventricle (Matson & Ingraham, 1951). The lumbosacral lipoma may be subcutaneous or combined with malformation of spinal cord and present as lipomyelomengocele.

Tethered cord syndrome is a rather recently recognized syndrome belonging to the group of occult spinal dysraphism. It consists of a low-situated spinal cord with a thick filum terminale associated often with other anomalies, and it coincides regularly with spina bifida. Sarwar et al. (1984) postulated its origin as local dysmorphogenesis in the lumbosacral area, involving three germinal layers. The short and thick filum terminale may disturb the ascent of the spinal cord, and adhesions and lumbosacral lipoma may also play a role in this process. According to Raghavan et al. (1989), the tip of the conus, in the majority of cases, is located below the middle of the L2 body. Individual signs including club foot, scoliosis, disturbances of gait, urologic complications, and motor and sensory deficits occur in this syndrome (Bode et al., 1985; Flanigan et al., 1989). For diagnosis, x-ray examination, myelography and CT and MRI are all useful (Bode et al., 1985; Raghavan et al., 1989). Treatment is surgical and often results in marked improvement. Tethered cord syndrome may appear as a late complication due to secondary adhesions after operation for a meningomyelocele (Tamaki et al., 1988).

Sacral agenesis consists of aplasia of the caudal part of the vertebral column, involving most often the coccyx, but sometimes also the superior parts, reaching even the thoracolumbar level (Sarnat et al., 1976). According to Sarnat (1992c), this anomaly is due to abnormal differentiation of the caudal part of the chordamesoderm involving derivatives of caudal eminence (Norman et al., 1995). In cases with extensive bony defects, dysplastic changes of the spinal cord are evident in its ventral part, and sometimes, meningomyelocele may occur. Lipoma of the conus medullaris and filum terminale, abnormalities within the spinal ganglia and nerve roots were also described (Towfighi & Hausman, 1991). The morphological abnormalities result in neurological, motor rather than sensory syndromes (Sarnat et al., 1976). Visceral anomalies and in the most severe cases, even abnormalities of the legs may coincide with sacral agenesis and have received the name 'syndrome of caudal regression' (Passarge & Lenz, 1966; Towfighi & Hausman, 1991). Maternal diabetes mellitus was found to play a predisposing role for this malformation in humans (Cousins, 1983), but a genetic factor was found in mice (Frye et al., 1964).

Klippel–Feil anomaly, although presenting as a vertebral defect, has to be mentioned with neural tube defects because it often coincides in complex syndromes. Klippel–Feil anomaly consists of fusion of vertebral spines, including only C2–3 or C5–6 vertebra or all at the cervical and upper thoracic level, eventually located at different levels of the spinal column. The anomaly may be asymptomatic and may only limit neck movements, but it could also coincide with various types of spinal dysraphic anomalies. Those may cause different clinical symptoms (Cochrane et al., 1990; Whiting et al., 1991).

Midline malformations

The principal events seen in morphological observations that occur within the anterior prosencephalon from the end of the first gestational month concern the appearance of hemispheric vesicles, introducing bilateral symmetry of the brain. The further formation of cerebral hemispheres prompts the connections between them by a consecutively arising commissural system (Sidman & Rakic, 1982; Müller & O'Rahilly, 1989). The abnormal course of these processes leads to malformations of various degrees, ranging from the lack of hemispheric division to mild commissural defects. The traditional thinking is to consider the midline prosencephalic malformations a separate group including holoprosencephaly, agenesis of corpus callosum (ACC), septo-optic dysplasia, and other anomalies of this area (Leech & Shuman, 1986).

Despite the different time and mechanism in which midline malformations arise (Müller & O'Rahilly, 1989), we think presenting them in a common chapter is justified. It may help to realize how many disturbances occurring consecutively from the early stage of CNS development and in different manners may affect the structures located in close proximity although belonging to several components of the telencephalon and diencephalon.

Holoprosencephaly – arhinencephaly

Holoprosencephaly (HPE), known since the last century particularly because of Kundrat's description (1882), presents as face and brain anomalies of various degrees and severity. When it consists of impaired division of the telencephalon, it presents as a single ventricle, lack of interhemispheric commissures (anterior commissure, CC, and usually the fornix), fusion of subcortical gray structures, and abnormal position of the hippocampus. Yakovlev (1959) considered the failure of the prosencephalon to divide into symmetrical halves as a basic defect for such malformation and proposed the name holotelencephaly or holoprosencephaly (DeMyer & Zeman, 1963). The latter is generally used now. The rhinencephalic structures, arising at a level similar to the prosencephalon anterior, are also often involved in an abnormal developmental process. The terms holoprosencephaly or arhinencephaly were used for both anomalies, comprising a univentricular telencephalon and a usual lack of peripheral olfactory structures. The term arhinencephaly was proposed by Kundrat (1882), who considered the lack of olfactory bulbs and tracts an important component of this malformation. Nevertheless, further observations demonstrated olfactory aplasia without any other CNS malformations, and univentricular brain without such anomaly. It is more appropriate to designate arhinencephaly a separate form of CNS malformation that could be more precisely named 'olfactory aplasia' (Friede, 1989); the originator of the first term did not take into account the cerebral component of rhinencephalon.

According to the degree of pathologic changes, three types of HPE can be distinguished (DeMyer & Zeman, 1963). (1) The most severe type is alobar HPE. In this anomaly, the brain is very small, without division into two hemispheres, resulting in a single ventricle. The neocortex is hy-

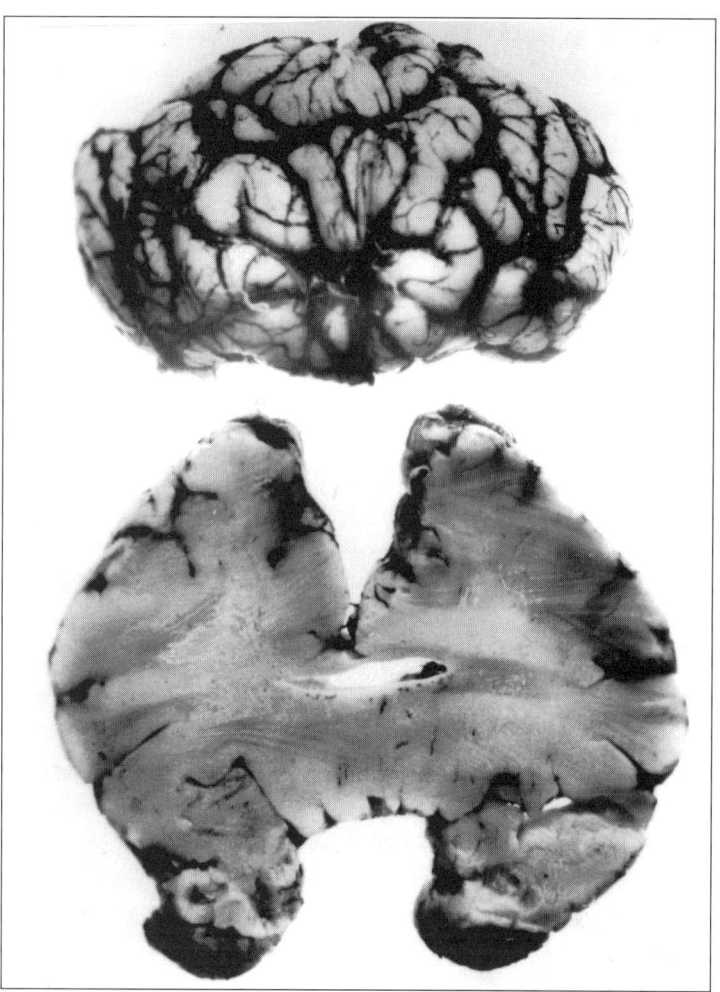

Fig. 66. Holoprosencephaly without division of frontal poles and a single ventricle.

poplastic, which is most accentuated in the nearly missing frontal cortex. Cortical organization is disturbed proportionally to the severity of malformation. Because so many factors impair their development, particular cortical areas can be 'sui generis', according to Norman et al. (1995). (2) A less severe type is semilobar HPE, with partial lack of hemispheric division, restricted to only the frontal level (Fig. 66). The single ventricle on the frontal level is often divided into two parts, with two temporal and posterior horns. The subcortical gray structures present most often as an undivided mass in which the striatal structures are usually lacking and the third ventricle does not exist. (3) Lobar holoprosencephaly has a rather normal division of hemispheres, but a single ventricle on the frontal level with midline continuity of the cerebral cortex instead of lacking the CC. The frontal lobes are often hypoplastic, even in this less severe type of malformation.

The brain stem and cerebellum are generally normal, except for secondary changes resulting from hemispheric anomalies. Sometimes, there is only a single cerebellar peduncle (Friede, 1989).

The bones of the skull base usually present some traits of developmental impairment. The facial deformities that coexist with HPE are of various types, but they do not correspond exactly to the severity of the brain malformation. They may present as various features, such as cyclopia with total or partial fusion of orbits; ethmocephaly, with the nose replaced by a proboscis, with single or paired nostrils; cebocephaly, with a narrow space between the orbits and one or two nostrils; premaxillary agenesis, with hypotelorism and some features of underdevelopment of the intermaxillary segment of the face; or only less severe facial dysmorphic traits (Currarino & Silverman, 1960; Bishop et al., 1964; DeMyer et al., 1964; Cohen et al., 1971; Rowlatt & Pruzansky, 1980; Cohen, 1982). Anomalies of the lateral parts of the face and also involving the ears, although rare, have been described (Carles et al., 1987). The absence, or aberrant position, of adrenohypophisis and other endocrine dysgeneses were also observed in HPE (Haworth et al., 1961; Siebert et al., 1987; Ikeda et al., 1987). Various CNS malformations of the dysraphic type may also coincide with HPE (Jellinger et al., 1981).

The complex cerebro-cranio-facial abnormalities that occur in cases of HPE can be explained by the close embryologic relation between mesenchymal, facial, and nerve system components and the known role of the prechordal mesoderm in anterior tube formation (Sulik & Johnston, 1982). Abnormalities of the embryonic, particularly prechordal, mesoderm, inducing the forebrain structures and perhaps also appearing within the neural plate, lead to a defect at the anterior end of the neural plate. They result in defects of the mediobasal prosencephalon (O'Rahilly & Müller, 1989). These authors described the sequence of developmental disturbances within this area starting at day 18 (stage 8) of embryonal life. They result in failure of hemispheric formation at week 4 of development (stage 13) and can be involved in the formation of cyclopia, arhinencephaly, and other related anomalies of the skull and face. The etiology of HPE is unknown. Many teratogens have been found to induce it in experimental animals, but in humans, a teratogen has not yet been identified. It has been observed that maternal diabetes increases risk (Barr et al., 1983). HPE occurs with trisomy 13, but also in 18 p-syndr, 13 p-syndr, trisomy 19, and triploidy (Leech & Shuman, 1986) and is possible with other associations. Nevertheless, HPE also occurs in cases with normal, verified karyotypes. This malformation is seen in Meckel–Gruber syndrome and in several others and may appear as familial with autosomal dominant or recessive inheritance. In families with this syndrome, minor traits may be visible in some family members (Berry et al., 1984). The incidence of HPE is difficult to evaluate, but it was reported to range from 6–25 cases per 100,000 births (Warkany, 1971; Jellinger et al., 1981). The clinical course depends on the severity of CNS and other malformations. Many stillborns and infants with HPE who die during early infancy are those with the most severe malformations; others may survive with only moderate behavioral abnormalities. Diagnosis by ultrasonography, even prenatal, computed tomography, and MRI is important for all such cases.

Developmental anomalies of commissural system

Agenesis of the corpus callosum (ACC) can occur as part of CNS dysgeneses, but it can also be the unique anomaly in an otherwise normal brain (Fig. 67) (Jellinger et al., 1981; Jeret et al., 1987; Aicardi et al., 1987). ACC was described as an autopsy finding (Reil, 1812) and can even now appear as an accidental or postmortem discovery. It may involve the CC in total or only partially (Fig. 68) (Loeser & Alvord, 1968; Unterharnscheidt et al., 1968).

In partial agenesis, the anterior parts (genu and rostrum) usually are present and the posterior parts are missing. According to the conviction of rostral to caudal (anteroposterior) development (Ettlinger, 1977) of this commissure, the rare cases in which the only posterior part of the CC was seen were considered atrophy of the anterior part due to the lack of vascular supply by the anterior cerebral artery. The more precise opinion is that 'the mechanisms governing formation of human CC are unknown' (Norman et al., 1995). Thus, it is possible to consider ACC as occurring only when developmental disturbances lead to a situation of insufficient or lack of crossing of the midline by axons. When the interhemispheric part of the CC is lacking, the longitudinal bundles (unless they are persistent

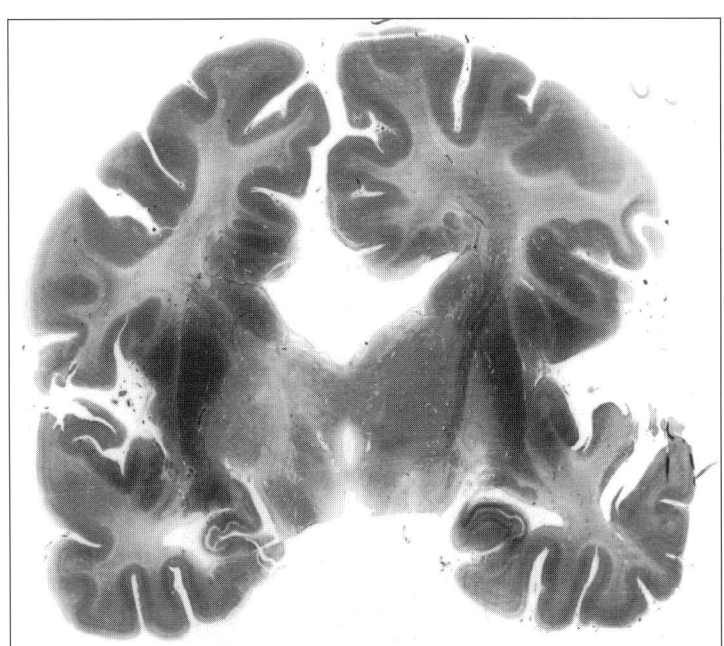

Fig. 67. Agenesis of corpus callosum. HE, × 2.

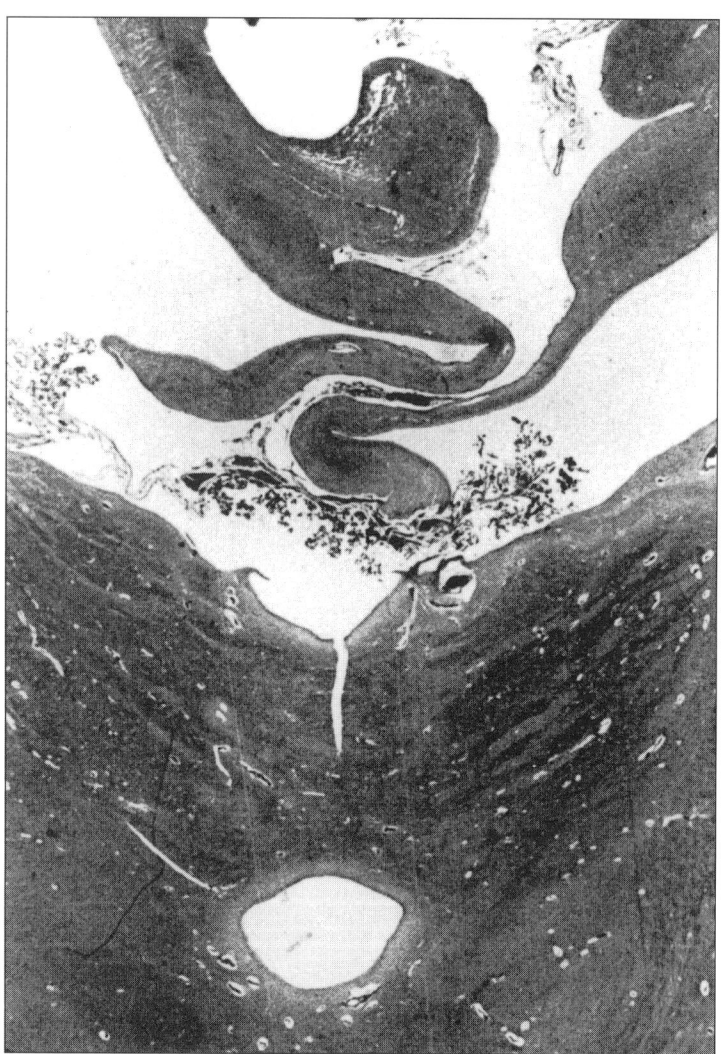

Fig. 68. Hypoplasia of corpus callosum. HE, × 4.

ipsilateral fibers) described by Probst (1901) as callosal fibers, run in the sagittal fronto-occipital direction in both hemispheres. ACC coincides with the lack of the cingulate gyrus. In cases with ACC, the ventricular system had a particular shape, depending on the position or eventual absence of the fornix and septum pellucidum. The leaves of the septum could be distended between the fornix and Probst bundles in both hemispheres. The third ventricle and the occipital horns of the lateral ventricles are usually enlarged.

ACC is combined with many dysgenetic syndromes, some of which are usually associated with ACC: (1) Aicardi syndrome, consisting of a typical triad – ACC, infantile spasms, ocular anomalies (see Chapter 6, on Cortical malformations and dysplasia (p. 118)); (2) Anderman syndrome, in which ACC coexists with sensimotor neuropathy and mental retardation (Anderman, 1981; Labrisseau et al., 1984); (3) Shapiro syndrome, in which ACC occurs with recurrent hypothermia (Shapiro et al., 1969); (4) acrocallosal syndrome, a combination of ACC with macrocephaly craniofacial and limb anomalies with mental retardation – probably with autosomal recessive inheritance (Schinzel & Kaufmann, 1986; Schinzel, 1988); (5) Apert syndrome (acrocephalosyndactyly), with face and skull anomalies, often including craniosynostosis and ACC with other CNS anomalies; and (6) Menkes syndrome, which presents as an autosomal recessive syndrome with partial agenesis of CC, mental retardation, and seizures (Menkes et al., 1964). ACC also appears in relation to exogenic factors such as fetal alcohol syndrome or postirradiation lesions and in metabolic diseases, including Krabbe, Leigh, or mucolipidosis types II or IV; and many others entities. On the other hand, such findings as dystrophic anomalies, cortical malformations, microcephaly, and hydrocephaly can be found on neuropathological examination of ACC. Finally, ACC can be combined with a variety of pathologic syndromes (Wiśniewski & Jeret, 1994).

Similarly, ACC's etiology is variable: it is heterogenous and multifactorial. Recent investigations revealed ACC with many chromosomal abnormalities such as trisomy 13, 18, 8, 112 and 17–18 (Inagaki et al., 1987; Serur et al., 1988). ACC is a rather rare malformation. Among children with developmental disabilities, it occurs in 2.3 per cent of cases (Jeret et al., 1986). It is difficult to define this malformation in the general population, because absence of the CC does not provoke any symptoms, and symptoms that are observed are instead due to associated pathologic diverse entities, as described above. Because diagnosis of ACC is more possible with neuroimaging techniques, the number of cases for clinical observations will multiply.

Other anomalies of midline structures

Septo-optic dysplasia (De Morsier syndrome), the third midline dysgenetic syndrome, is defined as a syndrome of ophthalmological abnormalities with hypothalamic dysfunctions (De Morsier, 1956; Wilson *et al.*, 1978). It presents as a triad of clinicopathological symptoms: (1) hypopituitarism, (2) optic anomalies, including aplasia of optic discs with nystagmus, or hemianopia; and (3) absence of the septum pellucidum (Friede, 1989). In some cases, the features of mental retardation are also observed. Despite agreement on the basic manifestations of this syndrome, we must admit to its great variability. The neuropathological findings confirm changes justifying the variability of clinical manifestations: the changes were found on various levels of the optic pathways; the topography and degree of pituitary gland changes vary from case to case; and aplasia of the supraoptic and periventricular nuclei were seen. Even anomalies belonging to other groups, such as encephalocele, were seen together with septo-optic dysplasia (Leech & Shuman, 1986; Roessmann *et al.*, 1987). This syndrome requires further observation, particularly when coexisting, as in many cases, with destructive lesions; Norman *et al.* (1995) chose to discuss it among syndromes with disruption.

Additional anomalies, including those of structures of this area, have to be mentioned. The differences in degree and the coexistence of various anomalies of the midline structures described above extend to a great number of anomalies that could not be included in the described syndromes, but nevertheless belong to the same group of CNS dysgeneses. The septum pellucidum could be absent because of primary aplasia, which is sometimes difficult to differentiate from secondary lesions (Gross & Hoff, 1959). The pituitary gland abnormalities including aplasia may appear within or separate from the syndromes described above, even as a familial syndrome. The midline dysgeneses may be present in combination with various other anomalies, such as those of the dysraphic group (Lemire *et al.*, 1975; Aicardi *et al.*, 1987; Friede, 1989).

Aprosencephaly/atelencephaly. The existence of aprosencephaly as a separate neuropathological entity is controversial. Sometimes it is considered a synonym of anencephaly (Sarnat, 1992) and classified as an early developmental anomaly within the lamina terminalis. Such cases described under the name aprosencephaly presenting with oculo-facial defects are compatible with this suggestion (Lurie *et al.*, 1980; Kim *et al.*, 1990). Observations of cases with a lack of prosencephalic structures, but with a well-developed cranial vault, inclined some authors to assign the term aprosencephaly to them. Such cases with a greater amount of nervous tissue and some rudimentary fragments of the brain recognizable (Kim *et al.*, 1990) even with fragment of polymicrogynic cortex (Iivanainen *et al.*, 1977) were also reported. Therefore, aprosencephaly/atelencephaly is sometimes considered an extreme form of microencephaly with 'common features' with anencephaly and HPE (Harding, 1992) or 'an intermediate position' only to anencephaly (Friede, 1989).

In the majority of descriptions, gliosis, proliferation of mesodermal elements, and calcifications are suggested as primary features, with the encephaloclastic lesions (Siebert *et al.*, 1986, 1990) arising earlier, but similar to in hydranencephaly (Della Giustina, 1987). Even disruptive changes, among which Norman *et al.* (1995) classify aprosenencephaly, occurring in addition to primary malformations, were taken into account. Finally, the pathomechanism of this severe anomaly appears to be heterogenous. At present, all questions presented above as to the pathomechanism and the classification of aprosencephaly/atelencephaly are under discussion.

Cortical malformations and dysplasia

Development of the cerebral cortex is a particularly long-lasting process that begins early during gestation and continues beyond birth. The abnormalities of its course may arise at each phase of the consecutive, but partly overlapping processes coinciding with formation of a cortical ribbon. Therefore, final results may be differentiated as sequalae of the abnormal course of one or more of these processes. The first one, neuronal migration (see Part One), may be abnormal when, among other, causes interactions between cell surfaces and extracellular matrix, or formation of growth cones, and its mechanisms are disturbed (Rakic, 1988, Norman et al., 1995). Formation of the glial-pial barrier is another important factor of control for neuronal migration (Choi & Matthias, 1987). Vascularization of the hemispheric wall paralleling neuronal migration (Kuban & Gilles, 1985; Norman & O'Kusky, 1986) also plays a role in proper formation of the cortex. Finally, the formation and maturation of cortical layering may be abnormal due to the disturbance of the mechanisms mentioned above, but anomalies of the course of programmed cell death, dendritic arborization, and parallel synaptic elimination are also very important at this phase of development.

The classification and resultant means of identification of such a wide and varied group of malformations was proposed following different criteria. The most common criterion is to classify according to the morphological picture of malformation (Barth, 1987; Friede, 1989; Rorke, 1994). Findings from clinical techniques such as electrophysiology and particularly, neuroimaging can be correlated with morphological examination for evaluation of the types of cortical anomalies (Raymond et al., 1995).

The classification of cortical dysplasia according to time of onset was proposed as useful, while correlating with the severity of lesions (Mischel et al., 1995). The identification of cortical malformations according to etiologic factors (Norman et al., 1995) was also introduced as approaching the morphological and clinical diagnosis and emphasizing the diversity of anomalies.

We believe that traditionally, morphology presents the best basic parameter for characterization of changes and allows correlation with clinical evaluation and with the most probable time of their onset. Classification, taking into account those three aspects of examination for cortical anomalies, appears to be useful for interdisciplinary diagnosis of this non-uniform group of malformations. The etiology of these malformations is often multifactorial and reveals the complex character of changes not fitting with typical forms of cortical dysplasias. This reminds us that all malformations differ from one case to another, and their final picture depends on the time and type of damaging-factor activity that interferes with developmental processes and results in a large variety of changes. The chromosomal abnormalities, autosomal or single gene-dependent inheritance, and environmental factors causing cortical malformation will be taken into account. We would like to emphasize that their numbers change and that they multiply constantly.

Cortical, early-occurring dysplasia

Cortical, early-occurring dysplasia is mentioned first when we take into account the time of onset of cortical anomalies. The term dysplasia is often used in a broad sense to define developmental anomalies. We would like to restrict this term here to those anomalies with abnormal differentiation of neuroectodermal cells. They are characterized by the presence of neurons with abnormal shape and size, abnormal dendrite arborization, and some of them of balloon type. Cells with abnormal features were also observed among glial cells (Mischel *et al.*, 1992; Prayson & Estes, 1993). The type of changes permits us to consider them as very early-arising. Such faulty differentiated cells are often seen at an abnormal position with or resulting in abnormal organization of a cortical stripe with disturbed layering (Taylor *et al.*, 1971; Raymonds *et al.*, 1995; Norman *et al.*, 1995). Such changes appear as focal or more extended. Therefore, the position of this type of cortical abnormalities between primary dysplasias and migratory disorders is not clear. Palmini *et al.* (1991) observed cases near to 'forme fruste' of tuberous sclerosis. We consider this early-arising, moderately dysplastic anomaly between cortical malformations and on the other hand, include hemimegalencephaly, which represents other similar cellular anomalies, together with tuberous sclerosis, in the group of neuromesodermal dysplasias – Ph (Chapter 5). One sequence of pathologic events must be mentioned when the borderline syndromes of cortical dysplasia are discussed, concerning the eventuality of arising dysembryoplastic tumors or gangliogangliomas within cortical dysplastic changes (Raymond *et al.*, 1995).

Cortical dysplasia is observed in cases of mental retardation and commonly with epileptic seizures (Moreland *et al.*, 1988). Recently, this dysgenesis was diagnosed in cases with intractable seizures and treated by surgical resection (Mischel *et al.*, 1995). For such cases, the neuroimaging technique can indicate focal or more diffuse changes, the final diagnosis is restricted to microscopic examination.

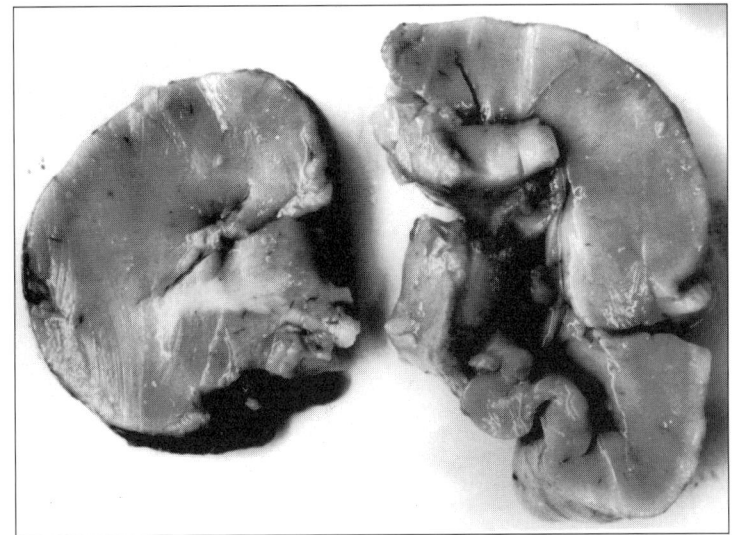

Fig. 69. General view of an agyric brain.

Agyria and pachygyria (lissencephaly type I)

The most severe, macroscopically visible anomaly of the cortical mantle is lissencephaly, which can be diagnosed clinically by CT and MRI examination (Raymond *et al.*, 1995). This macroscopic aspect of brain hemispheres may be the sequence of different anomalies of cortical stripe organization. Therefore, we consider it useful to distinguish two types of lissencephaly: lissencephaly type I and lissencephaly type II.

Lissencephaly type I belongs to the group of generalized dysgeneses and is characterized by the flat appearance of the brain hemispheres (Fig. 69) and also by the absence of gyri and sulci on microscopic examination.

The most frequently identified type of agyria has a four-layered structure of hemispheric wall (Fig. 70) consisting of the following layers: (1) molecular, (2) cellular containing mainly pyramidal neurons, (3) sparsely cellular, reaching into the nerve fibers, and (4) deep neuronal, separated from the ventricular wall by a thin sheath of white matter. Another type of agyria has a pallium with a more or less continuous mass of neurons under a thin molecular

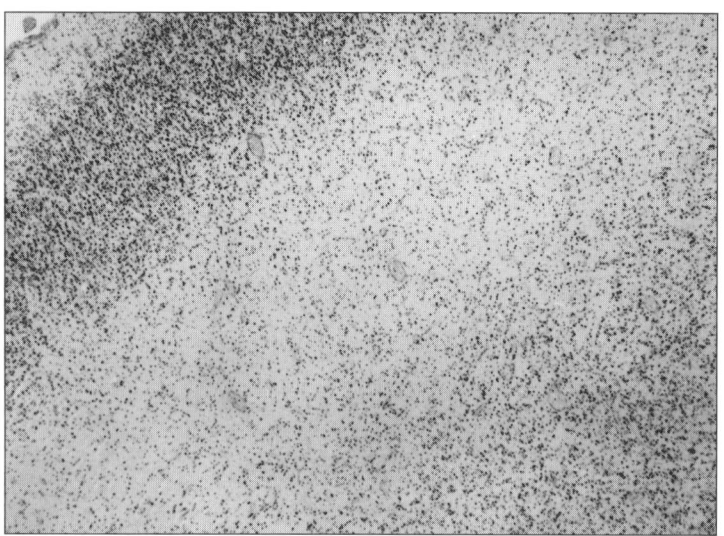

Fig. 70 (above). Four-layered structure of hemispheric wall in agyria. Cresyl violet, × 100.

Fig. 71 (below). Unilayered agyric cortex. Cresyl violet, × 100.

layer with a poorly demarcated borderline between internal and external parts containing neurons appearing to be arrested in migration (Fig. 71). Although, we agree with Ferrer *et al.* (1982), and consider the cytoarchitectonic analysis of eventual 'migration' changes as often insufficient and even misleading; we consider agyria/pachygyria as resulting from the arrest of neuronal migration.

The four-layered agyria appears to arise between the 11th and 13th week of development (Jellinger & Rett, 1976; Friede, 1989), when the second wave of migrating cells is in progress. For the agyria with a continuous mass of neurons without division into four layers within the cerebral wall, Friede (1989) supposed that before the onset of myelination, the layer rich in nerve fibers would be hard to distinguish and the four-layered structure could not be easily recognizable. Despite this possibility, some cases with this type of agyria (Miller, 1963; Daube & Chou, 1966; Dąmbska & Schmidt-Sidor, 1971) that were not younger than others with a four-layered pallial wall confirm the occurrence of this morphological type of agyria. It was also observed by Jellinger and Rett (1976), who suggested that for this anomaly the arrest of neuronal migration occurred at 10–11 weeks of development, the time at which the first great wave of migrating cells ends. In the agyric cortex, the neurons not segregated properly into layers are often found in an aberrant position, some of them with principal dendrites inverted (Fig. 72). This phenomenon, also observed in other cortical anomalies, may be interpreted to be a result of the absence of normal interneuronal connections (Bordarier *et al.*, 1986; Takada *et al.*, 1984). In some cases, both types of agyria were observed in regions differing in time of cortical development.

Pachygyria is a more attenuated anomaly of the same type. It presents as broad, abnormal gyri with a four-layered or six-layered structure and may appear in earlier-developing regions of brain hemispheres when other later-developing regions are agyric. In particular, the coincidence of different morphological types of this cortical malformation appear to indicate the time of their onset. The areas of transition between normal and pachygyric cortex were also observed, demonstrating that only the external layers were seen as the continuity of normal cortex, and the deep cellular layer corresponded in subcortical areas. This observation is an indirect morphological confirmation of the arrest of neuronal migration in agyria/pachygyria.

Pachygyric cortex may also be found in brains with large periventricular heterotopias (see below). The arrest of migration of many nerve cells results in a restricted number of neurons reaching the cortical stripe and finally leads to abnormal cortical organization and its abnormal folding.

Brains with agyric pallium commonly have large ventricles, and other CNS structures display some anomalies corresponding to cortical malformations by developmental connections or by time of origin. Absence of claustrum and capsula interna, disturbances within thalamic structures, heterotopias in inferior olivary nuclei, and anomalies of dentate nucleus and sometimes of cerebellar cortex may be observed. Hypoplasia of cerebrospinal tracts is a consequence of cortical maldevelopment.

Agyria/pachygyria belongs to a group of rare malformations. It has been observed as a familial syndrome (Miller, 1963; Dieker et al., 1969; Norman et al., 1976; Jellinger & Rett, 1976) and in sporadic cases (Munhoff & Noetzel, 1965; Dąmbska & Schmidt-Sidor, 1971; Stewart et al., 1975; Dobyns et al., 1985). The most extensively analyzed lissencephaly is Miller–Dieker syndrome, although it occurs in a minority of cases of agyria (Aicardi, 1991). This syndrome is characterized clinically by microcephaly, profound mental retardation, and craniofacial defects (micrognathia, ear abnormalities, anteverted nares, bitemporal growing of the forehead). Anomalies in internal organs have also been seen. It was observed that children who failed to thrive and experienced seizures, spasticity and epistotonic position rarely survived more than 2 years (Dobyns et al., 1985; Izmeth & Parameshwar, 1989). Investigations performed during the last several years established

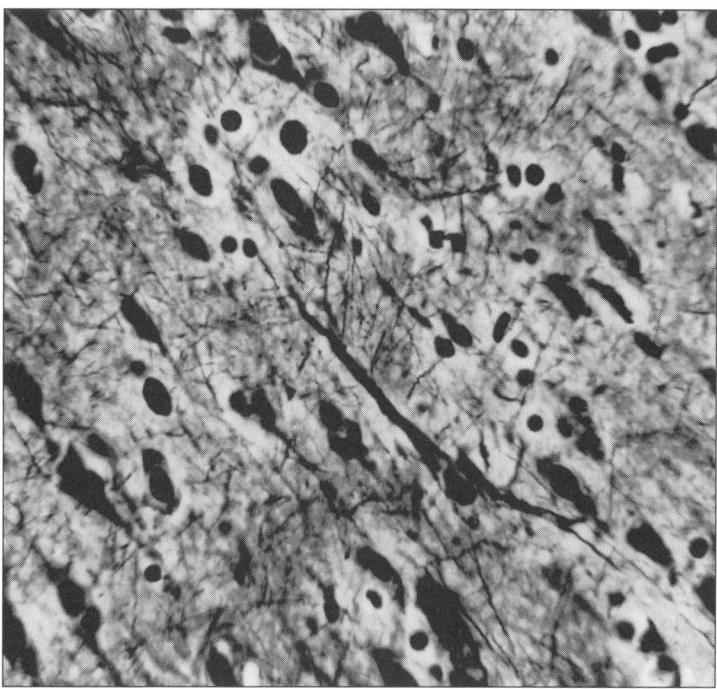

Fig. 72. Aberrant position of neurons in agyric cortex. Bodian, × 400.

that this syndrome is associated with chromosomal abnormalities of the LIS 1 gene located at chromosome 17p 13.3 (Dobyns et al., 1983; van Tuinen et al., 1988; Kwiatkowski et al., 1990).

Other than Miller–Dieker lissencephaly, familial syndromes with agyria/pachygyria (Pavone et al., 1990) and isolated non-familial cases with this cortical malformation have until now been less clearly defined. Among them, some cases reveal particular features. Norman–Roberts syndrome (Norman et al., 1976) is proposed as a distinct form of lissencephaly type I (Iannetti et al., 1993a). The primary case was microcephalic and had experienced seizures since birth; the hemispheres were agyric and four-layered, and periventricular heterotopia were abundant. Lack of the external granular layer and poor cells in the cortex were observed in the cerebellum. It appears that the syndrome was transmitted via autosomal recessive trait. Two familial cases with severe microencephaly and extreme neopallial hypoplasia described by Barth et al. (1982) displayed great malfor-

Fig. 73. Microcephalic brain with (a) lissencephalic; (b) agyric neocortex; Cresyl violet, × 120.

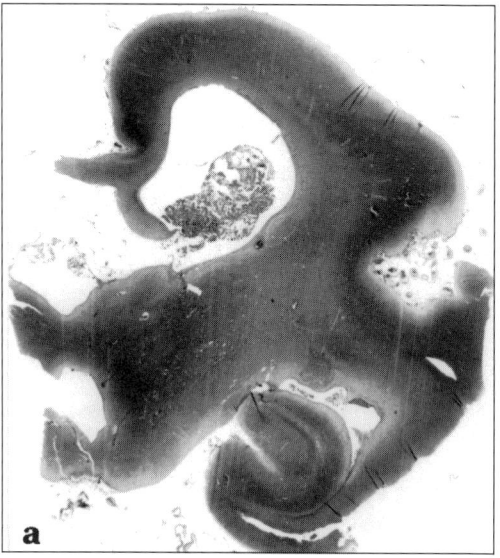

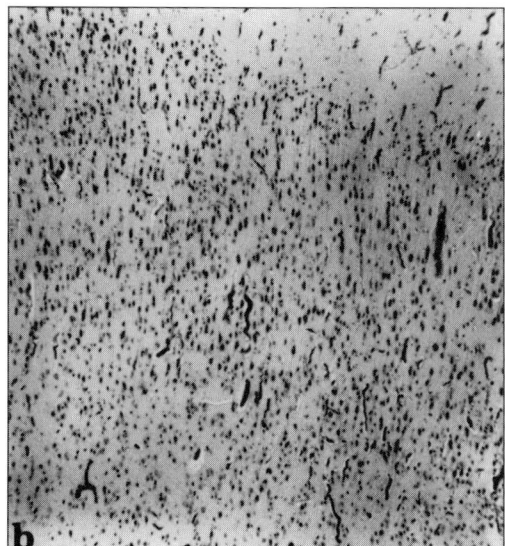

Fig. 74. CT scan of a brain with lissencephalic neopallium.

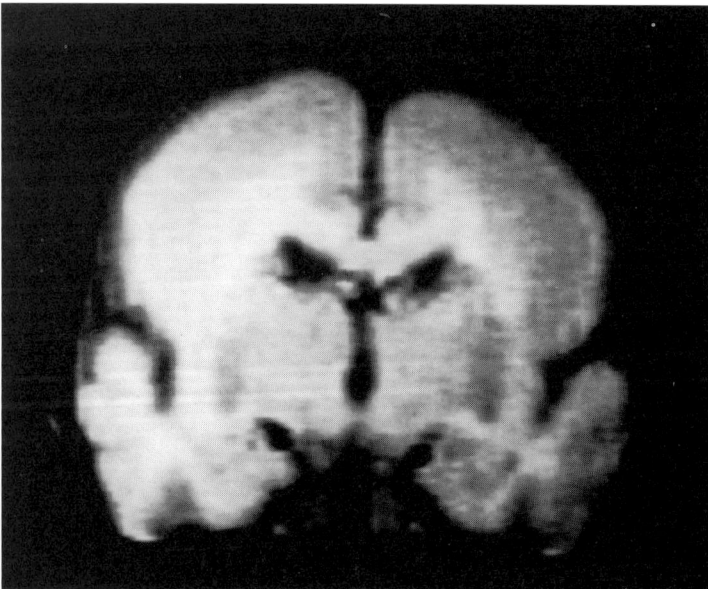

mations of the brain stem and cerebellum. Therefore, they have been named the cerebro-cerebellar syndrome. In addition, twins observed by Dąmbska *et al.* (1993) with even more advanced neopallial hypoplasia in microencephalic brains (weighing 56 and 60 g) presented anomalies restricted to a neocortical subform of its agyric appearance (Fig. 73).

Agyria/pachygyria syndrome has recently received more clinical attention and is recognized as less rare than was previously considered, as a result of CT and MRI examination allowing the diagnosis of such gross morphological changes in living individuals (Kuzniecky, 1994). Nevertheless, Raymond *et al.* (1995) use this term in neuroimaging diagnosis only to describe the brain devoid of gyri, leaving the precise differentiation of types of anomaly to histologic examination (Fig. 74).

Subcortical heterotopia

Subcortical heterotopia must be reviewed in relation to cortical abnormal development belonging to the same group of malformation. They are observed as laminar, which belong to the group of generalized dysgenesis, or as nodular.

Laminar heterotopia present as a subcortical layer of cells arrested in migration, separated by layers of white matter from the ventricular wall and from the cortex. This cortex could display a normal or a disturbed lamination and gyrification. Laminar heterotopia are usually bilateral. Rare cases with transitional changes between laminar heterotopia and pachygyria were mentioned in the literature (Jacob, 1936). Therefore, this type of heterotopia, although considered a distinct type of malformation, could be classified as similar to pachygyria as an example of disturbed neuronal migration, a rare type of developmental anomaly. They are recognized by MRI as a so-called 'double cortex,' which is considered one of the possible causes of epileptic seizures (Barkovich et al., 1989; Palmini et al., 1991; Rici et al., 1992; Iannetti et al., 1993b; Prayson et al., 1995).

Nodular heterotopia are more common. They present as clusters of neurons, often located around the corners of lateral ventricles, and are separated from each other by bundles of myelinated nerve fibers (Fig. 75). They include neurons and glial cells, sometimes at different levels of maturation (Dąmbska et al., 1996), but not presenting with the dysmorphic features necessary to consider the changes dysgenetic. Nodular heterotopia may occur in combination with various types of CNS malformations, in microcephalic as well as megalencephalic brains, and with an abnormal, often polymicrogyric cortex. Heterotopia may be induced by exogenous factors, as has been observed in some infants' brains (Choi et al., 1978) and confirmed in experimental animals after X-irradiation (Ferrer et al., 1984). Heterotopia are also suspected to be familial (Lott et al., 1979). It is important to distinguish the great masses of heterotopic nerve tissue from small neurons or groups of neurons scattered between the cortex and ventricular wall (see below).

Polymicrogyria

Polymicrogyria (PMG), formerly called micropolygyria and microgyria, presents as an excessive folding of all or the external cortical layers and the absence of the separation of gyri. The result is an abnormal surface of hemispheres with broad gyri, but sometimes also narrow gyri, increased in number. It is important not to mistake the small, narrow gyri with well-developed layering that are shrunken because of necrotic changes and consecutive scarring (ulegyria), with disturbed gyrification re-

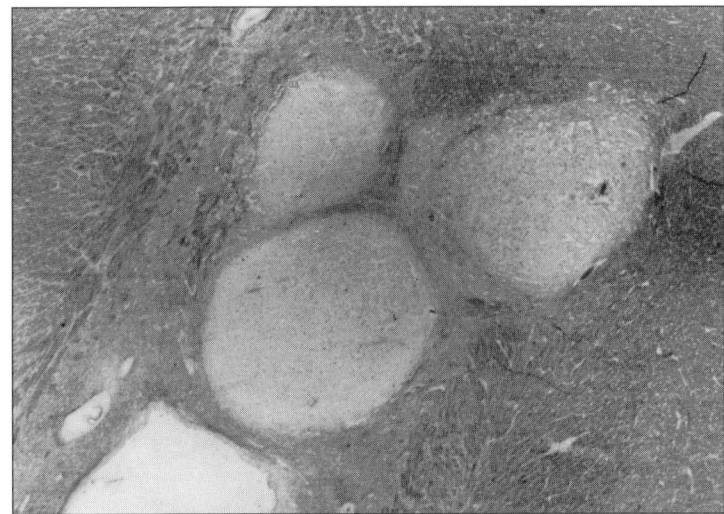

Fig. 75. Nodular heterotopias around the anterior horn of lateral ventricle. Cresyl violet, × 6.

sulting from abnormal cortical development, as is evident in PMG. PMG may occur as a more or less generalized cortical malformation of one or both hemispheres, but more often is observed as a focal lesion.

Two principal types of PMG may be seen: unilayered or four-layered. Unilayered PMG presents as an excessive folding of the cortex, containing a single cortical layer fused with the next one by their external surfaces (Fig. 76). This fusion is usually

Fig. 76. Unilayered polymicrogyria (PMG). Cresyl violet, × 100.

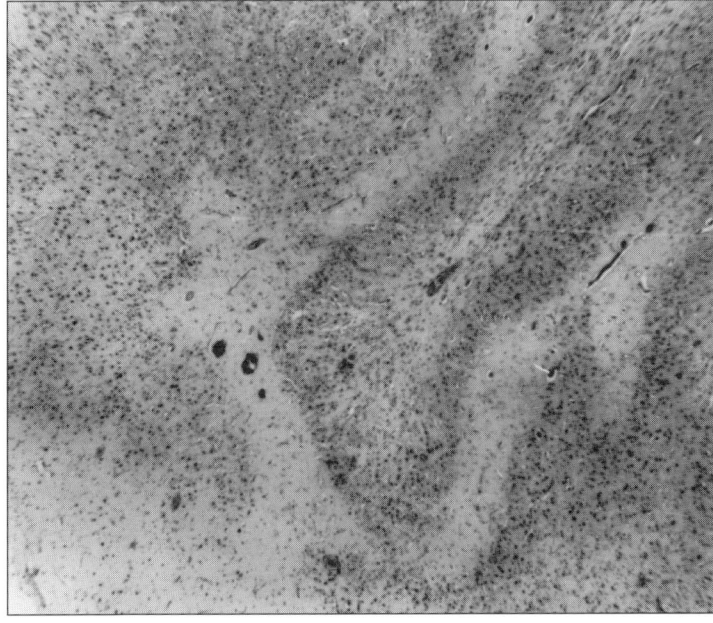

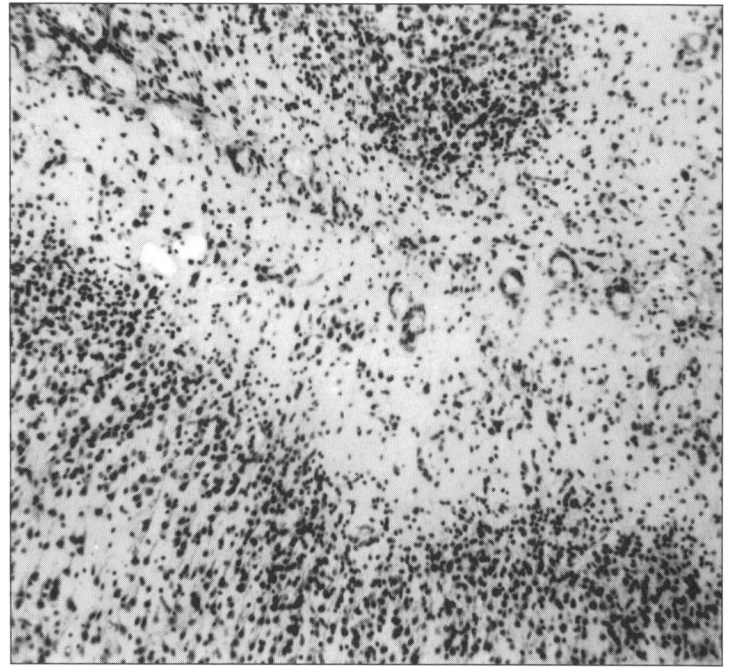

Fig. 77 (above). Fusion of cortical convolutions in polymicrogyric cortex marked by profiles of vessels. Cresyl violet, × 120.

Fig. 78 (below). Four-layered PMG. Cresyl violet, × 100.

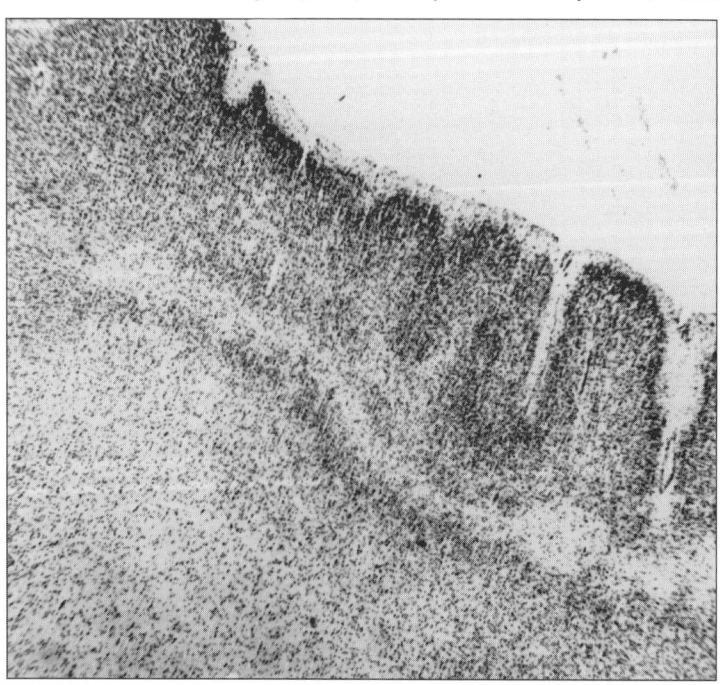

marked by a line of profiles of vessels (Fig. 77). The four-layered PMG comprise (1) a molecular layer, (2) an upper-cell layer, (3) a cell-sparse layer, and (4) a deep-cell layer (Fig. 78). The structure of four-layered PMG often demonstrates that the folding of the external and internal layers is different. Layers I and II, with rather preserved neuronal density, demonstrate abundant folding; the cell-sparse layer III and the layer IV, with less dense cellularity, are partially unfolded. The subpial plexus of myelinated fibers is seen in several cases as overlying the polymicrogyric cortex. In other cases, a break of the glial-pial barrier leads to formation of glio-neuronal heterotopias (GNH) into meninges. The role of lesions of the glial-pial barrier in the pathomechanism of cortical maldevelopment is discussed below.

When observed, the border between polymicrogyric and normal cortex makes evident the abnormally folded layers that correspond to layers I to III of normal cortex, and the cell-sparse layer III corresponding to the neocortical layer IV.

In the pathomechanism of PMG formation, the lesions occurring during the last phase of the migratory process and cortical lamination must be considered (de Leon, 1972; Larroche, 1977; Barth, 1987). The important role of perfusion failure has been noted for many years (Richman *et al.*, 1974; Levine *et al.*, 1974). The hypothesis that the arising of partial necrosis (Fig. 79) before the end of neuronal migration to the external cortical layers may result in PMG was verified experimentally in rats by Dvorak *et al.* (1978) and Dvorak and Feit (1977).

Our own case, age 22–23 weeks of development and presenting a formative stage of PMG closely related topographically to thick inflammatory infiltrations of meninges, confirms the role of focal perfusion failure in the observed anomaly (Fig. 80). The developing cortex is vascularized (as was previously described) by meningeal vessels forming an appropriate vascular bed for each cortical layer (Kuban & Gilles, 1985). The pathologic changes within the meninges may disturb this process.

A similar pathomechanism may be suspected in cases with vascular abnormalities within the meninges (Fig. 81) and even in rare cases of leptomeningeal lipomatosis (Scherer, 1935a; Dragojevic et al., 1973), when it is evident that meningeal changes overlay the cortical segments with polymicrogyric structure.

It is not uncommon to find PMG in brains with intrauterine CMV infection (Friede & Mikolasek, 1978; Dąmbska et al., 1983a). It is possible for an infection and PMG to exist by coincidence. The infection may occur in a brain with an anomaly, but may also cause malformation (Friede & Mikolasek, 1978). The PMG may be found in cortical regions where more or less severe necrotic changes in subcortical white matter are observed. They may be due to the lesions of distal terminal blood vessels. The cortical maldevelopment in this situation may be induced by the damage of radial glial fibers involved in the last phase of neuroblast migration (Ferrer & Catala, 1991).

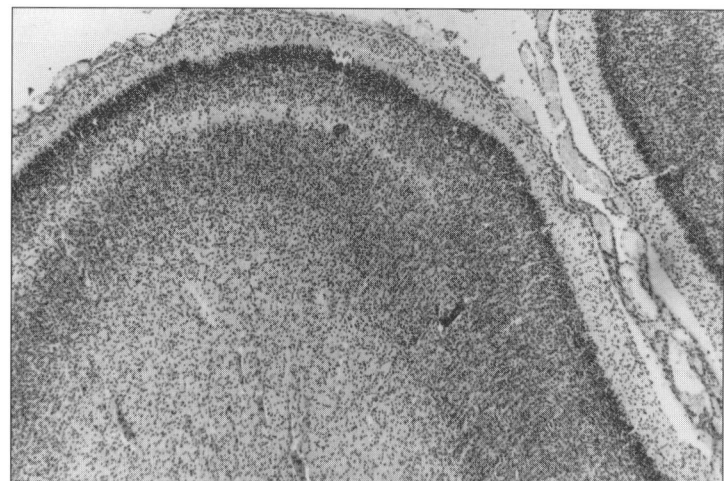

Fig. 79 (above). Partial necrosis of IV cortical layer, 22 WG. Cresyl violet, × 100.

Verification by many observations is necessary to determine how often the pathomechanism of focal changes described above occurs, and how often a transient generalized perfusion failure induces PMG formation (Marques-Dias et al., 1984). In cases with changes in the cerebral as well

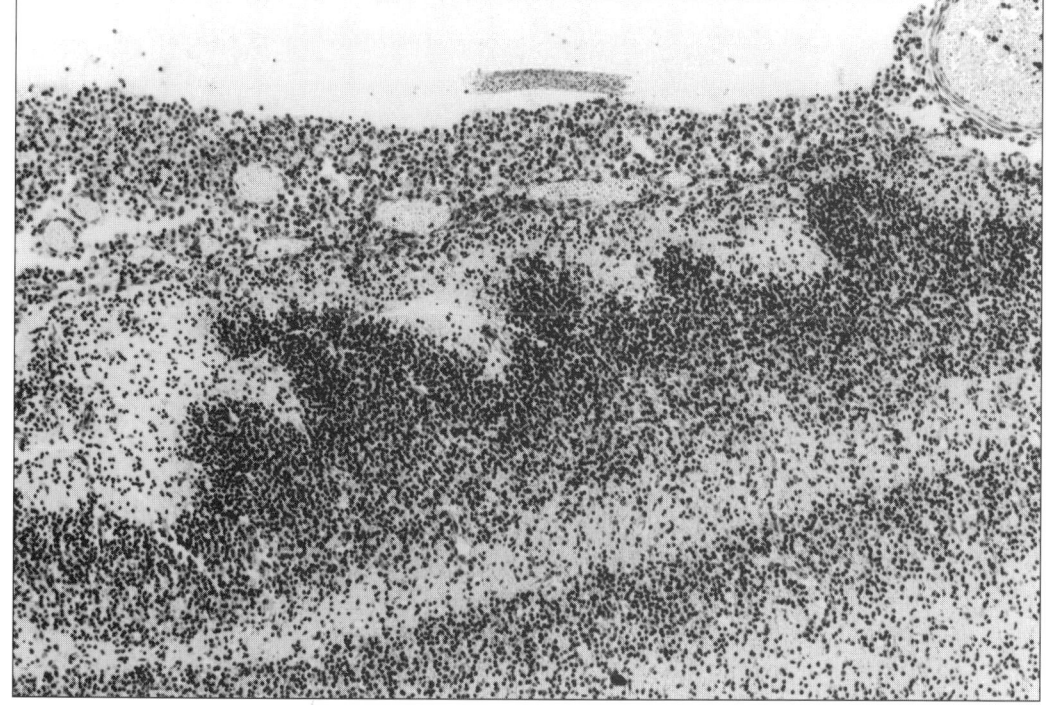

Fig. 80 (left). Formation of four-layered PMG in a case with intrauterine meningitis 23 WG.

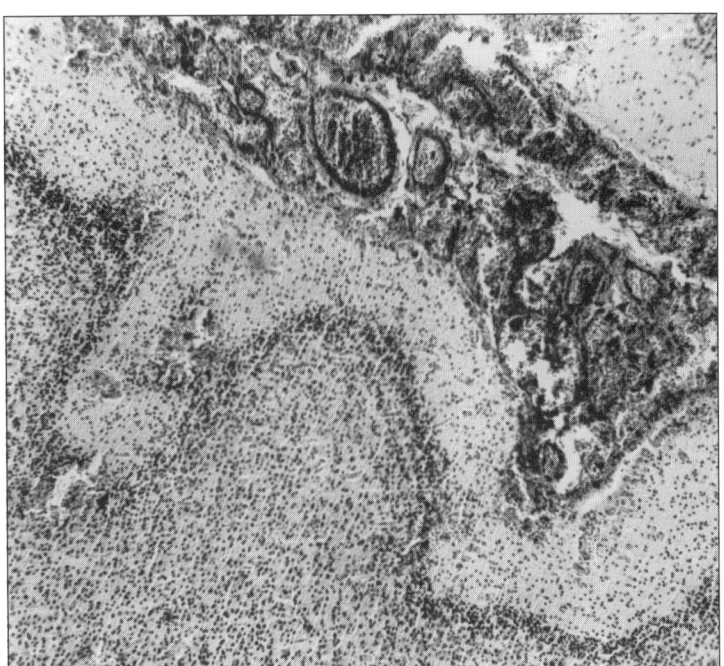

Fig. 81. Anomalies of cortical strip in areas with vascular anomalies within the meninges. Cresyl violet, × 100.

as the cerebellar cortex, a general insult is particularly suspected. The role of perfusion failure during the final period of intracortical neuronal migration in four-layered PMG has been confirmed by many authors (Levine et al., 1974; Williams et al., 1976; McBride & Kemper, 1982; Marques-Dias et al., 1984). The presence of both types of PMG in the same case and in coincidence with laminar cortical necrosis, as observed in our own case, demonstrates the possibility of the same pathomechanism for both types of PMG. Studies by Ferrer (1984) and Ferrer and Catala (1991) also led to the final conclusion that unilayered PMG may be produced by circulatory failure.

In concluding our considerations about the pathomechanism of PMG, the role of a break in the glial-pial barrier must be mentioned. The type of lesions observed in several cases of PMG resulting in excessive migration of glial and even nerve cells into the meninges appears to facilitate the fusion of abnormally folded cortical convolutions.

The time of formation of both types of PMG was analyzed many times in relation to pathologic events in pregnancy and their comparison with the rate of cortical development. According to such observations, it appears that unilayered PMG may arise after trauma between 14 and 19 WG (Norman, 1980; Barth, 1987; Ferrer & Catala, 1991), and four-layered PMG is the sequel of lesions occurring one month later (20–24 weeks) (Hallervorden, 1949; Bankl & Jellinger, 1967). The presence of both types of PMG in one case appears to reflect the topographic differences at the time of cortical development.

The etiology of PMG appears to be even more complicated than its pathomechanism. It is neither possible nor necessary to describe extensively all syndromes in which PMG may be found, but it is worthwhile to mention briefly such instances. PMG presents either as a developmental abnormality, which may be observed in genetic-metabolic or other familial diseases as a principal brain malformation, or as only a part of a wide spectrum of CNS malformations, as in Meckel syndrome (Paetau et al., 1985). PMG was observed in neonatal adrenoleukodystrophy (Barth, 1987; Friede, 1989), in Aicardi syndrome combined with other cortical anomalies, which are summarized below (Ferrer et al., 1986), and in several others. The examples cited above and those concerning other eventual cases lead to the conclusion that this cortical anomaly appears in many brains with various pathogeneses (as far as of genetic and as far as exogenic origin). Among exogenous factors, intrauterine infections, including CMV (as discussed above), play an important role. The principal role has to be reserved for perfusion failure, but it is evident that such failure could be provoked by various factors and in various mechanisms.

For in-vivo diagnosis of polymicrogyria, CT and MRI examination are helpful (Fig. 82) but are subject to restriction and possible misidentification of such anomaly as pachygyria (Aicardi, 1991).

Disorganized cortical structure (lissencephaly type II)

Lissencephaly type II presents as cortex deprived of macroscopically visible gyri and sulci, with a flat surface of the cerebral hemispheres. The result is a gross diagnosis of lissencephaly (Fig. 83). The cortical stripe is thick and deeply disorganized. The clusters and island of pyramidal and small nerve cells are intermixed. They are divided by stripes of glial tissue and by abnormal-looking vessels traversing the cortex. Some of the neurons are too immature for the age of the patient. No cortical lamination is detectable (Fig. 84). Rarely, fragments of the cortical stripe present the polymicrogyric structure and often only in the form of islands of cells surrounded by cell-sparse areas, which may be considered as transversely cut convolutions of unilayered PMG. In the majority of observed cases, the glial-pial barrier revealed damage over long segments of the cortical surface. Thus, GNH were observed (Fig. 85). According to previous observations (Dąmbska et al., 1986), this type of most advanced cortical disorganization correlates with particularly abundant GNH. Choi and Matthias (1987), analyzing the pathomechanism of this type of cortical mantel abnormality, emphasized the principal role of the damage of the glial-pial barrier in early development. The same suggestion was derived from observation of a fetus at 20 weeks of development presenting this type of abnormality (Squier, 1993). Damage to the glial-pial barrier may lead to aberrant migration to the molecular layer and into meninges and to consecutive disorganization of cortical layering. The structure of the abnormal cortex in several cases previously observed presented intracortical proliferation of glial and mesodermal elements, giving the impression of a scar. Single cases were also observed by Norman et al. (1976) and our own unpublished case, with or no or, only minimal disruption of the glial-pial barrier. Also taking into account the fragments of polymicrogyric structure in lissencephaly type II brains, we must consider destructive processes within the cortex during development as another possible or additional mechanism of this cortical anomaly.

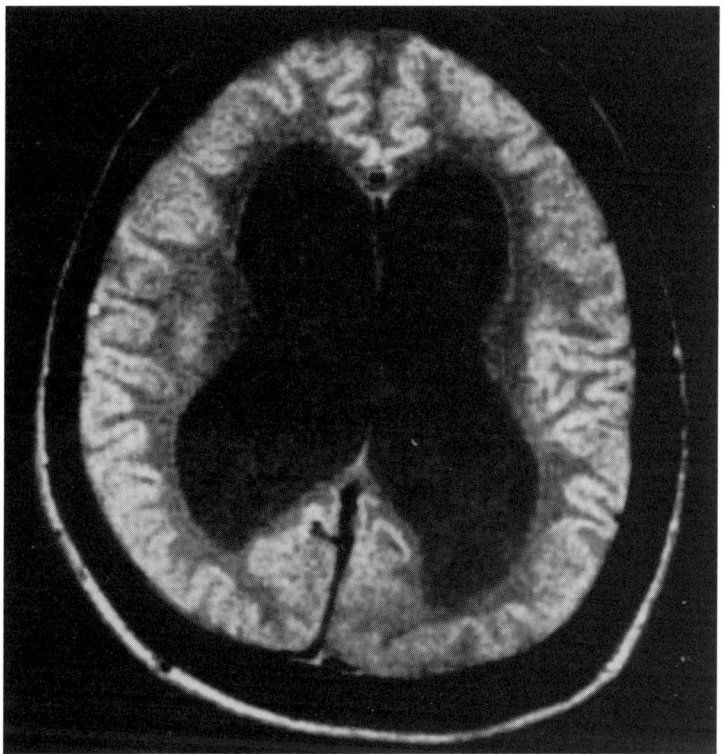

Fig. 82. MRI picture of a case with hydrocephaly and PMG.

The time of its formation has to be prolonged because the cortical layering is generally disturbed. The glial-pial barrier is mature before the end of the second month of development, and vascularization of cerebral hemispheres begins at a similar time. It seems that the most plausible teratogenic time for lissencephaly type II could be between the third and seventh month of development, during the active migration and vascularization of the cortical stripe. It is important to emphasize the differences between lissencephaly type I and type II (Dąmbska et al., 1983b). The general term 'lissencephaly' should be used only when clinical examination prevents a differential diagnosis. The diagnosis agyria/lissencephaly type I or lissencephaly type II can be precise when the type of cortical malformation is known.

Fig. 83 (right). Flat surface of cerebral hemisphere in lissencephaly type II. Cresyl violet, × 3.

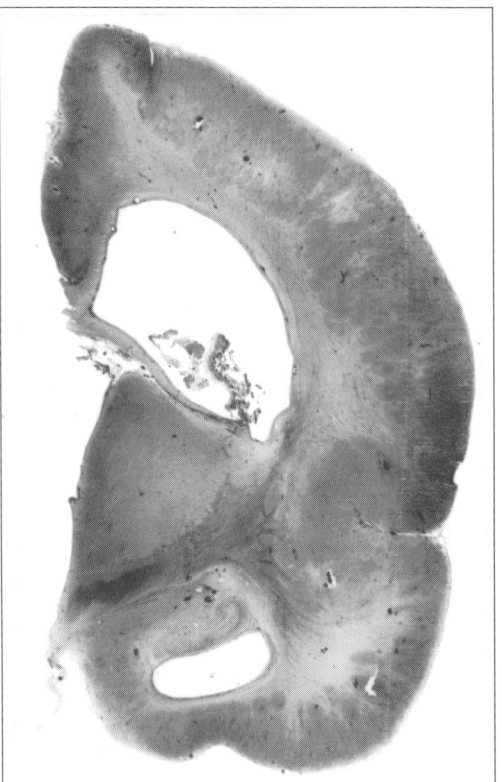

Lissencephaly type II corresponds to the type of cortical dysgenesis described by Walker (1942) and is known to occur in Walker–Warburg syndrome, also known as HARD + E syndrome (hydrocephalus, agyria, retinal dysplasia + encephalocele). Individuals with those syndromes do not survive more than a few months; they are microcephalic, with mental retardation, occipital encephalocele in 30 per cent of cases, retinal and other eye anomalies, several malformations among other extremities, and skeletal muscle pathology (Warburg, 1987; Dobyns *et al.*, 1989). Within the CNS, cerebellar abnormalities such as the absence of vermis (Lyon *et al.*, 1993) and the presence of cortical anomalies are observed. The cerebral hemispheres are smooth, and the cortex demonstrates a disorganized structure, as presented above. Williams *et al.* (1984) attempted to distinguish external and deeper zones in the cerebral mantle, but the zones are not similar to normal cortical layering.

Fig. 84 (right). Disorganized cortical structure in lissencephaly type II. Cresyl violet, × 100.

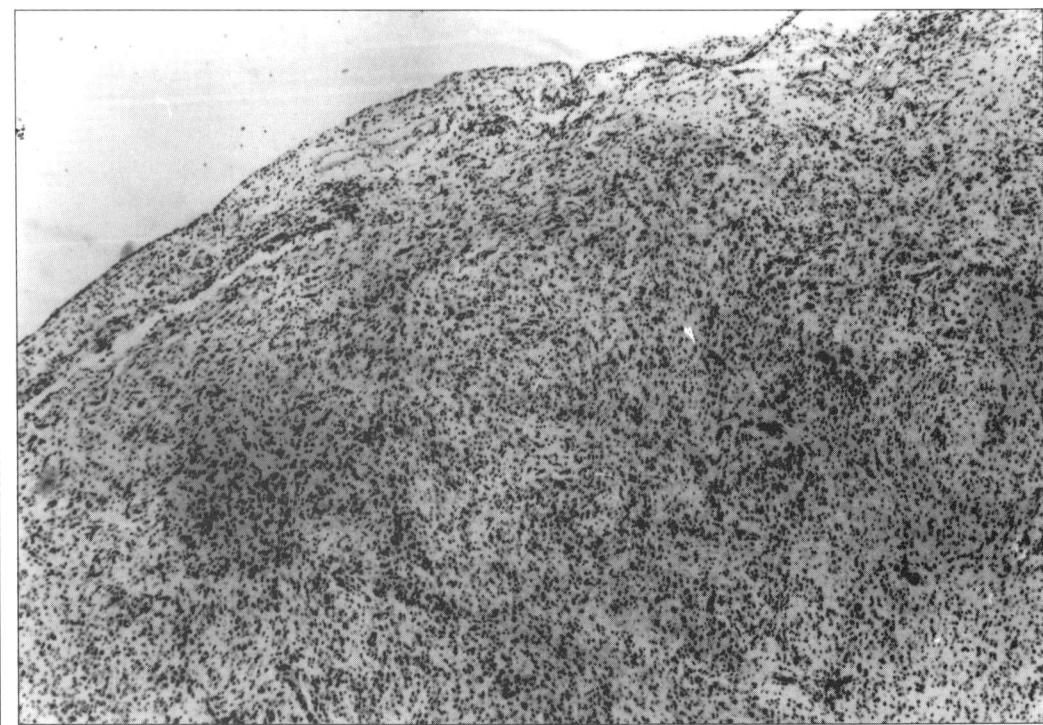

In Fukuyama syndrome (Fukuyama congenital muscular dystrophy = FCMD), lissencephaly type II also occurs (Dąmbska et al., 1982b). This disease is usually progressive and occurs, with hypotonia, muscular dystrophy, mental retardation, and eye and CNS developmental anomalies. In more severely affected cases (Krijgsman et al., 1980; Dąmbska et al., 1982b), all features of lissencephaly type II are present; in cases with less advanced cortical changes, unilayered PMG prevails, and most moderate cases demonstrate only cortical verrucosus dysplasia, analyzed below (Takada et al., 1984). In the most advanced changes, vascular anomalies are observed.

A genetically conditioned etiology according to clinical observation has been proposed for both syndromes. Recently, the specific gene 9 q 31–32 was identified for Fukuyama disease (Toda et al., 1993), and the coexistance of FCMD and WWS in one family suggests the genetic identity of both syndromes (Toda et al., 1995).

Muscle-eye-brain disease of Santavuori (Santavuori et al., 1989) seems to be a similar, but less severe, entity than those described above. All of the described syndromes appear to be closely related variants within a great group of complex malformations (Dobyns et al., 1985, Heyer et al., 1986; Heggie et al., 1987; Takashima et al., 1987; Kimura et al., 1993).

In vivo CT and MRI techniques sometime permit distinction of type II from type I lissencephaly (Kuzniecki, 1994), but errors occur. In such cases, correlation with EEG findings may be helpful for differential diagnosis (Aicardi, 1991).

Other cortical anomalies

Laminar and focal cortical developmental anomalies

Laminar and focal cortical dysplasias present changes usually suggesting the disturbances in the late or even the final phase of neuronal migration, which is partially combined with damage of glial-pial barrier. Recently, such anomalies were most commonly observed in cases with intractable epilepsy treated by cortical resection (Raymond et al., 1995; Mischel et al., 1995; Prayson et al., 1993). Some types of anoma-

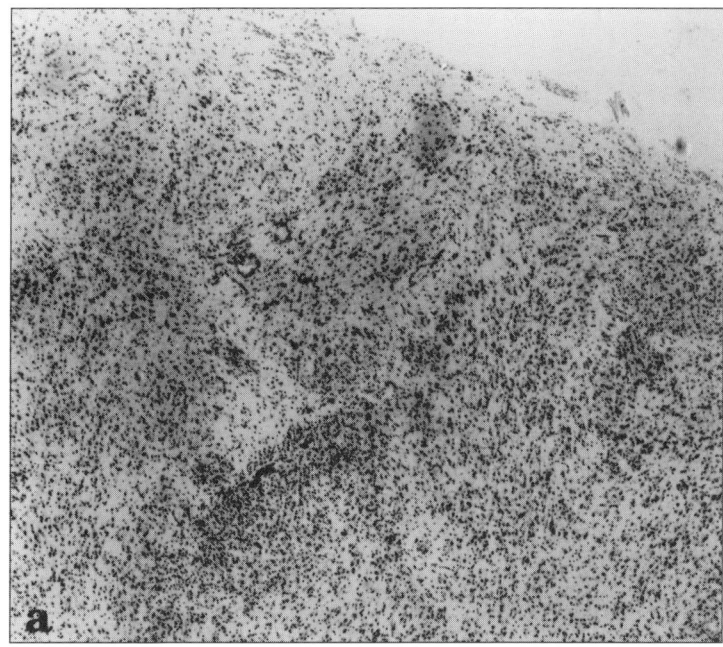
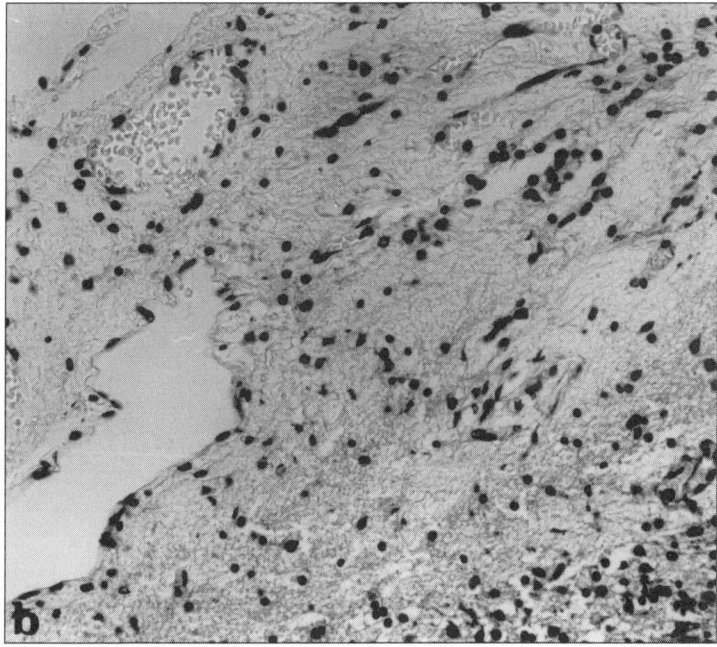

Fig. 85. Glioneuronal heterotopias on the surface of cortical stripe. Cresyl violet; (a) × 100; (b) × 400.

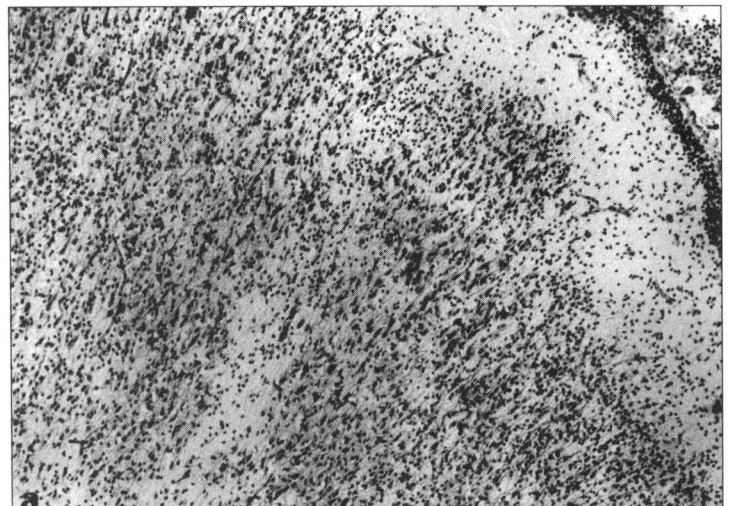

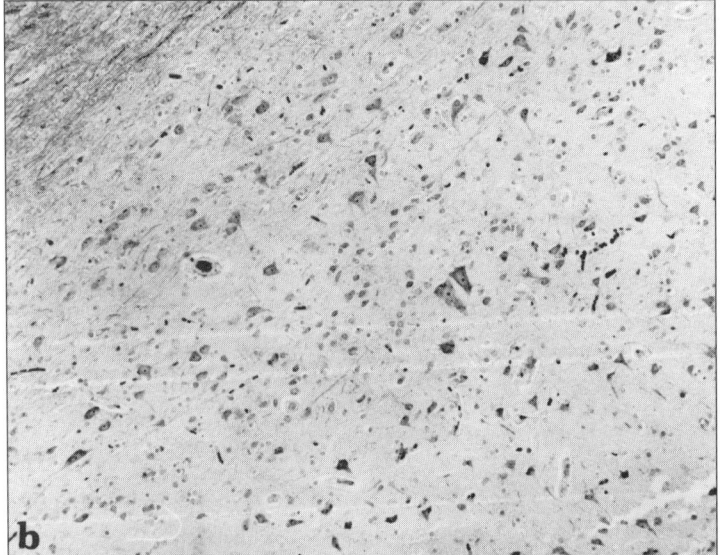

Fig. 86. Disturbed cortical lamination with neuronal clustering. Cresyl violet; (a) × 100; (b) × 300.

other eventual clinical symptoms deserves further studies. Leonard et al. (1993), who examined subjects with learning disabilities by MRI, concluded these individuals reveal a variation of anomalies of cortical cerebral structures with higher incidence than in control cases.

The radial arrangement of cortical neurons, a distinct type of cortical anomaly, appears as a very immature cortical organization lacking the formation of normal layering. Developmental abnormality is indicated by such radial arrangement when identified in neonates and small children.

Neurons disseminated subcortically within the intermediate zone, at the time by which migration should be accomplished and the subplate zone exhausted, may appear as a result of lesions within the radial glia. The number of such heterotopic neurons may depend on the number of affected glial cells (Sarnat, 1992).

According to the description of Jacob (1940) typical forms of 'brain warts' or *'dysgenesie nodulaire de l'ecorce'* (Morel & Wildi, 1952; Grcevic & Robert, 1961) consist of small protrusions of the external cortical layers into cortical layer I, which is thin at the apex of the protrusion. The nodules contain in their center a bundle of myelinated fibers. They may appear without other cortical abnormalities but may coincide with focal anomalies of the adjacent cortex, as described above.

Neurons in the molecular layer may also appear in evidently increased numbers as another minor anomaly. It is speculated that these neurons may come from migration waves transgressing the normal target area or may arise from the subpial granular layer. Persistence of the subpial granular layer may also be seen focally often coinciding with disturbances of cortical maturation (Mischel et al., 1995) or with glio-neuronal heterotopias (GNH). GNH, present as intrusions of glial and some nerve cells into meninges. They may be focal or more diffuse, effacing the borderline be-

lies may be specified in this group of cortical anomalies.

Laminar architectural disorganization is observed as a focal or more diffuse anomaly (Kazee et al., 1991). The disruption of cortical lamination with neuronal clustering and irregular arrangement (Fig. 86) is rarely found in routinely examined cases, except cases with epileptic seizures. The question of an eventual causal relation between minor, or focal, cortical anomalies and dyslexia (Galaburda et al., 1985; Kaufmann & Galaburda, 1989; Cohen et al., 1989) and

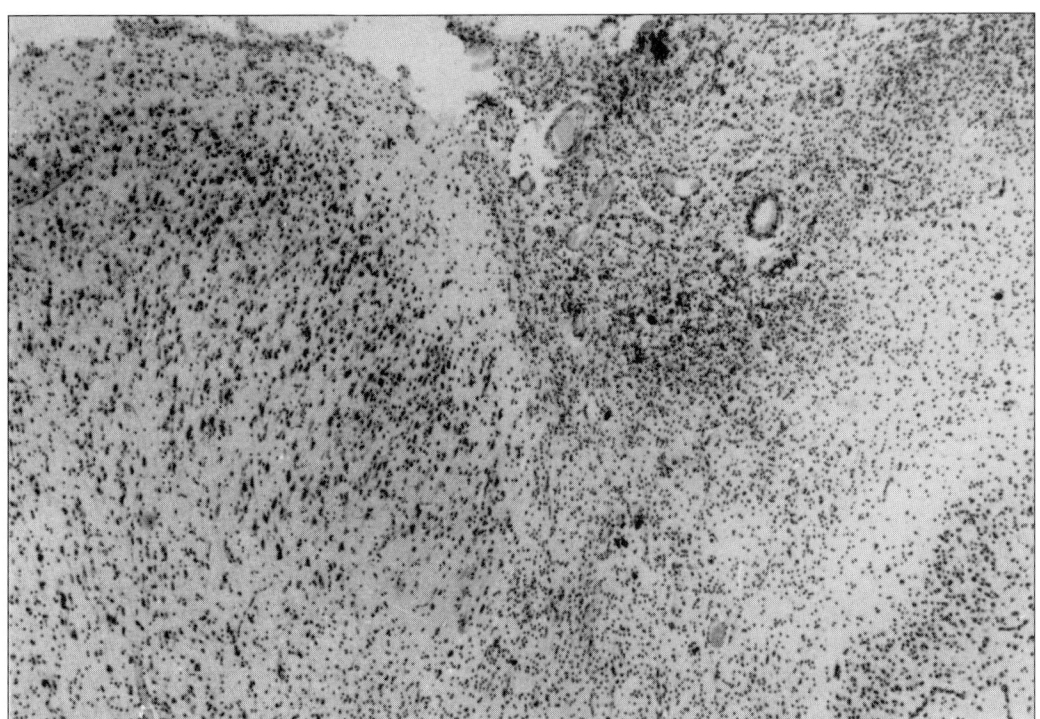

Fig. 87. Focal GNH effacing the border of cortical layer I. Cresyl violet, × 100.

tween the nerve tissue and meninges (Fig. 87). They may coincide with cortical malformation, suggesting the disruption of the glial-pial barrier in formation of those anomalies. In such cases, the disruption should appear earlier than when GNH occur without disturbances in cortical organization, indicating relatively late damage of this important barrier (Dąmbska et al., 1986). They may be combined with the persistence of horizontal Cajal–Retzius cells, which may be found in various cortical dysplasias as well as in normal brains.

Particular or complex cortical anomalies

We reviewed cortical dysplasias occurring during the time of cortical development. The cortical developmental abnormalities are difficult to include in any morphological classification, as they sometimes present a coincidence of various types of cortical malformations. They can be observed in some complex congenital syndromes involving, among others, the CNS.

We would like to present some characteristic examples of this type of malformation.

The cerebrohepatorenal syndrome of Zellweger includes an inborn error of metabolism represented by an increased very long chain of fatty acids in plasma (Dimmick & Applegarth, 1993). Children with this syndrome survive no more than 2.5 years, with failure to thrive, dysmorphic face, deafness, cataracts, glaucoma, liver cirrhosis, renal cysts, and the following CNS changes: the abnormal shape of the cortical gyri; PEGS often within the insular cortex; radially striated appearance of other cortical areas; subcortical heterotopia; dysgenetic nerve and glial cells; hypomyelination of the white matter; and heterotopia of Purkinje cells, constituting a picture of the borderline between inherited malformation of neuronal migration (Volpe & Adams, 1972) and dysgenetic changes. Inheritance of this syndrome is autosomal recessive.

Aicardi syndrome (Aicardi et al., 1965) occurs in girls; characteristics include sei-

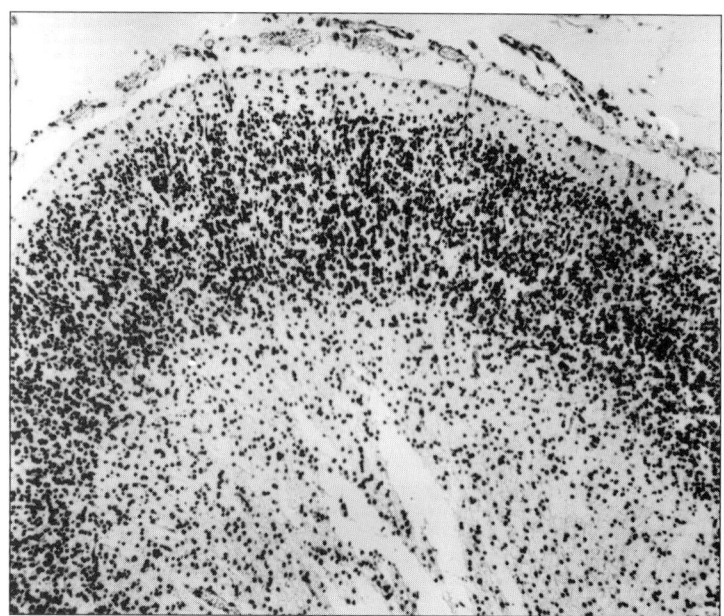

Fig. 88 (above). Immature cortical organization without normal layering in a mature newborn. Cresyl violet, × 100.

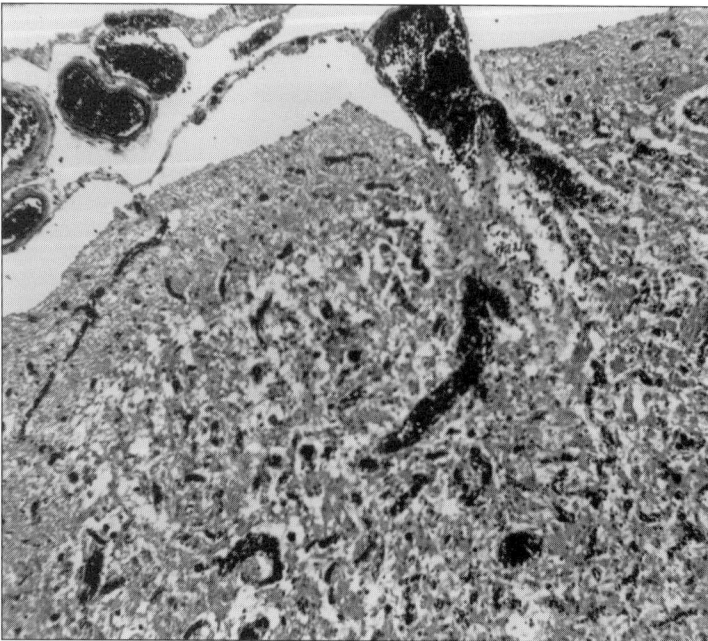

Fig. 89 (below). Proliferative vasculopathy in the cortex. Cresyl violet,

zures, mental retardation, choroid cysts, and ACC. Sometimes severe brain malformations also are seen (Takada *et al.*, 1984). Migration disorders in the CNS result in periventricular heterotopia, with disturbed lamination of the cortex, described by Ferrer *et al.* (1986) as 'unlaminated' and focal with PMG appearance.

Galloway–Movat cerebrorenal syndrome occurs with autosomal recessive inheritance and is characterized by congenital nephrosis, with protein loss in the urine and with micrencephaly, including cortical malformations (Kozłowski *et al.*, 1989). The cortex is poorly stratified and in large part appears immature for age. Focally, PMG features (Robain & Deonna, 1983), focal neuronal calcification, and meningeal glioneuronal heterotopias also are observed.

Ostrovskaya and Lazjuk (1988) described Neu–Laxova syndrome, which presents as an immature cortex, similar to that during the fifth to sixth month of development. This rare, lethal, autosomal recessive disorder, with cataracts and deformation of limbs, may be a third type of lissencephaly.

Immaturity of the neocortex was also observed sometimes in sporadic cases (Laure-Kamionowska & Majdecki, 1982) (Fig. 88).

Another type of cortical anomaly is observed in an autosomal-recessive, lethal syndrome of proliferative vasculopathy with hydranencephaly-hydrocephaly. Abnormal vessels penetrating the cortex, with a deficit of nerve cells, suggest disturbances of neuronal migration as characterizing the observed anomaly (Norman & McGillivray, 1988) (Fig. 89).

Cerebellum: primitive and secondary developmental abnormalities

Cerebellar aplasia and hypoplasia, including Dandy–Walker malformation

Cerebellar congenital anomalies are difficult to describe for several reasons. The period of development of the cerebellum is very long, lasting from the fifth week of postconception until some months after birth. During this time, many factors can disturb formation of the just-differentiating cerebellar components, pushing toward maturation in a wrong way. At this time, the primary malformation and disruption are particularly difficult to differentiate. The close developmental, topographical, and functional relation between the cerebellum and other parts of the CNS also may induce developmental anomalies secondary to those previously arising elsewhere. Cerebellar defects found together with an occipital encephalocele may present such types of complex malformation (Caviness & Evarard, 1975; Smith & Huntington, 1977). The developmental anomalies of both the cerebral and cerebellar cortex also belong to such types of changes (Dąmbska et al., 1983b). More or less well-determined complex syndromes, which will be discussed below, also are observed.

Agenesis of the cerebellum

Agenesis of the cerebellum is a most severe but very rare anomaly when occurring alone (Sternberg, 1912; Macchi & Bentivoglio, 1977) and is not known as total, except as described in a case by Larroche (1981). In other cases, small amounts of the remaining cerebellar tissue, often from flocculonodular lobes, were found. Total agenesis of the cerebellum (Larroche, 1981) was described, with hydrocephaly. Severe cerebellar hypoplasia was observed as a part of severe dysgeneses of the CNS such as anencephaly, dysraphic syndromes with meningo- and meningoencephaloceles (Karch & Urich, 1972), or basal ganglia midline malformations. The absence of only one cerebellar hemisphere (hemispheric aplasia) was observed rarely. Some reports are very old; others appear from time to time. We would like to quote only those of Neuburger and Edinger (1898) and of Mackiewicz (1935). When the foci of disorganized heterotopic elements of the cerebellar cortex were found instead of one cerebellar hemisphere, it was suggested that hypoplasia of one cerebellar hemisphere may be the result of a severe disorder in the contralateral cerebral hemisphere.

Aplasia of the cerebellar vermis

Aplasia of the cerebellar vermis may present as total or partial agenesis of this compound of cerebellum. It occurs in some known syndromes or in other instances, described below.

Dandy–Walker malformation. Dandy–Walker malformation is fairly common among the various types of vermis atrophies. It is characterized by a trio of symptoms including (1) complete or partial agenesis of the vermis, (2) cystic dilatation of ventricle IV, and (3) enlargement of the posterior fossa (Fig. 90).

Elevation of the tentorium cerebelli, lateral and transverse sinuses, and hydrocephalus also were stressed, but they are not observed in every case. This syndrome was described by Dandy and Blackfan (1914) and then defined once more by Taggart and Walker (1942), whose results were in acceptance of its eponym (Benda, 1954). Neuropathological examination in Dandy–Walker malformation revealed the continuity of remnants of the vermis with the roof of ventricle IV. The roof membrane contains glial and ependymal elements within its inner part.

The choroid plexus is observed in the lateral recesses of the enlarged ventricle, and posteriorly along the border between the medulla and roof membrane. The foramina of Luschka and Magendie are more often open, but in many cases, they are found to be closed. The lateral ventricles in Dandy–Walker malformation are sometimes evidently enlarged, but more often, hydrocephaly is moderate or even minimal. The clinical picture includes an enlarged dolichocephalic skull and neurological symptoms, including ataxia, nystagmus, and cranial nerve palsies. Mental retardation often coexists. Other types of neurological deficits depend on the existence of increased intracranial pressure and concomitant lesions. Among them, seizures, hemiparesis, and visual and hearing impairment were observed. Diagnosis is pos-

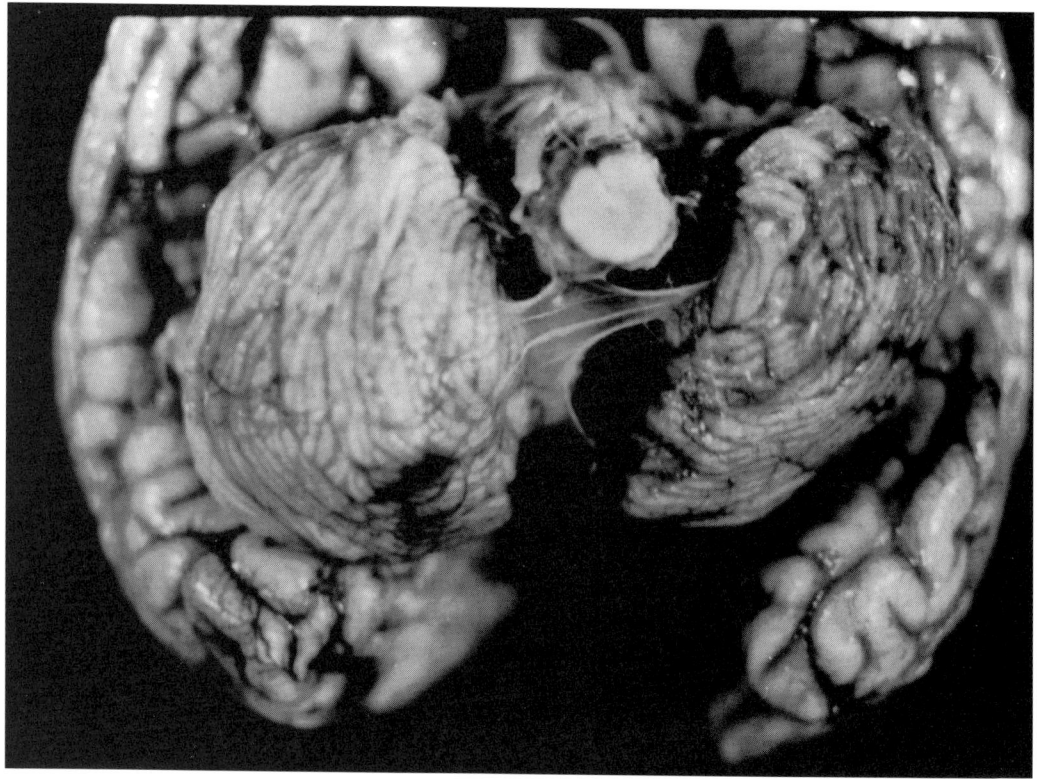

Fig. 90. Dandy–Walker malformation.

sible, even prenatally, by ultrasonography (Newman et al., 1982), and after birth, CT scan and MRI are the best methods to be used. Additional x-rays may confirm the posterior fossa anomalies, and angiography, vessels abnormalities. Some variants of MRI would even suggest use of the term Dandy–Walker complex (Barkovich et al., 1989).

The principal features of Dandy–Walker malformation are in most instances accompanied by a great variety of malformations. Most evident are the brain stem anomalies, including olivary nuclei and crossing of the spino-cortical tracts. Malformations can be moderate, but severe ones also were described (Lagger, 1979; Janzer & Friede, 1982). The cerebellar hemispheres may present cortical or dentate nucleus dysplasia or heterotopia, all of which were described previously in classical studies of this syndrome. The brain hemispheres may also reveal various anomalies such as cortical dysplasias, ACC, aqueduct stenosis, or microcephaly (Hart et al., 1972; Tal et al., 1980). Visceral anomalies also coexist.

The teratogenic time and pathomechanism of Dandy–Walker malformation have been discussed many times. Comparison with the timing of posterior fossa structure development allows agreement that this syndrome arises before the third month of postconceptional age. The most convincing explanation for its mechanism, which is supported by experimental studies on mice, is the arrest of development of rhombocephalic structures (Friede, 1989). This situation suggests the need for analysis of each case to determine which anomalies are secondary to the principal triad and which may suggest a longer teratogenic period. The last unsolved problem concerns the etiology of Dandy–Walker malformation. Some observations concerning its appearance in siblings encourage further studies (Jenkyn et al., 1981).

Joubert syndrome

Severe hypoplasia or agenesis of the cerebellar vermis in cases with respiratory abnormalities comprise Joubert syndrome (Joubert, 1969). Norman *et al.* (1995) indicated that this diagnosis is inappropriate in many cases with vermis hypoplasia, but without respiratory disturbances. They also stress that several clinicopathological changes, including retinal dysplasia and oculo-motor abnormalities, were attributed to this syndrome without concern for the existence of its basic traits. On the other hand, to what degree different changes may coincide with classic ones in Joubert syndrome is an open question. Under this hypothesis, heterotopias in the cerebellar white matter, abnormal stripe of dentate nuclei, moderate changes within the brain stem, and occipital encephalocele were reported. Clinically, abnormal eye movements and mental retardation were added to ataxia and respiratory disturbances (Fried & Boltshauser, 1978; King *et al.*, 1984). Inheritance of the syndrome is considered autosomal recessive (Laverda *et al.*, 1984), but also is believed to be recessive X-linked (Lindhout & Barth, 1985).

Tectocerebellar dysraphia

This defect also is in coexistence with the vermis aplasia. Occipital encephalocele evidently contains the cerebellar cortex, and the tectum is severely deformed.

Rhombencephalosynapsis

This condition involves lack of the vermis and fusion of the cerebellar hemispheres (De Morsier, 1955; Gross & Hoff, 1959b). The fused cerebellar hemispheres contain only a single horseshoe-shape dentate nucleus. This type of malformation also may be associated with other anomalies within the brain stem and cerebral hemispheres (Schachenmayr & Friede, 1982; Michaud *et al.*, 1982). Other combinations of vermis aplasia with various structural anomalies also were reported (Warkany & Bofinger, 1975; Bordarier & Aicardi, 1990); included among these anomalies was Warburg syndrome (Bordarier *et al.*, 1984).

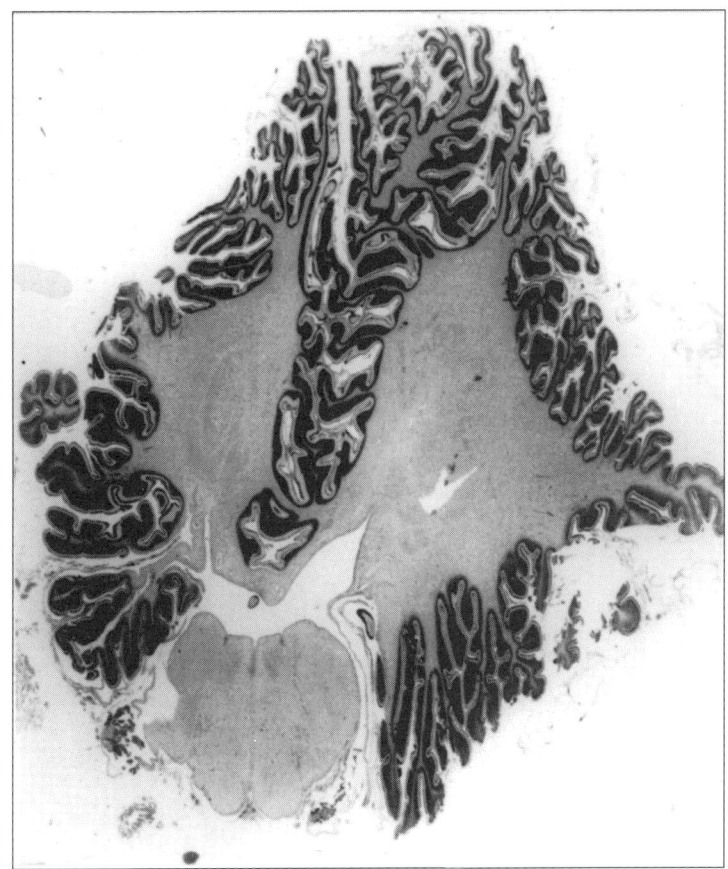

Fig. 91. Hypoplasia of the cerebellum. Cresyl violet, × 3.

Hypoplasia of the cerebellum

Hypoplasia of the cerebellum (Vogt & Astwacaturow, 1912; Sarnat & Alcala, 1980) represents an even more controversial entity. It can involve the entire cerebellum or some parts of it (Fig. 91), most often neocerebellar ones. Therefore, it is generally known as neocerebellar hypoplasia (Brun, 1917, 1918a,b). Nevertheless, this anomaly may affect both neocerebellar and paleocerebellar components (Rubinstein & Freeman, 1940). In such cases, the cerebellar cortex includes underdeveloped gyri; other cases show disorganized cortical structure, but also areas of cortical atrophy. The den-

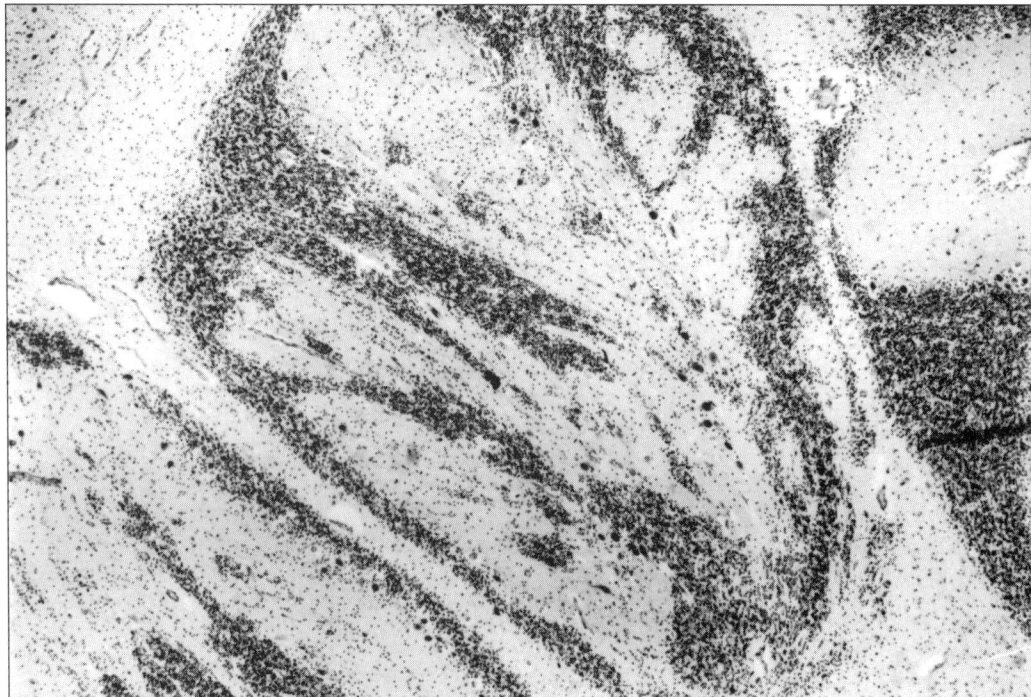

Fig. 92. Subcortical heterotopy within the cerebellar hemisphere. Cresyl violet, × 100.

tate nucleus also may be disorganized. Hypoplasia of the cerebellum was observed with a lack of neurons in the pons, as pontocerebellar atrophy (Colan et al., 1981) or even olivopontocerebellar atrophy. The question arises as to whether this hypoplasia is a congenitally-acquired disease or a developmental failure (Gadisseux et al., 1984). The differences observed between well-preserved vermis and underdeveloped neocerebellar structures suggest a developmental anomaly (Barth et al., 1990). Cases with anomalies as microencephaly also were observed with particularly small subtentorial structures, and among them, the most diminished were the cerebellar hemispheres. The cerebellar cortex looked particularly dysplastic, with abnormal dentate nuclei. The pontine nuclei and olives also were found to be hypoplastic or dysplastic. The observed cases had mental retardation, revealed motor disturbances and convulsions, and survived only a few years (Harding et al., 1988). Discussion concerning the character of changes in such pontoneocerebellar syndromes is particularly difficult because they present a combination of dysgenetic and degenerative changes (Urich, 1976). Pontocerebellar changes also were found to be associated with anterior horn cell atrophy. It has been proposed that such cases be considered as a rare syndrome of amyotrophic cerebellar hypoplasia (de Leon et al., 1984).

Malformations of the cerebellar cortex

Dysplasias of archicerebellar and neocerebellar gray structures present some particularities because their development is based on neuronal migration from two separate sources of neuroepithelial cells; moreover, they occur in different developmental periods. Migration from the periventricular area to roof nuclei, dentate nuclei, and Purkinje cell layer starts before the end of the second postconceptional month and is completed at about the fifth month, whereas migration from the external granular (Obersteiner) layer, giving neurons for the internal granular layer, occurs between the third month of gestation and the eigth to ninth month of life (see p. 34–35). In addition, the rate of migration to the paleocerebellar vermis and neocerebellar hemispheres differs considerably. Thus, there is a long-lasting period for exhibition of developmental failures. The dysplasias observed in cerebellar gray structures include the following.

The heterotopia contain neurons migrating from the rhombencephalic lip and sometimes also from the external granular layer. They may be located subcortically, more often in the cerebellar hemispheres than in the vermis. Some heterotopia are very small; others are larger and may contain all types of neurons characteristic for the cerebellar cortex, sometimes even looking like a well-organized cortex (Fig. 92). Other heterotopia include only the large neurons corresponding to Purkinje cells and neurons of cerebellar nuclei. Some heterotopia exist only temporally. They include immature round or spindle cells and are located within the dentate nucleus (sometimes also in the cochlear nucleus in the brain stem) (Fig. 93). They are seen in otherwise normal brains, but more often in brains containing malformations, in trisomies, or in Down syndrome (DS). They disappear within the ninth month of life. Heterotopia of spindle cells mixed with large ganglion cells are not rare in the nodulus and flocculus.

The cortical dysplasias present another type of anomaly observed in the cerebellar structures. They are focal or more diffuse and are often named cerebellar polymicrogyria. This term appears to be inappropriate. The picture of this anomaly is instead one of disintegration of the cortical structure with an intermixed group of neurons, proper for all cortical layers with only some scarring features (Fig. 94). On the other hand, the impression of fusion of molecular layers (de Leon et al., 1976), lack of sulci, and very small gyri in the deep of disorganized cortex partially justify this term. This type of change often coincides with malformation of the cerebral cortex, as with lissencephaly type II in Walker–Warburg syndrome (Dąmbska et al., 1982b). Similar changes also are found with severe defects of the cerebral hemispheres such as porencephaly (Friede, 1989). Minimal anomalies in Purkinje cell position within the internal granular layer as a result of a migration disorder also are sometimes observed (Fig. 95).

Finally, *some anomalies* may appear in the *internal granular layer*. Aplasia of the in-

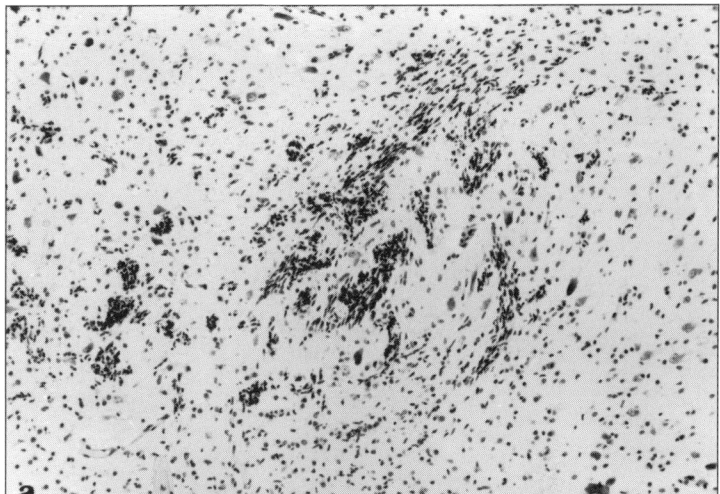
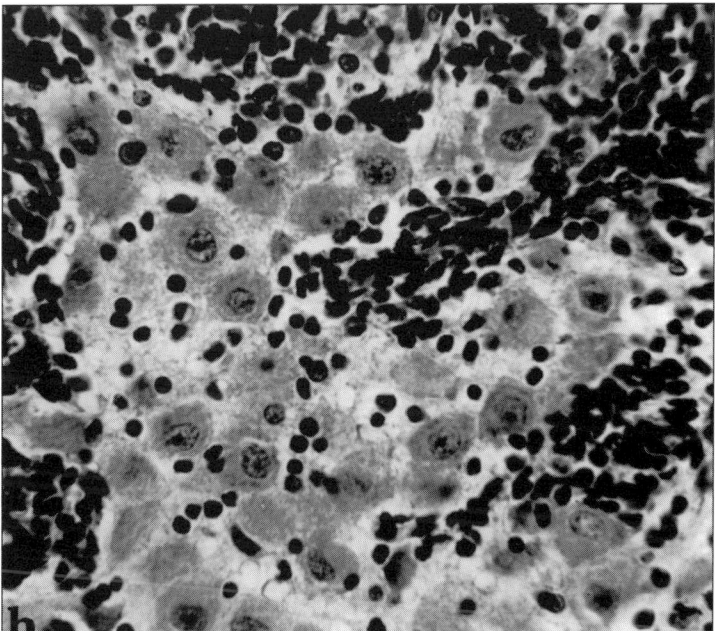

Fig. 93. Spindle-cell heterotopy:

(a) within dentate nucleus. Cresyl violet, × 100.
(b) within cochlear nucleus. Cresyl violet, × 200.

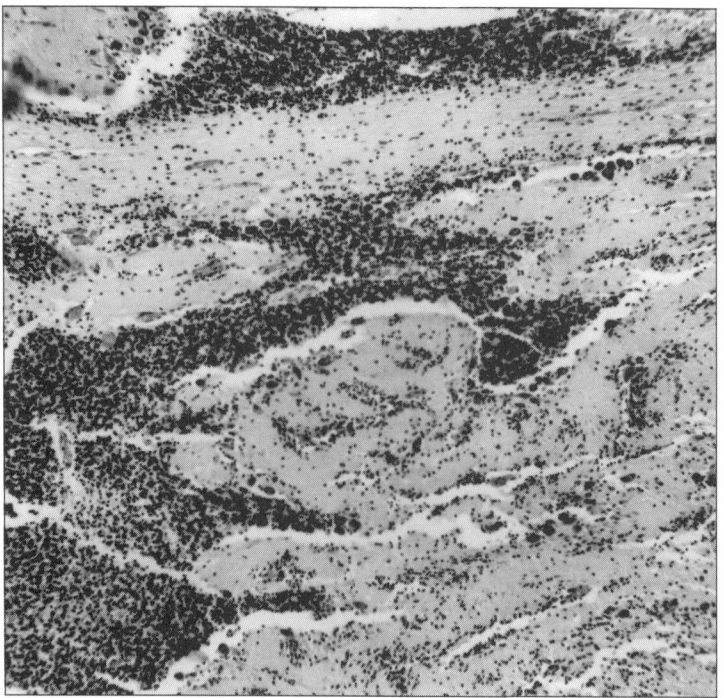

Fig. 94. Dysplasia of the cerebellar cortex. Cresyl violet, × 100.

ternal granular layer presents a particular developmental anomaly, arising when the external granular layer, the source of migrating neurons, was damaged. In such cases, the Purkinje cells that migrated earlier are present in the cortex, but sometimes in the wrong positions. The cortical gyri deprived of granular cells look shrunken. This is finally the aplasia of a distinct cortical layer, and its picture allows us to differentiate between the developmental anomaly and secondary atrophy of the cerebellar cortex. Such changes were described in children as sporadic, but also in siblings (Jervis, 1950). They also were seen after radium irradiation during the fifth to sixth month of gestation (van Bogaert & Radermecker, 1955). They are manifested clinically by ataxia and mental retardation. The ectopic granular cells found in a deep stratum of molecular layer present a particular variant of the external granular layer aplasia observed by Friede (1983).

Diffuse hypertrophy of the cerebellar cortex (Lhermitte–Duclos) should be mentioned because its classification – dysgenesis, neoplasm, or even belonging to Ph – is contro-

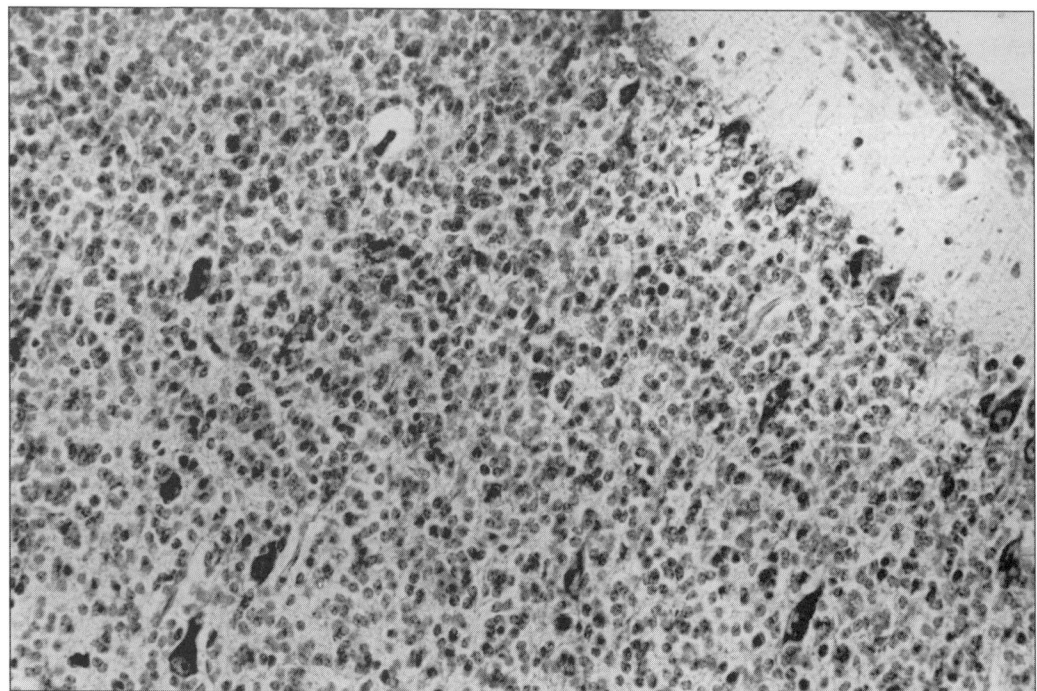

Fig. 95. Purkinje cells in the internal granular layer. Cresyl violet, × 400.

versial. The terms Purkingeoma, gangliocytoma, gangliocytom dysplasticum, and myelinated neurocytoma were used. We also describe this disease with the mesodermal dysplasias. (p. 98)

Micrencephaly and megalencephaly

Microcephaly means abnormal smallness of the cranial vault for age, whereas micrencephaly means abnormal smallness of the brain. It is appropriate to use the latter term when abnormal size of the brain, often mainly of the cerebral hemispheres, constitutes the leading developmental anomaly (Friede, 1989). Microcephaly may be recognized when head circumference is lower by 2–3 SD for age and sex. It is more a descriptive term of a particular clinical sign than a nosologic entity. Microcephalic heads are fairly common. In one study, 55 cases with head circumference too small by −2 SD were examined by MRI, and 34 of them were diagnosed as bearing congenital anomalies that were mainly migratory and the result of intrauterine or postnatal damage of the developing brain (Sugimoto et al., 1993).

Micrencephaly may occur as much as a result of genetic impedance of neuronal multiplication and migration as of environmental factors that disturb developmental processes at different stages (Cowie, 1987). It can be diagnosed ultimately as a static feature of the brain, but it is still impossible to define which level of brain volume reduction would be labeled as microencephalic. Warkany and Dignan (1973) proposed differentiation of three types of micrencephaly on the basis of etiology: those due to (1) gene mutation, (2) chromosomal changes, and (3) environmental influence. Ross and Frias (1977) proposed emphasizing the importance of morphological differences between micrencephaly with malformations and without malformations. It seems most convincing to take into account two large groups of micrencephaly caused by (1) genetic and (2) environmental factors. The great majority of cases within the first group and several from the second group can be diagnosed morphologically as primary micrencephaly. In other cases, the great majority of which are caused by environmental factors, the features of impaired early development coincide with destructive processes and secondary dysgenesis. Such cases may constitute parts of given syndromes, but on the other hand, the too-small-for-age brain constitutes so dominant a trait that we decided to discuss them jointly as the group with the static form of microencephaly (Table 5).

Table 5. Micrencephaly – static form of brain too small for age

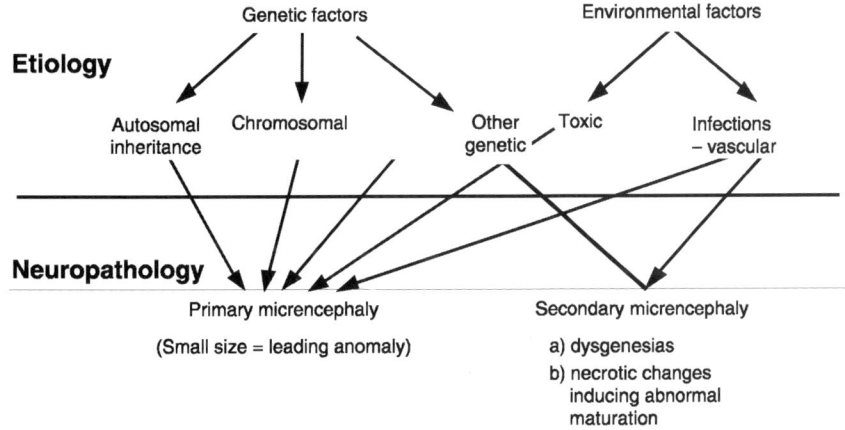

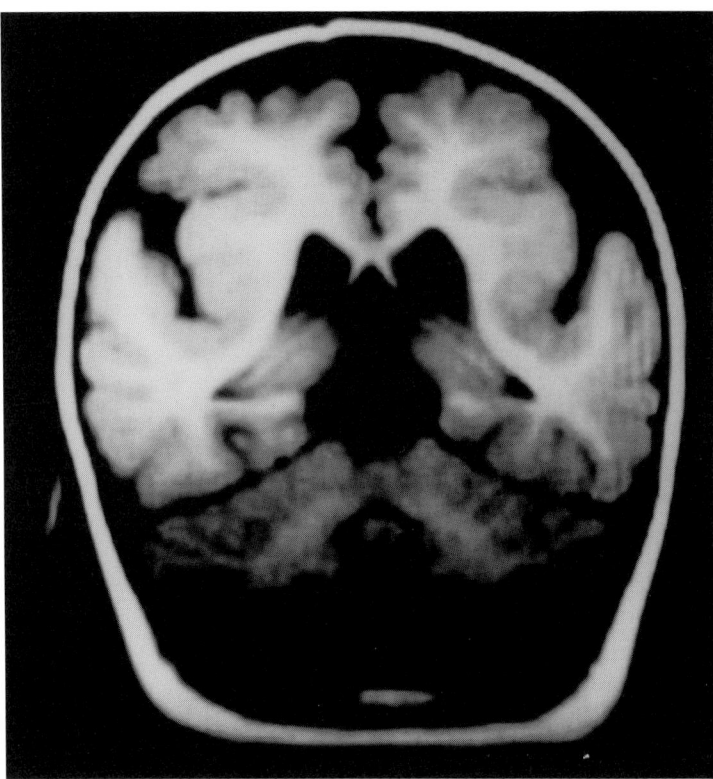

Fig. 96. Primary micrencephaly MRI-scan in a case of autosomal dominant inheritance.

Micrencephaly caused by genetic factors

This type of micrencephaly is of autosomal-recessive inheritance. If neuropathologically verified, it may correspond to 'true micrencephaly' (Giacomini, 1885). Its incidence is 1:40,000 live births (Qazi & Reed, 1975). In adults, the brain weight may be around 500 g, which corresponds to the brain weight of a 2-month-old infant. The brain hemispheres are very small, and the cerebellum and brain stem are relatively better developed (Fig. 96).

The underdevelopment of brain hemispheres consists of diminished size of the cortico-subcortical area. The cortical gyri may have a simplified, poorly differentiated topography. The cortex, in part, presents as a normal, six-layered structure and reveals moderate anomalies such as columnar arrangement of neurons (Robain & Lyon, 1972) or focal disorganization of cortical layering (Haslam, 1987). Periventricular heterotopia also are often found. This familial micrencephaly is seen with short stature, small and slanting forehead, and prominent ears and nose. Seizures and neurological signs are observed often, and severe mental retardation usually coexists.

Autosomal dominant inheritance

Micrencephaly may appear also as autosomal dominant in individuals more or less normal and with normal karyotype (Haslam, 1987; Hennekam, 1992). This form appears to be a specific familial trait, rather than a pathologic condition. Nevertheless, in a fetus diagnosed by ultrasonography in a pregnant micrencephalic mother, some features of micrencephaly with pachygyria were suspected (Persutte et al., 1990).

Autosomal recessive inheritance

Microcephaly and micrencephaly may occur in various nonchromosomal dysgenetic syndromes, often with autosomal recessive inheritance. Their frequency is still growing. Friede (1989) cited 39 of them, but we can expect that some of them will be recognized as occurring secondary to precise etiologic factors.

Chromosomal abnormalities

The too-small brain also is common in chromosomal abnormalities. In such genetically conditioned impairment as DS, the small size of the brain may be due to failure of neuronal multiplication and resulting from abnormally programmed CNS development (Chapter 7). In other chromosomal anomalies, severe malformations may be found, resulting in small brain and head, but in such cases, it is more appropriate to consider micrencephaly as a part of severe dysgenesis.

Micrencephaly induced by environmental factors

Micrencephaly induced by environmental factors constitutes a large group. The list of such factors is long in both experimental and human pathology. Micrencephaly was induced in rats by cycasine (Spatz & Laqueur, 1968), azacytidine (Langman & Shimada, 1971), or methylazoxymetanol (Dąmbska et al., 1982a) injection. The last produced a dose-dependent degree of lesions. Among the agents well known as influencing cell multiplication, X-irradiation has been known in experimental studies for a long time (Hicks, 1953, 1954; Altman et al., 1986). In humans, micrencephaly was observed after atomic bomb radiation in Japan and after exposure to X-irradiation, with frequency depending on the dose given before the third trimester of intrauterine life (Yamazaki, 1966; Wood et al., 1967; Blot & Miller, 1973). Malnutrition may not only cause low brain weight in infants, but also may induce true micrencephaly (Dobbing & Sands, 1971).

Among maternal factors inducing microcephaly and micrencephaly in fetuses, exposure to some drugs during the first half of pregnancy is observed. The injurious role of antiepileptic treatment (Gaily et al., 1990) and exposure to cocaine and heroine (Fulroth et al., 1989) was confirmed. Microcephalic fetuses also were seen in mothers with phenylketonuria, and with uncontrolled biochemical abnormalities (Haslam, 1987; Levy et al., 1992). Many such cases were diagnosed by brain imaging. It appears that their precise neuropathological classification requires further study. Fetal alcohol syndrome includes micrencephaly with developmental delay and with a great variability of CNS anomalies ranging from minimal to severe (Wiśniewski et al., 1983).

Among other factors responsible for micrencephaly in human pathology, special attention must be paid to prenatal HIV infection. It was found that 50 per cent of children who die of AIDS before two years of age have micrencephalic brains. The degree of brain weight deficit is variable, but it is possible to find some cases with weight 40 per cent of the weight proper for a given age. The cerebral hemispheres are normally more affected than the subtentorial structures (Kozłowski, 1995). HIV micrencephaly did not correlate with HIV encephalitis. Its pathomechanism is not clear, like the progressive atrophy observed in adult patients (Everall et al., 1993; Masliah et al., 1994). We can assume that in infant brains, both processes are induced by HIV infection: abnormal development and progressing atrophy overlap each other, but the mechanism of their influence has not been detected (Dambska et al., 1997).

Diminished brain size and consecutively small head circumference occurs in many other intrauterine infections, leading to damage of the developing brain at different stages of this process. The general rule that the type and degree of changes depend on the time of lesion can be applied. The changes may result from the primary diminished number of neurons, focal necrotic lesions, and cortical anomalies occurring secondary to them and in various correlations. Such changes were observed in rubella (Rorke & Spiro, 1967), CMG, toxoplasmosis, and other infections (Bignami & Appicciutoli, 1964).

Megalencephaly

Megalencephaly means brain that is too large and too heavy. It was described by Fletchner (1900) as true hyperplasia of brain tissue. To diagnose megalencephaly, it is indispensable to exclude other causes of overweight in the examined brain, such as hydrocephalus or brain edema. The heavy brain also may be associated with some metabolic diseases, including Canavan's and Alexander's diseases. The question as to when we are authorized to consider a brain as megalencephalic is still discussed. DeMyer (1986) proposed that megalencephaly can be recognized when the brain size and weight exceed the mean by more than 2 SD. Friede (1989) considers an adult brain megalencephalic if its weight is greater than 1600 g, and Escourolle and

Poirier (1973), if it is greater than 1800 g. Neuropathologically, in megalencephalic brains, gyri were observed as bulky, and sometimes, selectively more advanced hyperplasia of some parts of the brain was reported (Friede & Briner, 1978).

Megalencephaly may appear as a benign, familial anomaly without neurologic deficits, despite eventual slow development, with autosomal dominant inheritance (DeMyer, 1986), or it may show some neurologic deficit also with autosomal dominant or recessive inheritance. It also is observed in cases with generalized gigantism. Unilateral megalencephaly is a part of hemihypertrophy of the body always occurring at the same side (Matsubara et al., 1983). Another type of hemimegalencephaly, with abnormalities of neuronal shape and structural abnormalities of hypertrophied hemisphere, may be considered part of the group of Ph (see Chapter 5).

Anomalies of the brain stem and spinal cord

An attempt to present dysplasia of the brain stem and spinal cord demonstrates that primary developmental anomalies of these structures are infrequent (except for the previously described neural tube defects of the dysraphic type) in comparison with the large group of secondary abnormalities. Such anomalies occur after early-arising CNS malformations or after destructive lesions, or they eventually constitute an element of complex developmental anomalies. Dysplasia within the brain stem often involves the inferior olivary nuclei. They appear as heterotopia arising in the course of neuronal migration, destined for olives from the rhombic lip, or as disturbances of the shape and the convolution's pattern of olivary ribbon. They are observed in cases with complex anomalies, including cerebellar malformations; hemispheric migration disorders such as agyria, holoprosencephaly in trisomies 13 and 18; or without chromosomal aberration, and eventually in the autosomal-recessive Zellweger syndrome.

Other anomalies observed in the brain stem are those of the corticospinal tracts. They include a lot of anomalies secondary to those involving the upper part of the corticospinal pathways (e.g. anencephaly, holoprosencephaly) or to similarly localized early-arising destructive lesions (e.g. hydranencephaly). The primary anomalies involving topography of pyramidal tracts and of their decussation may be seen from time to time. It is important to remember that, according to the investigations of Yakovlev and Rakic (1966), decussation of pyramidal tracts very often presents some variants because decussation is partly asymmetric. From time to time, the asymmetry reaches the degree of a developmental anomaly, for instance, when anterior or lateral pyramidal tracts are missing (Larroche, 1977).

Moebius syndrome (congenital facio- and ophthalmoplegia) has an uncertain nosology and course. In describing this syndrome, Moebius (1988) included congenital manifestations of ophthalmoplegia and facial dysplasia. Later, a lot of brain stem and other even extra-neural anomalies were attributed to the same syndrome, dividing them even into four groups (Towfighi et al., 1979; Friede, 1989). Finally, Norman et al. (1995) accepted an opposite point of view, suggesting restriction of the term Moebius syndrome to bilateral paralysis of nerves VI and VII. Theoretically, the syndrome may be secondary to hypoxic-ischemic changes occurring in the maturing brain stem. Taking into account the course of nerve VII axons encircling the nucleus of nerve VI, and their proximity to a part of reticular formation particularly susceptible for damage, such changes are possible (Norman, 1972). Nevertheless, according to our experience, such focal bilateral lesions with only minimal involvement of other brain stem centers should be exceptional not only during chronic fetal asphyxia (Dąmbska et al.,

1987), but also during an eventual accident of deep hypoperfusion (Dąmbska et al., 1976). Norman et al. (1995) also agree that the course of this congenital syndrome is unknown, thus warranting our discussing it among the brain stem dysplasias.

Another controversial position has to be attributed to the arthrogryposis congenital multiplex, considered by Moessinger (1983) as 'fetal dyskinesia deformation sequence'. The description of its peculiar and complicated symptoms, concurrent with multiple curved joints arising during fetal development, is beyond the scope of our presentation of developmental abnormalities of the CNS. We will only mention that within this large group, a neurogenic form, including dysplasia of the spinal cord and brain stem, was isolated (Friede, 1989).

Hydrocephalus

The definition of hydrocephalus must be precise. It is necessary to determine which type enlargement of the ventricular system is present, and all space filled with an excessive amount of CSF (Shaw & Alvord, 1995) warrants this diagnosis. Recent progress in detecting a dilated ventricular system by use of ultrasonography, CT, and MRI (Fig. 82) examination can lead to the tendency to accept that the presence of abnormally large ventricles, despite the coexistence of characteristic pathophysiological and morphological features, is sufficient for diagnosis of hydrocephalus.

As a result of more precise evaluation, the inclination is to diagnose as hydrocephalus the sequelae of disorganized CSF flow dynamics, resulting in dilatation of the CSF space (Russell, 1968; Friede, 1989; Gross & Goldberg, 1995; Norman et al., 1995). These sequelae may be due to developmental failures or various pathological processes. For all of them, the increased-pressure hydrocephalus constitutes a secondary effect on the brain. The sequel of early-arising changes during development of hydrocephalus causes disturbances in the course of the further maturation processes of the CNS.

On the other hand, developmental anomalies or postnecrotic lesions exist that lead to enlargement of the CSF space as a result of abnormalities in the shape and volume of brain structures. They participate in formation of ventriculomegaly without impairment of CSF flow, a kind of hydrocephalus *ex vacuo*, which will not be taken into account in our description. Holoprosencephaly and some types of lissencephaly may serve as an example of such changes. All types of CNS malformations occurring with CSF space enlargement are described in the appropriate chapters.

Taking into account the correlations between CNS development and formation of hydrocephalus, only early-arising hydrocephalus will be discussed. Referring the evaluation of CNS growth and maturation to morphological criteria visible in macroscopic and light-microscopic examination, we will confine our presentation to hydrocephalus arising until around the end of the second year of life. Originating often during fetal life, hydrocephalus can be considered congenital, despite it also being genetic or acquired. We will discuss some aspects of the pathomechanism and final clinical and neuropathological result of increased-pressure hydrocephalus in fetuses, infants, and small children. For correlations with developmental data concerning the ventricular system, choroid plexus, and CSF, see Chapter 3, on Prosencephalon (p. 35).

Hydrocephalus is not rare within the brain pathology of infants and is considered a relatively common birth defect. Blackburn and Fineman (1994) found it in their material of 934 cases with an incidence of 0.7 per 1,000 live births and stillbirths. Because it arises during fetal development, hydrocephalus cannot be diagnosed earlier than around the middle of gestation, when CSF production and circulation reach an appropriate level of development.

Hydrocephalus may potentially occur in various ways, such as increased production, reduced absorption, and impaired circulation of CSF. The last mechanism is the most common. The first pathomechanism, increased production of CSF, occurs chiefly in cases of choroid plexus papilloma, sometimes seen in small infants. McComb and Davis (1990) even considered that such overproduction was not observed in cases without plexus papilloma. The pathomechanism observed most often is impaired CSF circulation, which depending on the level at which the CSF flow is hindered, may result in non-communicating or communicating hydrocephalus.

Non-communicating

Non-communicating hydrocephalus starts by obstruction of the foramina of Monroe. Such obstruction results in unilateral or bilateral distension of the lateral ventricles, depending on the topography of changes. Unilateral hydrocephalus is rather rare (Pfeiffer & Friede, 1984). For differential diagnosis, the asymmetry of ventricles due to plexus papilloma in one of them must be considered (Cohen et al., 1984). More often, bilateral changes are seen, and at each level, the CSF circulation may be disturbed by intracranial tumors. Among them, craniopharyngioma may induce obstruction of the foramina of Monroe. Bilateral distension of the lateral ventricles also appears as the result of fetal and perinatal hemorrhages and eventually of inflammatory changes (Segall et al., 1974). Both of these types of pathological processes may disturb CSF flow, leading to enlargement of the ventricular system. Nevertheless, the problem of hydrocephalus sometimes occurring after germinal matrix hemorrhages is not clear. Such bleeding disruption of the ventricular wall within the anterior horn results in hemocephalus (Dąmbska et al., 1971; Paneth et al., 1994), but clearly visible thrombi blocking the CSF pathways were not found (Gilles et al., 1986).

The aqueduct is the most common level at which the obstruction of CSF flow occurs. Its obstruction may be total (atresia) or partial (stenosis) and may occur early during fetal life, but also later after birth. All exogenous factors may play a role in this process, and genetically conditioned syndromes also are known.

Sex-linked aqueductal stenosis is the most common form of inherited hydrocephalus, and it affects only boys. In the majority of cases, the aqueduct is not completely closed; therefore, hydrocephalus may be moderate. Holoprosencephaly, agenesis of the corticospinal tract, and other anomalies were found as coexisting with such changes, leading to neurological deficit. Among other characteristics, spasticity and poor intellectual functioning were observed. For this syndrome, the gene encoding the L1 neural cell adhesion molecule was found (Jouet & Kenwrick, 1995). A mutation in axon 28 of the L1 CAM gene in one family was additionally detected as responsible for the coexistence of sex-linked hydrocephalus and mental retardation – aphasia – shuffling gait – abducted thumles (MASA) syndrome (Fransen et al., 1994).

Subtentorial obstruction of CSF circulation leading to hydrocephalus may occur as a result of obstruction of the foramina of Luschka and Magendie and herniation of the subtentorial structures into the foramen magnum. Dandy–Walker and Chiari malformations, and infratentorial retro-cerebellar, cerebello-pontine angle, or other leptomeningeal cysts (Gilles et al., 1971) may play a crucial role in such changes.

Communicating

Communicating hydrocephalus may be caused by obliteration of the subarachnoid space. The abundant glioneuronal heterotopia, other meningeal and vascular anomalies (Norman et al., 1981), and meningeal lipomatosis were described as blocking the subarachnoid space. Nevertheless, the fibrotic organization of purulent inflammatory changes is reported more often as inducing the obstruction of the subarachnoid space. The failure of resorption also may play a role in this type of lesion. Such changes were, in many cases, recognized as responsible for hydrocephalus in infancy. Impairment of CSF absorption as a cause of hydrocephalus also is admitted as possible in the course of pathologic changes within arachnoid granulations, as was described by Gilles and Davidson (1971). Impaired absorption also may be functional, occurring as a sequel of increased venous pressure when surpassing the pressure of CSF (Friede, 1989). Such conditions have to be taken into consideration in diagnosis and treatment of intracranial vascular malformations and cardio-circulatory pathology. In addition, communicating hydrocephalus was described as a new syndrome, with endocardial fibroelastosis and cataract (HEC) being suspected to be genetically determined (Devi et al., 1995).

The genetic and exogenous factors responsible for hydrocephalus that is congenital or arises in early infancy are not definitively known. Progress in molecular genetics has led to the discovery of many genes responsible for the appearance of syndromes, including hydrocephalus. It was reported that a gene on chromosome 8 q causes brachio-oto-renal syndrome, Duane syndrome, a dominant form of hydrocephalus, and trapeze aplasia (Vincent et al., 1994). Hydrolethal syndrome with autosomal recessive inheritance and with hydrocephalus and other malformations within the internal organs also was described (Salonen et al., 1981).

In addition to the various bacterial, viral, and parasitic infections and circulatory-hemorrhagic lesions mentioned above, many teratogens, including hypo- and hyper-vitaminosis A and X-irradiation, have been reported as playing a causative role in communicating hydrocephalus. The pathologic changes that occur in increased-

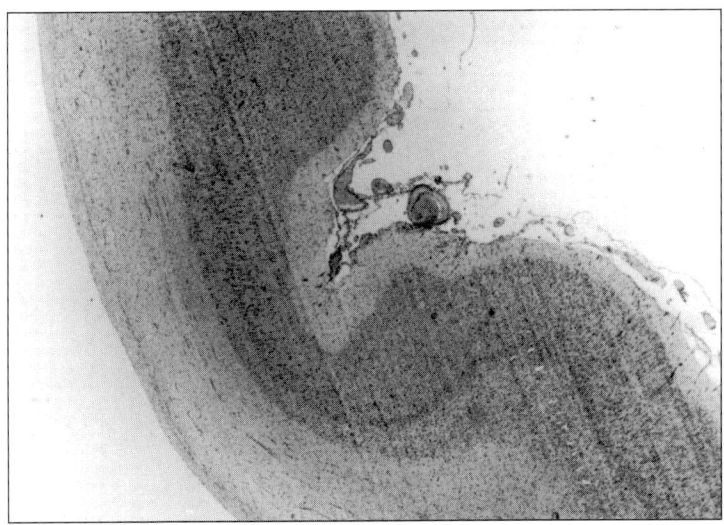

Fig. 97. The hemispheric wall in a hydrocephalic brain. Cresyl violet, × 20.

pressure hydrocephalus before the end of CNS maturation disturb this process.

The enlarged ventricles are covered only in part by ependymal cells and to a greater degree by subependymal glia. The increased pressure of the CSF and secondary damage of the ventricular wall lead to penetration of the CSF into the periventricular nerve tissue, resulting in chronic edema and, finally, gradually progressing atrophy. The atrophic subcortical white matter becomes narrow. Friede (1962) observed and evaluated in such infantile cases a rather normal process of myelination, but degeneration of myelin sheaths and nerve fibers also was seen in infantile hydrocephalus (Weller et al., 1972). The cortex covering the distended hemispheres presents with typical changes. The convolutions are irregular because of increased hemispheric surface, but the basic topography and microscopic structure of the cortical stripe are chiefly normal in the majority of cases (Fig. 97).

Some rather minor cortical anomalies, if observed, testify as to the start of the pathologic process within the hemispheres (Fig. 98). The extension of the cortex over the large hemispheres results in very shallow sulci, with the intra-sulcal cortex on the brain surface. The focal cortical lesions observed in more severely damaged cases consists of cortical infarcts.

Clinical diagnosis of early-arising hydrocephalus may even be accomplished prenatally, during the second half of gestation, by using ultrasonography. Repeated examination is necessary to obtain the diagnosis of progressive fetal hydrocephalus. The possibility of fetal shunting is permissible for treatment. After birth and in small infants, the increase in skull circumference, widened (if not closed at the time of examination) cranial sutures and fontanelle, and optic atrophy in more severe cases are the elements of diagnosis, confirmed by neuroimaging techniques. Neurological deficit is absent in many cases. In untreated cases, the wide spectrum of symptoms from mild to severe increases along with progressing intracranial pressure and brain atrophy. Intellectual and motor problems may appear, but no gross correlations were observed between intellectual level and degree of brain changes (Lonton, 1984).

Changes related to vascular, skull bone and meningeal anomalies

Vascular anomalies

The vascular malformations arising during development of the CNS may coincide with its anomalies, or influence secondary brain lesions. In the following short review, we will look at vascular anomalies from this perspective.

The first anomaly to be mentioned is the persistence of fetal meningeal vessels. It was described by Karch and Urich (1972) in a case with dysraphic changes (occipital encephalocele). Fetal vessels within the meninges occur most often together with this type of malformation. The abundant plexus of vessels presenting early embryonic stages of development may be seen in the area cerebrovasculosa in anencephaly, meningomyelocele, or encephalocele, even over the tissue not primarily malformed. On the other hand, it is possible that a persistent vascular net may play a role in impaired vascularization of the underlying part of the cortical ribbon, leading to its abnormal development. We observed a case with occipital meningoencephalocele in which the segments of the polymicrogyric cortex were found at the parietal lobe, covered by abnormal primitive meningeal vessels.

Arteriovenous malformations are circumscribed focal changes, including abnormal arteries and veins. They present as developmentally abnormal structures of vessel walls (such as thick or absent elastic lamina, abnormal media, sometimes as an aneurysmatic enlargement of their lumen). They are localized rather supratentorially (Kondziolka et al., 1992), often within the cerebral hemispheres, and submeningeally (Garcia & Anderson, 1991). Calcifications, thrombi on vessel walls, and gliosis within surrounding nerve tissue were observed in children who were older than six years of age, with such vascular anomalies (Takashima & Becker, 1980). Although arteriovenous malformations may be formed when vascularization of the CNS starts even at the third WG (Warkany & Lemire, 1984), their clinical manifestations occur instead in adulthood and very rarely in small infants. A case with changes at the spinal cord level in a neonate was described by Park et al. (1986). Older cases between nine and 14

Fig. 98. Cortical anomaly in early-arising hydrocephalus. Cresyl violet, × 20.

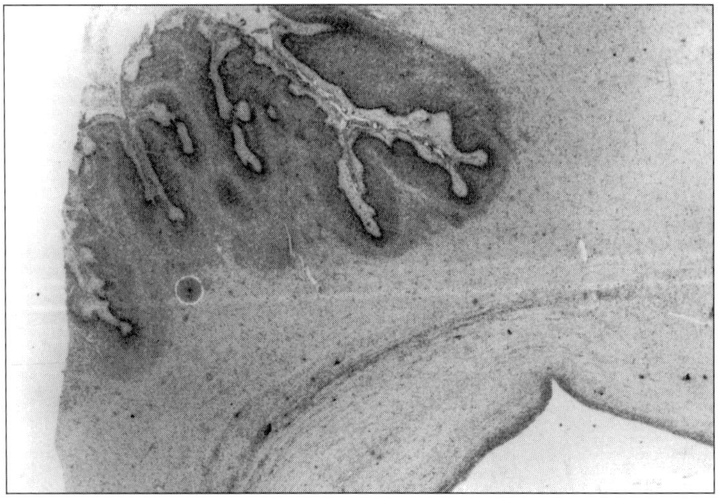

years of age, dying from intracranial hemorrhages, were observed by Byard et al. (1991) and Norman and Ludwin (1991). In cases with arteriovenous malformations within the CNS, focal neurologic symptoms, headache, and seizures may appear. CT and MRI are helpful for diagnosis, but angiography is still important for recognizing abnormal feeding and draining vessels, which is necessary for the final decision concerning treatment in particular cases: neurosurgery or embolization.

Arteriovenous aneurysm of the vein of Galen presents a particular type of arteriovenous malformation (Norman et al., 1995). This congenital anomaly consists of dilatation of the great vein of Galen due to shunting into it of cerebral arteries, most often the posterior cerebral, but also the anterior cerebral rather bilateral than unilateral. Shunting of the middle cerebral artery is very rare. Other arteries – basilar, carotid and vertebral – often are enlarged. Infants with arteriovenous aneurysm of the vein of Galen combined with congestive heart failure most often die in the neonatal period. Severe CNS damages, cortical or periventricular, often are observed in such cases (Hirano & Solomon, 1960; Norman & Becker, 1974). Less severely affected are those with mild heart failure, but with hydrocephalus due to compression of the aqueduct by an abnormal vein of Galen. Such changes result often in craniomegaly (Amacher & Sillito, 1973). Individuals with arteriovenous malformation of the vein of Galen who, being least affected, survive several years, may suffer from headache and have other neurological symptoms. Subarachnoidal and intracerebral hemorrhages also may occur (Vinters, 1995).

The vascular developmental anomalies described above are not all late-appearing ones. Persistence or agenesis of some arteries supplying the blood to the CNS is seen from time to time. Most cases are asymptomatic; only occasionally are focal neurologic symptoms seen. Other anomalies also are rare (Madonick & Ruskin, 1962). They are found rather accidentally and are even controversial in respect to their developmental or necrotic origin. The meningocerebral angiodysplasia is such a controversial anomaly. Jellinger et al. (1966) described a case, in which the brain was covered by a net of abnormal vessels. Severe cortical and white matter lesions were seen together with abnormal, small, sometimes mineralized intracerebral vessels; other cases with similar changes also were described, and Friede (1989) accepts these separate types of vascular dysplastic changes. Norman et al. (1995) consider them not special types of changes, but as occurring secondary to destructive lesions or belonging to the group of arteriovenous malformations of the vein of Galen.

Capillary telangiectasia may be found rather accidentally, being clinically asymptomatic. It occurs more often in the pons (Kuchna et al., 1994), and sometimes in the cerebral white matter (Garcia & Anderson, 1991). One difference between a telangiectasis and a capillary hemangioma of the brain is that a telangiectasis has normal neural tissue between the excessive small vessels, whereas a hemangioma has abnormal, gliotic neural tissue and no surviving neurons between the vessels.

Aneurysms in children are very rare, but they may be found in young patients, suggesting a developmental failure in the vascular wall.

Multiple neonatal angiomata, which also are very rare, were observed in the majority of cases with CNS involvement, in which angiomatous nodules are disseminated throughout brain tissue. Developmental anomalies also may affect the vessels of the choroid plexus. They may lead to subarachnoidal or intraventricular bleeding.

Skull bone anomalies

Skull bone anomalies, with the exception of those occurring with dysraphic CNS changes, may or may not coincide with brain anomalies. Therefore, it is worthwhile mentioning them as a consideration in differential, even prenatal, diagnosis by ultrasonography. Being variable from one case to another, they may be represented by the following types of changes:

Craniosynostosis. An abnormal, early fusion of cranial sutures, which may occur in many syndromes (Cohen, 1988). These include syndromes of known origin, those associated with chromosomal aberrations, or many others with unknown origin. Among them are Apert syndrome, which was already described and is sometimes associated with hydrocephaly (Collman *et al.*, 1988).

Aplasia or hypoplasia of the scalp and vault bone may appear in various forms. As aplasia cutis congenita localized on the scalp (Frieden, 1986), it occurs in several cases together with or without the absence of vault bones. The absence or hypoplasia of 'membrane bones of the skull' (Barr & Cohen, 1991), but with preserved skin, constitutes a separate type named acalvaria (or hypocalvaria), suggesting an early anomaly in membranaceous calvarium formation (Harris *et al.*, 1993).

Craniolacuniae are only focal thinning of cranial vault bones, which may occur in congenital hydrocephalus, but usually disappear during the first year of life.

Meningeal anomalies

Most of the rare meningeal anomalies consist of formation of arachnoid cysts and were described first by Scherer (1935b). Such cysts are located subdurally, between the outer and inner layers of the arachnoidal sheath. They are lined by tissue, similar to, but somewhat more dense than this sheath in normal arachnoid membrane. Collagen fibers are involved in this wall formation (Schachenmayr & Friede, 1979). According to Rengachary and Watanabe (1981), such cysts are formed probably by splitting of the arachnoid during formation of arachnoid cisterns. The cysts are localized intracranially within the Sylvian fissure, interhemispherically, over the cerebral convexity, in the cerebropontine angle, in the posterior fossa midline, supracollicularly within the third ventricle. They may also be clival, prepontine, basal or intraspinal (Rengachary & Watanabe, 1981; Friede, 1989). The cysts may expand, probably as a sequence of the hydrodynamic influence of CSF circulation. The nervous tissue compression may develop in such instances, and clinical symptoms of increasing intracranial pressure appear, requiring surgical treatment, usually by shunting the cyst.

Arachnoid cysts constitute the great majority of cysts on the convexity of brain hemispheres and around the spinal cord, where they share the retrocerebellar and supracollicular localization with glioependymal cysts. Such cysts, which are similar in appearance at the macroscopic level to arachnoid cysts, are demonstrated on microscopic and electron microscopic examination to have walls with epithelial lining often bearing microvilli and cilia. Epithelium is sometimes situated at the basement membrane, and in other cases, on glial tissue. Friede and Yasargil (1977), who analyzed the problem of the structure and origin of such cysts, suggest that they derive from displaced neuroectodermal tissue.

Chapter 7

Developmental Disturbances Due to Chromosomal Aberrations

Genetically induced disturbances of CNS development may, as we mentioned above (*see* Chapter 4 on Genetic factors (p. 89), result in major or minor malformations, at early stages of development, but also in long-lasting impaired brain maturation. In this chapter, we will briefly summarize the dysgeneses (described in detail in appropriate chapters), that appear in cases of two types of disturbed brain maturation – (1) the more common trisomies 13 and 18 and (2) trisomy 21 (DS) – and fragile X syndrome, which are examples of long-lasting impaired brain maturation.

Trisomy 13 (Patau syndrome)

From the clinical point of view, it is important to realize that most cases with trisomy 13 die before birth; the incidence of this syndrome is about 1:10,000 births. Fifty per cent of newborns with trisomy 13 did not survive the first months, and less than 20 per cent survived the first year of life (Norman *et al.*, 1995). Such infants present many abnormalities, the most characteristic among them appearing to be microcephaly and eye abnormalities such as microphthalmia, hypertelorism or cyclopia, and retinal dysplasia. Deformities of ears, cleft lip and palate, hemangiomas of the head or neck, polydactyly, and foot deformities also are seen, as are congenital heart defects and urogenital tract anomalies.

The most characteristic abnormality of the CNS present in trisomy 13 is holoprosencephaly. The presence of holoprosencephaly in persons with trisomy 13 was reported in 44 per cent of cases with this chromosomal aberration, and an additional 19 per cent revealed partial arhinencephaly (Norman *et al.*, 1995). According to Gullotta *et al.* (1981), about 63 per cent of trisomy cases presented with anomalies. Within cerebral hemispheres, polymicrogyria and neuroglial meningeal heterotopias, including muscle fibers, were seen (Johnson & Ludwin, 1984). In the cerebellum, the heterotopias, including germinal cells within the dentate nucleus, were particularly extensive, and other dysplasias of the cerebellar gray structures also were observed (Norman, 1966; Terplan et al., 1966). Even neural tube defects may appear in rare instances (Rodriguez et al., 1990).

Trisomy 18 (Edwards syndrome)

This syndrome, described by Edwards et al. (1960), occurs in about 1:8,000 newborns, (95 per cent of conceptuses affected by this syndrome are lost before birth). The advanced age of the mother is often noted in nonfamilial cases. Live-born infants die in great part before the end of the second month; some reach more than 15 years of life as children with profound mental retardation (Norman et al., 1995). They have a dysmorphic face and anomalies of hands and feet. Abnormalities such as congenital heart diseases or dysplasia of digestive and urogenital tract are present.

CNS dysgeneses may involve many structures. The lobar and gyral pattern of cerebral hemispheres may be altered, and the hippocampus and geniculate nuclei may be marked by dysplasia (Friede, 1989). The cerebellum and pons were observed as hypoplastic within the small posterior fossa (Nakamura et al., 1986a). Severe dysgeneses such as holoprosencephaly, arhinencephalu, ACC, Chiari II malformation, and neural tube defects also have been reported in this chromosomal aberration. The changes within the cerebellum and pons (as far as other severe defects mentioned above) may be visualized by computed tomography or ultrasonography. Unilateral choroid plexus cysts were observed (Ostlere et al., 1990) in 15.8 per cent of cases with this syndrome (Twining et al., 1991). When seen on an ultrasound scan, they may be considered as one of the markers for further examination for trisomy 18. Dendritic abnormalities also have been described in this syndrome (Jay et al., 1990).

Trisomy 21 (Down syndrome)

In Down syndrome (DS), the most frequent chromosomal disorder associated with developmental disability, the CNS is characterized by disturbed development and impaired maturation. Described by Down in 1866, this syndrome was recognized to be caused by aberrations of chromosome 21 by Lejeune in 1959. It is now known that it appears as a sequel of trisomy 21 in the majority of cases, and of mosaic trisomies or translocation of a part of chromosome 21, in others (Kemper, 1988). It was also established, using DNA analysis, that in trisomy 21, the extra chromosome 21 is of maternal origin in 95 per cent of cases (Antonarakis, 1991). DS occurs in approximately 1:600 newborns; before birth, the occurrence of spontaneous abortion of conceptuses with DS reaches 70 per cent. Its risk in nonfamilial cases increases with the mother's age. The dysmorphic features of individuals with DS are characteristic from birth. They have a small head, eyes with epicantal folds, often a large tongue, irregular dentition, and short hands with abnormal dermal ridge patterns. Congenital heart diseases and other anomalies of the internal organs are common in DS (Benda, 1971). Atlanto-occipital and atlanto-axial subluxation because of laxity of ligaments have been reported sporadically, with neurological sequelae (Chaudhry et al., 1987; Trumble et al., 1994). Susceptibility to various infections and increased incidence of leukemia also were observed in DS. Cognitive dysfunction and disturbed motor coordination characterize this syndrome. Children with DS have different degrees of developmental disabilities, and often reveal a friendly social behavior.

The brain sometimes reveals major but, more frequently, minor anomalies and an impairment of maturation. It is possible that an abnormal gene dosage is responsible for the course of this process (Opitz & Gilbert-Barnes, 1990; Wiśniewski, 1990). The major CNS malformations, such as holoprosencephaly, cerebellar dysplasia, and hypoplasia of the hippocampal structure, were seldom reported (Norman et al., 1995), and it is not clear how much the incidence of such anomalies surpasses that in the general population. Mineralization of the basal ganglia was reported on the basis of radiological (Iashima et al., 1984; Wiśniewski et al., 1990) and neuropathological (Takashima & Becker, 1985) findings. Nevertheless, within a representative group of cases of DS, the changes within brain structures were not started before midgestation. The electrophysically abnormal membrane properties in the fetal brain observed by Scott et al. (1982, 1983) were the first signs of abnormal brain function. The findings from their immunohistochemical investigations suggest that changes in reactivity to Bcl–2, synaptophysine, highly phosphorylated neurofilaments, and some other proteins may be involved in abnormal neurogenesis and synaptogenesis, which start during gestation (Wiśniewski & Kida, 1994, 1995). Neuropathological quantitative examination allowed finding essential changes at the cortical level from birth. The neuronal density was found to be lower in the occipital and frontal cortex (Wiśniewski et al., 1984, 1986), and ultrastructural studies also reveal lower synaptic density and changes in their morphological features (Wiśniewski et al., 1986). In the superior temporal cortex, although neuronal density did not reveal a decrease, abnormal lamination was seen, and the axonal and dendritic arborization demonstrated abnormalities (Golden & Hyman, 1994). The only minor morphological changes starting before birth became much more evident during postnatal life, correlating with developmental delay of DS infants increasing with age in comparison to that in control groups. Individuals with DS become microcranial and micrencephalic, the brain weight in midinfancy reaching 20–30 per cent of that of normal subjects (Crome et al., 1966; Wiśniewski et al., 1986). The brain also gains particular features because of the reduction of frontal lobes (Schmidt-Sidor et al., 1990) and the narrowing of superior temporal gyri (Friede, 1989; Wiśniewski et al., 1986), which are more evident than in fetal life (Bahado et al., 1992). The cerebellum and brain stem appear to be too small (Gullotta & Rehder, 1974; Wiśniewski, 1990). Such morphological abnormalities may be examined by MRI morphometry (Raz et al., 1995). Morphometric studies revealed the background of such changes. The neuronal density decreased consecutively in the examined areas, and cytoarchitectonic changes appeared to be caused particularly by the deficit of small neurons (Ross et al., 1984; Wiśniewski et al., 1986). The reduction of synaptic spines, synaptic length, and surface areas complete the picture of morphologic changes (Suetsugu & Mehrain, 1980; Wiśniewski et al., 1986; Becker et al., 1986). Myelination delay was seen in 22 per cent of examined DS cases, mostly in 'tracts with late beginning and protracted cycle of myelination' (Wiśniewski & Schmidt-Sidor, 1989).

Finally, CNS development in DS, except in rather rare cases with malformations, can be described as disturbed, leading to reorganization of cortical structures, but without evident focal lesions detected easily in routine neuropathological examination. The genetically programmed, disturbed, and retarded brain development may result in greater-than-normal elimination of the neuronal population by cell death. Patients with DS who survive until adulthood may demonstrate progressive dementia of the Alzheimer disease (AD) type. The changes described above will overlap during their life with premature aging. Neurofibrillary tangles and senile plaques, pathological hallmarks of AD, are typically observed in adult DS brains (Wiśniewski et al., 1985a; Cork, 1990; Mann & Esiri, 1989; Ferrer & Gulotta, 1990). Moreover, these changes appear in DS brains much earlier than in brains in the normal population and or in individuals with sporadic AD (Wiśniewski & Dąmbska, 1992; Wiśniewski et al., 1994). The topographic distribution of amyloid-associated proteins within Ab deposits in DS individuals is similar to that in AD brain (Kida et al., 1995; Wiśniewski et al.,

1995a,b). All these findings stress the similarities of these pathological changes and the putatively similar pathogenetic mechanisms underlying their formation in both AD and DS brains.

Fragile X syndrome

This syndrome is caused by a fragile site on the long arm of the X chromosome. It was found experimentally that low folic acid and thymidine concentrations may induce this fragile site (Brown et al., 1986). It was also shown that fragile X contains an unstable DNA sequence (Sutherland et al., 1991). The last result suggests that the fragile-X gene (FMR1) influences the function of cAMP. Its absence, inducing diminished cAMP production, may result finally in changes of cognitive function (Berry-Kravis et al., 1995). Fragile X syndrome is estimated to be the most common cause of inherited mental retardation (Hinton et al., 1991). This syndrome occurs in 1:12,000 male individuals. It is characterized by macroorchidism and dysmorphism of the face, which is narrow with prominent forehead and large ears (Turner & Jacobs, 1983; Opitz & Sutherland, 1984). Mental retardation (Wiśniewski et al., 1985c), although often mild, suggests morphological changes in the CNS. Nevertheless, the development of the hemispheric cortex was observed as normal around midgestation (Jenkins et al., 1984). In adults, neuropathological observations are rather scarce. Hagerman (1991) found single cases with heterotopia, myelin loss, and siderosis within the pallidum. In one clinically documented case, only the dendritic spine abnormalities and synaptic immaturity were found, indicating involvement of cerebral structures (Rudelli et al., 1985). Such changes are good examples of the only mild morphological traits within the CNS in chromosomal abnormalities characterized by mental retardation.

The fragile-X syndrome represents a new type of neurogenetic disorder that resulted from triplet expansion. A triplet of CGG repeats localized at 5'UTR of fragile-X gene, the FMR1 (Verkerk et al., 1991) was found to expand more than 200 in the fragile-X patients. However, there is only 5–50 repeats in the normal population (Fu et al., 1991). Although molecular mechanism of CGG expansion is not quite clear, imperfect interruption of AGG within the CGG repeat region appears to play a role (Zhong et al., 1995). Loss of AGG interruption allows CGG repeats unstable. The pathogenesis of the fragile-X syndrome is unknown yet. FMR1 encodes an RNA-binding protein, the FMRP, that consists of KH domains and RGG box. To understand the FMRP function will help to get insight into this syndrome.

Chapter 8

Late and Secondary Developmental Anomalies

Malformations of the CNS arising as a result of early disturbances in its structural development (resulting from genetic or exogenic factors) constitute a common group from the morphological point of view, as was previously emphasized. The influence of exogenic lesions should be considered a disruption of the normal developmental process (Harding & Copp, 1997), and the early incidents lead to formation of embryopathies in the form of defects independent of their etiology and entering into the group of malformations.

In the course of further development, the results of any disruptive changes that occur depend on the degree of CNS maturation. The successively appearing necrotic and reparative processes coincide, overlap and influence abnormalities of the final phase of CNS maturation. Sometimes, the sequence of events may be inverted – the early-arising malformations may facilitate the occurrence of ensuing necrotic lesions (Bargeton, 1959). The different rates of development within particular structures may lead to different types of changes induced by the same injurious factor, damaging the maturing organ. As an example, we would like to remember the classical observation of Hallervorden (1949) concerning the case deriving from a pregnancy complicated during the fifth month by carbon monoxide intoxication of the mother. In the newborn, necrotic changes were found within the brain stem, and cortical malformations within the brain hemispheres. They reflected the time of these structures' formation and maturation. Further observations revealed that focal necrotic or inflammatory changes may result in developmental failures within structures that are interdependent not only morphologically, but also functionally.

Although the syndromes that are sequelae of the damage of already-formed structures belong to fetopathies or even early-arising infantile encephalopathies, they often also reveal developmental changes affecting the late stages of maturation. The type and degree of such changes allows their classification in many cases at the borderline between malformative (e.g. minimal cortical anomalies, impairment, or only delay of myelination) and encephalopathic lesions. They deserve clinico-neuropathologic attention as the morphological background of infantile cerebral palsy.

We will discuss some of these abnormalities that occur secondary to relatively late disruption of normal brain development. Some of them deserve discussion concerning their pathomechanism.

Hydranencephaly

Hydranencephaly is an anomaly in which nearly all supratentorial structures are lacking and are replaced by a balloon-like bladder. According to the classic definition, its difference from an extremely distended hydrocephaly lies in the structure of its wall, which includes only mesodermal elements originating from meninges and glial scars, without the discernible remnants of hemispheric walls (Hallervorden & Meyer, 1956). In cases of hydranencephaly, some parts of the occipital and temporal lobes, owing their blood supply to the cerebral posterior arteries, are often preserved, whereas all structures with blood supply from the anterior, and especially middle cerebral arteries are lacking. Such topography of changes indicates the role of failure of the blood supply in the pathomechanism of hydranencephaly, although its direct morphological confirmation is difficult to obtain (Ajuriaguerra & Bonis, 1959). Sarnat (1992) considers even hydranencephaly as the last stage of internal carotid occlusion. Hydranencephaly was reported as a sequel of hemorrhagic lesions (Edmondson et al., 1992; Norman et al., 1995). The destruction of brain hemispheres resulting in formation of hydranencephaly may occur in the course of inflammatory/necrotizing processes, as was observed in herpes simplex (Parish, 1989), CMG infection (Norman et al., 1995) and congenital toxoplasmosis (Dąmbska et al., 1965; Laure-Kamionowska et al., 1982). In such cases, the small remnants of hemispheric structures did not correlate strictly with territories vascularized by particular arteries. On the other hand, the role of glial proliferation leading to aqueduct stenosis is evident. In hydranencephaly with partially preserved structures such as basal ganglia and thalamus, secondary neuronal damage was observed. Subtentorial structures are rather well preserved, but the associated lesions of cerebellum may occur. The secondary changes are observed in the descending corticospinal pathways. Clinically, hydranencephaly may be diagnosed during pregnancy by ultrasonography. If the cerebellum and brain stem are relatively preserved, the affected newborns may survive, and later, such children develop neurological and developmental problems including mental retardation, quadriparesis, endocrinological disturbances, and even seizures. Despite the degree of CNS damage, they may survive some years (Fergusson et al., 1974).

Schizencephaly and porencephaly

Schizencephaly was characterized by Yakovlev and Wadswords (1946a,b) as a failure of growth and differentiation of circumscribed 'areas of the cerebral wall during the first 2 months of the fetal life'. Such abnormality of the developmental process may result in formation of clefts in one or both hemispheres between their convexity and lateral ventricles (Fig. 99), cushioned with polymicrogyric cortex. Formation of this type of change was considered a developmental failure (Larroche, 1977), but also a result of the encephaloclastic process.

The second possibility was supported by further observations, among others the description of Klingensmith et al. (1986). Barth (1987) also emphasized that the anatomy of clefts suggests a destructive lesion. Finally, Friede (1989) proposed not using the term schizencephaly and classified such changes as porencephaly, being the result of encephaloclastic processes. Another term, 'mantle defect', was suggested by Gilles (1991). Norman et al. (1995) agree with the opinion of Friede and emphasize that when the damage in developing brain occurs early in development, during the migration of neurons (probably before 20 WG), the classic picture of schizencephaly may arise. Recognizing destructive changes as the pathomechanism of the majority of schizencephalic changes, we would like to describe one examined case with complex cerebro-oculo-cutaneous malformations suggesting the participation of developmental failure in some of them. In this case, the disturbances of neuronal migration resulted in the focal reduction of the hemispheric wall to the rather thin area filled by migrating cells, reaching and invading the subarachnoid space. The observed changes looked like they would lead, in case of longer survival, to formation of the morphological picture required by Yakovlev and Wadsworth (1946a,b) for schizencephaly (Dąmbska et al., 1996).

This term has until now been used by neuroradiologists for a given type of changes in children's brain. Among them, Robinson (1991) reported 'familial schizencephaly', and Hosley et al. (1992) mentioned its familial incidence, which supports the possibility that rare familial cases may appear, including developmental failures in their pathomechanism.

The classical form of porencephaly, presenting as damage of the full thickness of the hemispheric wall (Fig. 100), for which we have restricted this term (Barth, 1984; Friede, 1989), includes several developmental defects of the adjoining cortex. The cortical convolutions around the submeningeal top of the cavity covered only by pial/glial elements present with severe neuronal loss and damage and also more or less pronounced cortical anomalies, mainly of the polymicrogyric type.

In the pathomechanism of destructive changes resulting in porencephaly, the hypoxic and hemorrhagic lesions have to be taken into account. It is important to mention that neonatal thrombocytopenia was found in a case of porencephaly (Manson et al., 1988). When antenatal diagnosis of thrombocytopenia is possible (Reznikoff-Etievant, 1988), treatment is possible (Norman et al., 1995).

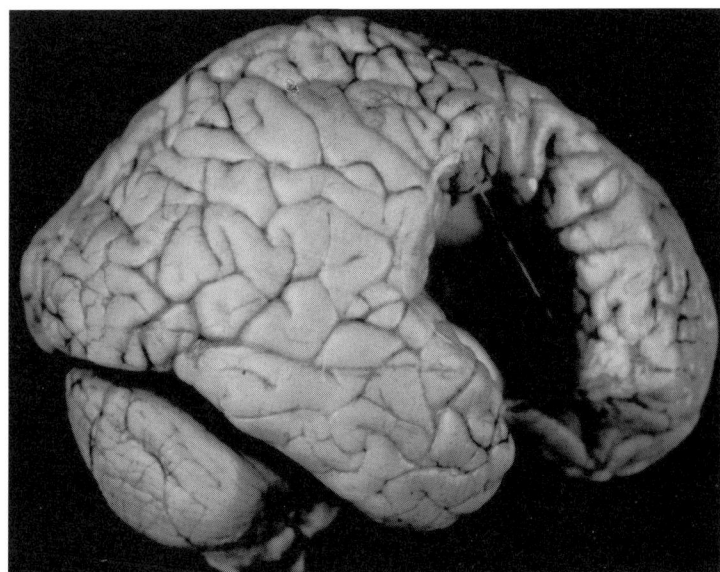

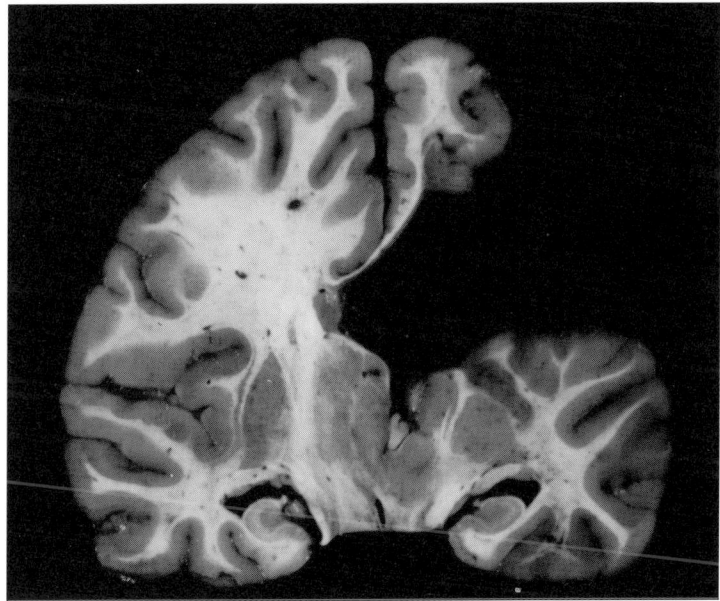

Schizencephaly can be detected *in utero* by color-flow Doppler imaging (Suchet, 1994), but more often it is diagnosed after birth. Children with unilateral or bilateral clefts within the hemispheric walls visualized by neuroimaging technique present with neurological symptoms corresponding to the topography of changes, retardation of psychosomatic development and often epileptic seizures.

Fig. 99 (upper). A cleft between cerebral convexity and lateral ventricles.

Fig. 100 (lower). The damage of full hemispheric wall.

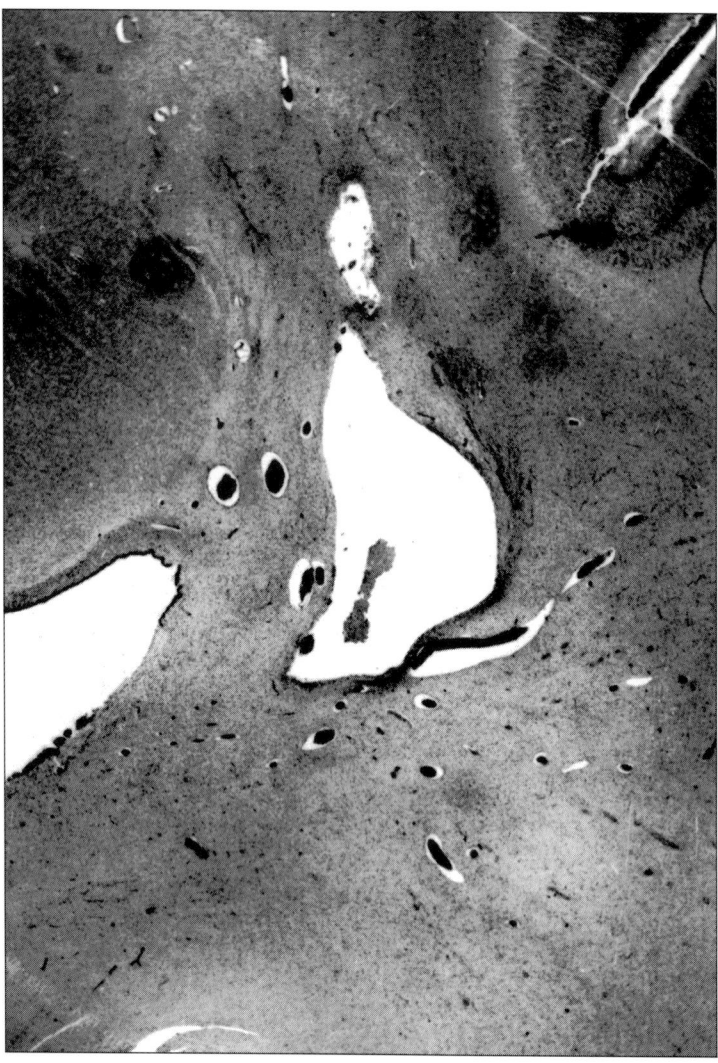

Fig. 101. A cyst arose after periventricular infarct.

Variants of cystic encephalopathy

In the group of encephaloclastic changes, we still have to review damage of the hemispheric white matter leading to disturbances of the last phases of brain maturation. The predilection for this topography of lesions in the developing brain (Kennedy et al., 1970; Lou, 1988; Rorke, 1992a,b) leads to some variants of cystic encephalopathy. Following the suggestions of Friede (1989) and Rorke (1992b), we think it is useful to differentiate the residual defects of periventricular infarcts (Fig. 101) and cystic encephalopathy restricted to the white matter, from multicystic encephalopathy, which also involves other cerebral structures. This term was already used by Crome (1958) and was accepted by Larroche et al. (1986). In such cases, the cortical changes of ulegyric type coincide with some anomalies of the last phases of cortical development, most often in the form of focal polymicrogyric-like changes (Dąmbska et al., 1994). Their topography corresponds usually with periventricular or subcortical white matter destructive lesions.

The majority of multicystic changes can be attributed to circulatory-hypoxic ischemic injuries, but the precise pathomechanism in particular cases is most often difficult to reconstruct (DeReuck, 1972; Nakamura et al., 1986b). In addition, it is necessary to mention that periventricular white matter is often involved and damaged, although not severely as when resulting in hydranencephaly, but significantly during inflammatory processes in the maturing brain (Norman, 1978). Secondary anomalies of the cortical structure, corresponding topographically to white matter, are the changes that are observed in such cases (Dąmbska et al., 1983a).

In infants with longer survival, all types of cystic lesions that arose in maturing white matter tend to disappear, suggesting their resorption and consecutive formation of diffuse glial scars (de Vries, 1988; Ferrer & Navarro, 1978; Dąmbska & Laure-Kamionowska, 1989). The hypomyelination of hemispheric white matter is the final result of this process. Despite this often-observed sequence of events, it is possible to observe, from time to time, brains of adults who survived perinatal brain damage with persisting cystic changes in the white matter.

Chapter 9

Delay of the CNS Maturation

The term 'maturation' used in the title of this chapter is required to be precise. Sarnat (1992) defines maturation as 'a composite of growth and development' and disorders of maturation as 'aberration of sequence of normal developmental process'. We would like to limit the topic of this chapter to the final phase of maturation, when developmental disorders do not result in more or less advanced malformations, but when above all, the retardation of normal maturation occurs. It is obvious that after the CNS structures obtain their definite morphological features, and multiplication of nerve cells is finishing, this complex organ still has much more development ahead, particularly adjustment of the number and connections of neurons, myelination of axons, and stabilization of biochemical composition and metabolism. We will discuss impairment of this phase of brain development, as evaluated by neuropathological examination. In preterm and term newborns, the estimation of the six parameters proposed for evaluation of CNS developmental age at the end of Part One may be useful. For brains of older infants, evaluation consists first of examination of cerebral and cerebellar cortex maturation, often by using Golgi impregnation and morphometric study (Takashima et al., 1980; Kuchna, 1994), level of myelination of hemispheric white matter (Body et al., 1987; Dąmbska & Laure-Kamionowska, 1990), and compatibility of these parameters with age.

Aberration of sequence and retardation of the final phase of brain maturation, particularly of myelination of axons occurring in various circumstances that impair their normal rate, can reach normal levels to a significant degree over time. Therefore, this problem justifies particular attention also from the clinical point of view. Retardation of brain maturation occurs in some genetically determined syndromes, as it is well documented in trisomy 21 (DS), see Chapter 7, on Trisomy 21 (Down syndrome), (p. 150). In such cases, delay of maturation, being expected, is detected most easily. Also in metabolic disorders not directly associated with myelin formation, such as phenylketonuria and other aminoaciduria, myelination may be delayed (Sarnat, 1992).

Other pathologies in which analysis of large groups of cases allowed diagnosis of the retardation of brain maturation are some maternal diseases during pregnancy. Retardation of brain maturation was found in 30 per cent of infants born to mothers with diabetes mellitus, despite the infants' great length and weight due to their particular carbohydrate metabolism (Laure-Kamionowska et al., 1980). Severe gestosis (preeclampsia), eclampsia also were recognized to cause retardation of fetal brain growth and maturation (Laure-Kamionowska, 1980). Despite the relative protection of the brain and kidneys (Larroche, 1977) in the course of fetal dystrophy, in cases with severe undernutrition, brain weight was found to be lower than normal for developmental age (Robain & Pansot, 1978; Winnick, 1974). Prolonged asphyxia also was suspected to be an injurious factor inducing, among other diseases, retardation of nerve cell maturation (Takashima et al., 1980). Disturbances of dendritic development were seen in fetal alcohol syndrome (Ferrer & Galofre, 1987) and even in cases with unclassified mental retardation (Purpura, 1975; Marin-Padilla, 1975).

Chronic hypoxia, nutritional deficiency, and other noxious agents inducing impairment of fatty acids and of the particular enzyme necessary for myelin formation lead particularly often to retardation of myelination of the CNS pathways (Robain & Pansot, 1978; Sarma & Rao, 1974; Wiggins, 1982; Bourre, 1989). Such delayed myelination was very evident in fetuses born of pregnancies complicated by gestosis (Laure-Kamionowska, 1980).

Observation of similar myelination delay in the course of other pathological syndromes in infants at the time of active myelination of brain hemispheres inclines us to propose that the course of myelination could be considered a parameter of normal or retarded brain maturation (Dąmbska & Laure-Kamionowska, 1990).

The observation of human material correlates well with results obtained in experimental studies. They were confirmed by Krigman and Hogan (1976) in studies on rats. After administration of phenobarbital to pregnant rabbits, retardation in CNS maturation also was observed, among other changes (Chmielik, 1996; Dąmbska et al., 1979b).

We will conclude our presentation of abnormal brain development with remarks concerning retardation of CNS maturation, because of its clinical aspect. The everyday practice of brain imaging by CT and MRI of newborns and infants permits, at times, observation of brains too small for age, with hemispheric-mantle convolutions that are too narrow, large sulci, and also the features of insufficient myelination. In such cases, it is necessary to perform differential diagnosis between brain atrophy and retardation of brain maturation.

References to Part Two

Ahdab-Barmada, M. & Claassen, D. (1990): A distinctive triad of malformations of the central nervous system in the Meckel–Gruber syndrome. *J. Neuropathol. Exp. Neurol.* **49**, 610–620.

Aicardi, J., Lefebvre, J. & Lerique-Koechlin, A. (1965): A new syndrome: spasm in flexion, callosal agenesis, ocular abnormalities. *Electroencephalogr. Clin. Neurophysiol.* **19**, 609–610.

Aicardi, J. & Goutieres, F. (1981): The syndrome of absence of the septum pellucidum with porencephalies and other developmental defects. *Neuropediatrics* **12**, 319–329.

Aicardi, J., Chevrie, J.J. & Baraton, J. (1987): Agenesis of the corpus callosum. In: *Handbook of clinical neurology*, eds. P.J. Vinken, G.W. Bruyn & H.L. Klawans, vol. 50, pp. 149–173. Amsterdam, New York: Elsevier Science Publishers, Elsevier Science Publishers Company.

Aicardi, J. (1991): The agyria-pachygyria complex: a spectrum of cortical malformations. *Brain Dev.* **13**, 1–8.

Ajuriaguerra, J. & Bonis, P. (1959): L'hydranencephalies. In: *Malformations congenitales du cerveau*, eds. G. Heuyer, M. Feld & J. Gruner, pp. 399–408. Paris: Masson.

Albrecht, S., Haber, R.M., Goodman, J.C. & Duvic, M. (1992): Cowden syndrome and Lhermitte–Duclos disease. *Cancer* **70**, 869–876.

Aleksic, S., Budzilovich, G., Greco, M.A., Feigin, I., Epstein, F. & Pearson, J. (1983): Iniencephaly: a neuropathological study. *Clin. Neuropathol.* **2**, 55–61.

Alexander, G.L. & Norman, R.M. (1960): The Sturge–Weber Syndrome. Bristol: John Wright and Sons.

Altman, J., Anderson, W.J. & Wright, K.A. (1968): Differential radiosensitivity of stationary and migratory primitive cells in the brains of infant rats. *Exp. Neurol.* **22**, 52–74.

Amacher, A.L. & Sillito, J. Jr (1973): The syndromes and surgical treatment of aneurysms of the great vein of Galen. *J. Neurosurg.* **39**, 89–98.

Andermann, E. (1981): Agenesis of the corpus callosum. In: *Handbook of clinical neurology*, ed. N.C. Myrianthopoulos, vol. 42, pp. 6–9. Amsterdam: Elsevier/North Holland Biomedical Press.

Anderson, C.E. (1995): The genetics of disorders of the developing nervous system. In: *Pediatric neuropathology*, ed. S. Duckett, pp. 41–53. Baltimore: Williams and Wilkins.

Anonymous (1993): Identification and characterization of the tuberous sclerosis gene on chromosome 16. The European Chromosome 16 Tuberous Sclerosis Consortium. *Cell* **75**, 1305–1315.

Anonymous (1988): Neurofibromatosis. Conference statement. National Institute of Health Consensus Developmental Conference. *Arch. Neurol.* **45**, 575–578.

Antonarakis, S.E. (1991): Parental origin of the extra chromosome in the trisomy 21 as indicated by analysis of DNA polymorphisms. *N. Engl. J. Med.* **324**, 872–876.

Aoki, S., Barkovich, A.J., Nishimura, K., Kjos, B.O., Machida, T., Cogen, P., Edwards M. & Norman, D. (1989): Neurofibromatosis types 1 and 2: cranial MR findings. *Radiology* **172**, 527–534.

Arnold, J. (1894): Myelocyste transposition von Gewebs, Gewebskenmen und Sympodie. *Beitrage zur Pathologischen Anatomie und zur Allgemeinen Pathologie* **16**, 1–18.

Baird, P.A. & Sadovnick, A.D. (1984): Survival in infants with anencephaly. *Clin. Pediatr. (Philadelphia)* **23**, 268–271.

Bahado-Singh, R.O., Wyse, L., Dorr, M.A., Copel, J.A., O'Connor, T. & Hobbins, J.C. (1992): Fetuses with Down syndrome have disproportionately shortened frontal lobe dimensions on ultrasonographic examination. *Am. J. Obstet. Gynecol.* **167**, 1009–1014.

Bamberger-Bozo, Ch. (1987): Chiari II malformation. In: *Handbook of clinical neurology*, ed. P.J.Vinken, G.W. Bruyn & H.L. Klawans, vol. 50, pp. 403–412. Amsterdam: Elsevier Science Publishers.

Bankl, H. & Jellinger, K. (1967): Zentralnervosa Schaden nach fetaler Kohlenoxydverfigtung. *Beitr. Pathol. Anat.* **135**, 350–376.

Bargeton, E. (1959): Les malformations tardives. In: *Malformations congenitales du cerveau*, eds. G. Heuyer, M. Feld & J. Gruner, pp. 361–376. Paris: Masson.

Barker, D., Wright, E., Nguyen, K., Cannon, L., Fain, P., Goldgar, D., Bishop, D.T., Carey, J., Baty, B., Kivlin, J. et al. (1987): Gene for von Recklinghausen neurofibromatosis is in the pericentric region of chromosome 17. *Science* **236**, 1100–1102.

Barkovich, A.J., Kjos, B.O., Norman, D. & Edwards, M.S. (1989): Revised classification of posterior fossa cysts and cyst like malformations based on the results of multiplanar MR imaging. *AJR Am. J. Roentgenol.* **153**, 1289–1300.

Barr, M. Jr., Hanson, J.W., Currey, K., Sharp, S., Toriello, H., Schmickel, R.D. & Wilson, G.N. (1983): Holoprosencephaly in infants of diabetic mothers. *J. Pediatr.* **102**, 565–568.

Barr, M. Jr. & Cohen, M.M. Jr. (1991): ACE inhibitor fetopathy and hypocalvaria: the Kidney-skull connection. *Teratology* **44**, 485–495.

Barth, P.G., Mullaart, R., Stam, F.C. & Slooff, J.L. (1982): Familial lissencephaly with extreme neopallial hypoplasia. *Brain Dev.* **4**, 145–151.

Barth, P.G. (1984): Prenatal classic encephalopathies. *Clin. Neurol. Neurosurg.* **86**, 65–75.

Barth, P.G. (1987): Disorders of neuronal migration. *Can. J. Neurol. Sci.* **14**, 1–16.

Barth, P.G., Vrensen, G.F.J., Uylings, H.B.M., Oorthuys, J.W. & Stan, F.C. (1990): Inherited syndrome of microcephaly dyskinesia and pontocerebellar hypoplasia: a systemic atrophy with early onset. *J. Neurol. Sci.* **97**, 25–42.

Becker, L.E., Armstrong, D.L. & Chan, F. (1986): Dendritic atrophy in children with Down's syndrome. *Ann. Neurol.* **20**, 520–526.

Bell, J.E., Gordon, A. & Maloney, A.F.J. (1980): The association of the hydrocephalus and Arnold-Chiari malformation with spina bifida in the fetus. *Neuropathol. Appl. Neurobiol.* **6**, 29–39.

Bell, J.E. & Green, R.J.L. (1982): Studies on the area cerebrovasculosa of anencephalic fetuses. *J. Pathol.* **137**, 315–328.

Benda, C.E. (1954): The Dandy–Walker syndrome or so-called atresia of foramen Magendie. *J. Neuropathol. Exp. Neurol.* **13**, 14–29.

Benda, C.E. (1971): Mongolism. In: *Pathology of the nervous system*, ed. J. Minckler, vol. 2, pp. 1361–1371. New York: McGraw-Hill Book Co.

Bentley, J.F.R. & Smith, J.R. (1960): Developmental posterior enteric remnants and spinal malformations: the split notochord syndrome. *Arch. Dis. Child.* **35**, 76–86.

Berry, A.D. & Patterson, J.W. (1991): Meningoceles, meningomyeloceles, and encephaloceles: a neuro-dermatopathologic study of 132 cases. *J. Cutan. Pathol.* **18**, 164–177.

Berry-Kravis, E., Hicar, M. & Ciurlionis, R. (1995): Reduced cyclic AMP production in fragile X syndrome: cytogenetic and molecular correlations. *Pediatr. Res.* **38**, 638–643.

Berry, S.A., Pierpont, M.E. & Gorlin, R.J. (1984): Single central incisor in familial holoprosencephaly. *J. Pediatr.* **104**, 877–880.

Beuche, W., Wickbold, J. & Friede, R.L. (1983): Lhermitte–Duclos disease B its minimal lesions in electron microscope data and CT findings. *Clin. Neuropathol.* **2**, 163–170.

Bignami, A. & Appicciutoli, L (1964): Micropolygyria and cerebral calcification in cytomegalic inclusion disease. *Acta Neuropathol. (Berl.)* **4**, 127–137.

Bishop, K., Connolly, J.M. & Carpenter, D.G. (1964): Holoprosencephaly: a case report with no extracranial abnormalities and normal chromosome count and karyotype. *J. Pediatr.* 1964, **65**, 406–414.

Blaauw, G. (1971): Defect in posterior arch of atlas in myelomeningocele. *Dev. Med. Child. Neurol.* (suppl.) **25**, 113–115.

Blackburn, B.L. & Fineman, R.M. (1994): Epidemiology of congenital hydrocephalus in Utah, 1940–1979: report of an iatrogenically related 'epidemic'. *Am. J. Med. Genet.* **52**, 123–129.

Blankenberg, T.A., Ruebner, B.H., Ellis, W.G., Bernstein, J. & Dimmick, J.E. (1987): Pathology of renal and hepatic anomalies in Meckel syndrome. *Am. J. Med. Genet.* (suppl.) **3**, 395–410.

Blot, W.J. & Miller, R.W. (1973): Mental retardation following in utero exposure to the atomic bombs of Hiroshima and Nagasaki. *Radiology* **106**, 617–619.

Bode, H., Sauer, M., Strassburg, H.M. & Gilsbach, H.J. (1985): Das Tethered-cord-syndrom. *Klin. Padiatr.* **197**, 409–414.

Bolande, R.P. (1984): Models and concepts derived from human teratogenesis and oncogenesis in early life. *J. Histochem. Cytochem.* **32**, 878–884.

Bordarier, C., Aicardi, J. & Goutieres, F. (1984): Congenital hydrocephalus and eye abnormalities with severe developmental brain defects: Warburg's syndrome. *Ann. Neurol.* **16**, 60–65.

Bordarier, C., Robain, O., Rethore, M.D., Dulac, O. & Dhellemes, C. (1986): Inverted neurons in agyria. A Golgi study of a case with abnormal chromosome 17. *Hum. Genet.* **73**, 974–978.

Bordarier, C. & Aicardi, J. (1990): Dandy–Walker syndrome and agenesis of cerebellar vermis diagnostic problems and genetic counseling. *Dev. Med. Child. Neurol.* **32**, 285–294.

Bourre, J.M. (1989): Developmental synthesis of myelin lipids: origin of fatty acids. Specific role of nutrition. In: *Developmental neurobiology*, eds. E. Evrard & A. Minkowski, pp. 111–154. New York: Raven Press.

Braffman, B. & Naidich, T.P. (1994a): The phakomatoses: Part I. Neurofibromatosis and tuberous sclerosis. *Neuroimaging. Clin. N. Am.* **4**, 229–324.

Braffman, B. & Naidich, T.P. (1994b): The phakomatoses: Part II. von Hippel–Lindau disease, Sturge–Weber syndrome, and less common conditions. *Neuroimaging. Clin. N. Am.* **4**, 325–348.

Bremer, W.F. (1927): Die pathologisch-anatomische Begrundung des Status dysraphius. *Deutsch. Zeitschr. Nervenheilk.* **99**, 104–123.

Brown, W.T., Jenkins, E.J., Krawczun, M.S., Wiśniewski, K., Rudelli, R., Cohen, I.L., Fisch, G., Wolf-Schein, E., Miezajeski, C. & Dobkin, C. (1986): The fragile x syndrome. *Ann. N.Y. Acad. Sci.* **477**, 129–150.

Brun, R. (1917): Zur Kenntnis der Bildungfehler des Kleinhirns. *Schweiz. Arch. Neurol. Psych.* **1**, 61–123.

Brun, R. (1918a): Zur Kenntnis der Bildungfehler des Kleinhirns. *Schweiz. Arch. Neurol. Psych.* **2**, 48–105.

Brun, R. (1918b): Zur Kenntnis der Bildungfehler des Kleinhirns. *Schweiz. Arch. Neurol. Psych.* **3**, 13–88.

Buchler, B.A., Delimont, D., van Waes, M. & Finnell, R.H. (1990): Prenatal prediction of risk of the fetal hydantoin syndrome. *N. Engl. J. Med.* **322**, 1567–1572.

Byard, R.W., Bourne, A.J. & Hanieh, A. (1991–92): Sudden and unexpected death due to hemorrhage from occult central nervous system lesions. A pediatric autopsy study. *Pediatr. Neurosurg.* **17**, 88–94.

Byrne, P.J., Silver, M.M., Gilbert, J.M., Cadera, W. & Tanswell, A.K. (1987): Cyclopia and congenital cytomegalovirus infection. *Am. J. Med. Genet.* **28**, 61–65.

Campbell, L.R., Dayton, D.H. & Sohal, G.S. (1986): Neural tube defects a review of human and animal studies on the etiology of neural tube defects. *Teratology* **34**, 171–187.

Carles, D., Serville, F., Mainguene, M. & Dubecq, J.P. (1987): Cyclopia-otocephaly association: a new case of the most severe variant of agnatia-holoprosencephaly complex. *J. Craniofac. Genet. Dev. Biol.* **7**, 107–113.

Caviness, V.S. & Evrard, P. (1975): Occipital encephalocele: a pathologic and anatomic analysis. *Acta Neuropathol. (Berl.)* **32**, 245–255.

Chaudhry, V., Sturgeon, C., Gates, A.J. & Myers, G. (1987): Symptomatic atlantoaxial dislocation in Down's syndrome. *Ann. Neurol.* **21**, 606–609.

Chaurasia, B.D. (1984): Calvarial defect in human anencephaly. *Teratology* **29**, 165–172.

Chiari, H. (1891): Uber Veranderungen des Kleinhirns, des Pons und der Medulla Oblongata infolge von kongenitaler hydrocephalic des Grosshirns. *Deutsch. Med. Wochenschr.* **56**, 825–836.

Chiari, H. (1896): Uber die Veranderungen des Kleinhirns, des Pons und der Medulla Oblongata infolge von kongenitaler hydrocephalic des Grosshirns. *Drukschriften der Akademie der Wissenschaften* **63**, 71–116.

Chmielik, J. (1996): Adverse effects in transplacental action of phenobarbital: experiment in rabbits. *Epilepsia* **37** (suppl.), 61 (Abstract).

Choi, B.H., Lapham, L.W., Amin-Zaki, L. & Saleem, T. (1978): Abnormal neuronal migration, deranged cerebral cortical organization, and diffuse white matter astrocytosis of human fetal brain: a major effect of methyl mercury poisoning in utero. *J. Neuropathol. Exp. Neurol.* **37**, 719–733.

Choi, B.H. & Matthias, S.C. (1987): Cortical dysplasia associated with massive ectopia of neurons and glial cells within subarachnoid space. *Acta Neuropathol. (Berl.)* **73**, 105–109.

Chou, T.M. & Chou, S.M. (1989): Tuberous sclerosis in the premature infant. A report of a case with immunohistochemistry on the CNS. *Clin. Neuropathol.* **8**, 45–52.

Cleland, J. (1883): Contribution to the study of spina bifida, encephalocele and anencephalus. *J. Anat. Physiol.* **17**, 257–292.

Cochrane, D.D., Adderley, R., White, C.P., Norman, M. & Steinbok, P. (1990): Apnea in patients with myelomeningocele. *Pediatr. Neurosurg.* **16**, 232–239.

Coffey, V.P. & Jessop, W.J. (1957): A study of 137 cases of anencephaly. *Brit. J. Prev. Soc. Med.* **11**, 174–189.

Cohen, M.M. Jr. (1982): An update on the holoprosencephalic disorders. *J. Pediatr.* **101**, 865–869.

Cohen, M.M. Jr. (1988): Craniosynostosis update 1987. *Am. J. Med. Genet. Suppl.* **4**, 99–148.

Cohen, M.M. Jr., Jirasek, J.E., Guzman, R.T., Gorlin, R.J. & Peterson, M.Q. (1971): Holoprosencephaly and facial dysmorphia: nosology, etiology and pathogenesis. *Birth Defects* **7**, (7) 125–135.

Cohen, M.D., Slabaugh, R.D., Smith, J.A., Jansen, R., Greenman, G.F., Macdonald, N. & Reider, J.I. (1984): Neurosonographic identification of ventricular asymmetry in premature infants. *Clin. Radiol.* **35**, 29–31.

Cohen, M., Campbell, R. & Yaghmai, F. (1989): Neuropathological abnormalities in developmental dysphasia. *Ann. Neurol.* **25**, 567–570.

Colan, R.V., Snead, O.C. & Ceballos, R. (1981): Olivopontocerebellar atrophy in children: a report of seven cases in two families. *Ann. Neurol.* **10**, 355–363.

Collmann, H., Sorensen, N., Krauss, J. & Muhling, J. (1988): Hydrocephalus in craniosynostosis. *Child's Nerv. Syst.* **4**, 279–285.

Conti, P., Conti, R. & De Luca, G. (1984): Observations on some rare cases of vertebra-medullar malformations associated with tumors. *J. Neurosurg. Sci.* **28**, 81–87.

Cooney, T.P. & Thurlbeck WM (1985): Lung growth and development in anencephaly and hydranencephaly. *Am. Rev. Respir. Dis.* **132**, 596–601.

Copp, A.J., Brook, F.A., Estibeiro, J.P., Shum, A.S. & Cockroft, D.L. (1990): The embryonic development of mammalian neural tube defects. *Prog. Neurobiol.* **35**, 363–403.

Copp, A.J. (1994): Genetic models of mammalian neural tube defects. *Ciba Found. Symp.* **181**, 118–134; discussion 134–143.

Cork, L.C. (1990): Neuropathology of Down syndrome and Alzheimer disease. *Am. J. Med. Genet.* Suppl. **7**, 282–286.

Cousins, L. (1983): Congenital anomalies among infants of diabetic mothers. Etiology, prevention, prenatal diagnosis. *Am. J. Obstet. Gynecol.* **147**, 333–338.

Cowie, V.A. (1987): Microcephaly: a review of genetic implications and its causation. *J. Ment. Defic. Res.* **31**, 229–233.

Crome, L. (1958): Multiocular cystic encephalopathy of infants. *J. Neurol. Neurosurg. Psychiatr.* **21**, 146–152.

Crome, L., Cowie, V. & Slayer, E. (1966): A statistical note on cerebellar and brain-stem weight in mongolism. *J. Ment. Defic. Res.* 10, 69–72.

Currarino, G. & Silverman, F.N. (1960): Orbital hypertelorism, arhinencephaly, and trigonocephaly. *Radiology* **74**, 206–217.

Cusmai, R., Curatolo, P., Mangano, P., Cheminal, R. & Echenne, B. (1990): Hemimegalencephaly and neurofibromatosis. *Neuropediatrics* **21**, 179–182.

Dąmbska, M. & Kansy, J. (1963): A morphological study on the central nervous system of an anencephalous fetus surviving 62 hours after birth. *Pol. Med. J.* **1**, 227–239.

Dąmbska, M., Krasnicka, Z. & Michalowicz, R. (1965): [Hydronencephalia in the course of congenital toxoplasmosis.] *Neuropatol. Pol.* **3**, 49–58. Published in Polish.

Dąmbska, M., Krasnicka, Z. & Mossakowski, M.J. (1970): [Contribution of blood vessels to the picture reflecting the developmental disturbances of the spinal cord.] *Neuropatol. Pol.* **8**, 279–286. Published in Polish.

Dąmbska, M., Szamborski, J. & Troszynski, M. (1971): [Peri-, and intraventricular hemorrhages in premature infants.] *Neuropatol. Pol.* **9**, 71–79. Published in Polish.

Dąmbska, M. & Schmidt-Sidor, B. (1971): Ceux cas d'agyrie et son rapport aux malformation du cerveau a l'incidence familiale. *Neuropatol. Pol.* **9**, 139–144.

Dąmbska, M., Dydyk, L., Szretter, T., Wozniewicz, J. & Myers, R.E. (1976): Topography of lesions in newborns and infant brains following cardiac arrest and resuscitation. Damage to brain and hemispheres. *Biol. Neonate* **29**, 194–206.

Dąmbska, M., Iwanowski, L. & Kozłowski, P.(1979a): The effect of transplacental intoxication with dichlorvos on the development of cerebral cortex in newborn rabbits. *Neuropatol. Pol.* **17**, 571–576.

Dąmbska, M., Brylko-Chmielik, J., Danielewicz-Kotowicz, A., Dydyk, L., Maślińska, D. & Onyszkiewicz, J. (1979b): [Comparison of transplacental effect of luminal and epileptic seizures in pregnant rabbits on the development of the nervous system.] *Probl. Med. Wieku. Rozwoj.* **9**, 319–323. Published in Polish.

Dąmbska, M. & Maślińska, D. (1981): Combined effect of phenobarbital and DDVP on the brain of young rabbit. *Acta Med. Pol.* **3**, 207–215.

Dąmbska, M., Haddad, R., Kozłowski, P.B., Lee, M.H. & Shek, J. (1982a): Telencephalic cytoarchitectonics in the brains of rats with graded degrees of micrencephaly. *Acta Neuropathol. (Berl.)* **58**, 203–209.

Dąmbska, M.,Wiśniewski, K., Sher, J. & Solish, G. (1982b): Cerebro-oculo-muscular syndrome a variant of Fukuyama congenital cerebromuscular dystrophy. *Clin. Neuropathol.* **1**, 93–98.

Dąmbska, M., Laure-Kamionowska, M. & Kozłowski, P.B. (1983a): Meningoencephalitis in newborns and infants as the cause of the central nervous system injury during its development. *Neuropatol. Pol.* **21**, 45–54.

Dąmbska, M., Wiśniewski, K. & Sher, J.H. (1983b): Lissencephaly: two distinct clinico-pathological types. *Brain Dev.* **5**, 302–310.

Dąmbska, M., Iwanowski, L., Maślińska, D. & Ostenda, M. (1984a): Blood–brain barrier in young rabbit brain after dichlorvas intoxication. *Neuropatol. Pol.* **22**, 129–137.

Dąmbska, M., Wiśniewski, K.E. & Sher, J.H. (1984b): An autopsy case of hemimegalencephaly. *Brain Dev.* **6**, 60–64.

Dąmbska, M., Wiśniewski, K.E. & Sher, J.H. (1986): Marginal glioneuronal heterotopias in nine cases with and without cortical abnormalities. *J. Child. Neurol.* **1**, 149–157.

Dąmbska, M., Laure-Kamionowska, M. & Liebhart, M. (1987): Brainstem lesions in the course of chronic fetal asphyxia. *Clin. Neuropathol.* **3**, 110–115.

Dąmbska, M. & Laure-Kamionowska, M. (1989): Early and late neuropathological changes in perinatal white matter damage. *J. Child Neurol.* **4**, 291–298.

Dąmbska, M. & Laure-Kamionowska, M. (1990): Myelination as a parameter of normal and retarded brain maturation. *Brain Dev.* **12**, 214–220.

Dąmbska, M.,Wiśniewski, K. & Scheinesson, G.P. (1993): Agyria with extreme microcephaly in twins. *Child's Nerv. Syst.* **9**, 125 (Abstr).

Dąmbska, M., Kuchna, I. & Nowicki, K. (1994): Neuropathological variants of cystic encephalopathy in infants. *Folia Neuropathol.* **32**, 31–35.

Dąmbska, M., Kuchna, I., Bobkiewicz, P. & Wiśniewski, K. (1996): Migration disorders leading to a wide spectrum of brain malformations in a case with multiorganic dysgeneses: A new syndrome? *Folia Neuropathol.* **34**, 11–15.

Dąmbska, M., Kozłowski, P. *et al.* (1997): The white matter changes in microcephalic HIV infected infants. A preliminary report. *Folia Neuropathol.* **35**, 145–148.

Dandy, W.E. & Blackfan, K.D. (1914): Internal hydrocephalus. *Am. J. Dis. Child.* **8**, 406–482.

Daniel, P.M. & Strich, S.J. (1958): Some observations on the congenital deformity of the central nervous system known as the Arnold-Chiari malformation. *J. Neuropathol. Exp. Neurol.* **17**, 255–266.

David, D.J. (1993): Cephaloceles: classification, pathology, and management – a review. *J. Craniofac. Surg.* **4**, 192–202.

David, D.J. & Proudman, T.W. (1989): Cephaloceles: classification, pathology and management. *World J. Surg.* **13**, 349–357.

Daube, J.R. & Chou, S.M. (1966): Lissencephaly: two cases. *Neurology* **16**, 179–191.

Dekaban, A.S. (1963): Anencephaly in early human embryos. *J. Neuropathol. Exp. Neurol.* **22**, 533–548.

Dekaban, A.S. & Bartelmez, G.W. (1964): Complete dysraphism in 14 somite human embryo. A Contribution to normal and abnormal morphogenesis. *J. Am. Anat.* **115**, 27–38.

Della Giustina, E. (1987): Microcephalic atelencephalique perspective pathogeniques. *Rev. Neurol.* **143,** 319 (Abstract).

de Leon, G.A. (1972): Observations on cerebral and cerebellar microgyria. *Acta Neuropathol. (Berl.)* **20,** 278–287.

de Leon, G.A., Grover, W.D. & Mestre, G.M. (1976): Cerebellar microgyria. *Acta Neuropathol. (Berl.)* **35,** 81–85.

de Leon, G.A., Grover, W.D. & D'Cruz, C.A. (1984): Amyotrophic cerebellar hypoplasia: a specific form of infantile spinal atrophy. *Acta Neuropathol. (Berl.)* **63,** 282–286.

De Morsier, G. (1955): Etudes sur les dysraphies cranio-encephaliques. II. Agenesic du vermis cerebelleux Dysraphic rhomencephalique mediane (rhomboschisis). *Monatsch. Psychiatr. Neurol.* **129,** 321–344.

De Morsier, G. (1956): Etudes sur les dysraphies cranio-encephaliques. III. Agenesic du septum lucielum avec malformation du tractus optique: la dysplasic septooptique. *Arch. Neurol. Neurochir. Psychiatr.* **77,** 267–292.

DeMyer, W. & Zeman, W. (1963): Alobar holoprosencephaly (arhinencephaly) with median cleft lip and palate: clinical, electroence-phalographic and nosologic considerations. *Confin. Neurol.* **23,** 1–6.

DeMyer, W., Zeman, W. & Palmer, C.G. (1964): The face predicts the brain diagnostic significance of median facial anomalies for holoprosencephaly (arhinencephaly). *Pediatrics* **34,** 256–263.

DeMyer, W. (1967): The median cleft face syndrome. Differential diagnosis of cranium bifidum occultum hypertelorism, and median cleft nose, lip and palate. *Neurology* **17,** 961–971.

DeMyer, W. (1986): Megalencephaly: types, clinical syndromes, and management. *Pediatr. Neurol.* **2,** 321–328.

De Reuck, J., Chattha, A.S. & Richardson, E.P. Jr. (1972): Pathogenesis and evolution of periventricular leukomalacia in infancy. *Arch. Neurol.* **27,** 229–236.

Devi,, A.S., Eisenfeld, L., Uphoff, D. & Greenstein, R. (1995): New syndrome of hydrocephalus, endocardial fibroelastosis, and cataracts (HEC syndrome). *Am. J. Med. Genet.* **56,** 62–66.

de Vries, L.S., Regev, R., Dubowitz, L.M.S., Whitelaw, A. & Aber, V.R. (1988): Perinatal risk factors for the development of extensive cystic leukomalacia. *Am. J. Dis. Child.* **142,** 732–735.

Dias, M.S. & Walker, M.L. (1992): The embryogenesis of complex dysraphic malformations: a disorder of gastrulation? *Pediatr. Neurosurg.* **18,** 229–253.

Dieker, H., Edwards, R.H., ZuRhein, G., Chou, S.M., Hartman, H.A. & Optitz, J.M. (1969): The lissencephaly syndrome. *Birth Defects* **5(2),** 53–64.

Dimmick, J.E. & Applegarth, D.A. (1993): Pathology of peroxisomal disorders. *Perspect. Pediatr. Pathol.* **17,** 45–98.

Dobbing, J. & Sands, J. (1971): Vulnerability of developing brain. IX. The effect of nutritional growth retardation on the timing of the brain growth-spurt. *Biol. Neonate* **19,** 363–378.

Dobyns, W.B., Stratton, R.F., Parke, J.T., Greenberg, F., Nussbaum, R.L. & Ledbetter, D.H. (1983): Miller–Dieker syndrome: lissencephaly and monosomy 17p. *J. Pediatr.* **102,** 552–558.

Dobyns, W.B., Gilbert, E.F. & Opitz, J.H. (1985): Further comments on the lissencephaly syndromes. *Am. J. Med. Genet.* **22,** 197–211.

Dobyns, W.B., Pagon, R.A., Armstrong, D., Curry, C.J., Greenberg, F., Grix, A., Holmes, L.B., Laxova, R., Michels, V.V., Robinow, M. *et al.* (1989): Diagnostic criteria for WalterBWerburg syndrome. *Am. J. Med. Genet.* **32,** 195–210.

Dom, R., Ho, C., Goffin, J., Joosten, E., D'Haen, V. & Lammens, M. (1990): Giant intracranial neurenteric cysts in an 82 year old man. *Acta Neurol. Belg.* **90,** 291–292 (Abstract).

Down, J.H.L. (1866): Observations on an ethnic classification of idiots. *Clin. Lect. Rep. London Hosp.* **3**, 259–262.

Dragojevic, S,, Mehraein, P. & Bock, H.J. (1973): Beobachtung eines Lipoms der Temporalregion mit Rindenmissbildung und Epilepsie. Klinisch-pathologische Studie. *Arch. Psychiatr. Nervenkr.* **217**, 335–342.

Dvorak, K. & Feit, J. (1977): Migration of neuroblasts through partial necrosis of the cerebral cortex in newborn rats B contribution to the problems of morphological development and developmental period of cerebral microgyria. Histological and autoradiographical study. *Acta Neuropathol. (Berl.)* **38**, 203–212.

Dvorak, K., Feit, J. & Jurankova, Z. (1978): Experimentally induced focal microgyria and status verrucosus deformis in rats B pathogenesis and interrelation. Histological and autoradiographical study. *Acta Neuropathol. (Berl.)* **44**, 121–129.

Editorial Progress in TS (1990): Progress in tuberous sclerosis. *Lancet* **336**, 598–599 (Editorial).

Edmondson, S.R., Hallak, M., Carpenter, R.J. Jr. & Cotton, D.B. (1992): Evolution of hydranencephaly following intracerebral hemorrhage. *Obstet. Gynecol.* **79**, 870–871.

Edwards, J.H., Harnden, D.G., Cameron, A.H., Crosse, V.M. & Wolff, O.H. (1960): A new trisomic syndrome. *Lancet* **1**, 787–790.

Emery, J.L. & MacKenzie, N. (1973): Medullo-cervical dislocation deformity (Chiari II deformity) related to neurospinal dysraphism (meningomyelocele). *Brain* **96**, 155–162.

Emery, J.L. & Lendon, R.G. (1973): The local cord lesions in neurospinal dysraphism (meningomyelocele). *J. Pathol.* **110**, 83–96.

Emery, J.L. (1974): Deformity of the aqueduct of sylvius in children with hydrocephalus and myelomeningocele. *Dev. Med. Child. Neurol.* (suppl.) **32**, 40–48.

Escourolle, R. & Poirier, J. (1973): Manual of basic neuropathology. (Translator: L.J. Rubinstein, Translation of *Manuel elementaire de neuropathologic*), Philadelphia: Saunders.

Ettlinger, G. (1977): Agenesis of corpus callosum. In: *Congenital malformations of the brain and skull*, Part I, Handbook of Clinical Neurology, eds. J.P. Vinken & G.W. Bruyn, vol. 30, pp. 285–297. Amsterdam: North Holland Publishing Co.

Everall, I., Luthert, P. & Lantos, P. (1993): A review of neuronal damage in human immunodeficiency virus infection: its assessment, possible mechanism and relationship to dementia. *J. Neuropathol. Exp. Neurol.* **52**, 561–566.

Faillace, W.J., Okawara, S.H. & McDonald, J.V. (1984): Neurocutaneous melanosis with extensive intracerebral and spinal cord involvement. Report of two cases. *J. Neurosurg.* **61**, 782–785.

Ferguson, J.H., Levinsohn, M. & Derakshan, I. (1974): Brain stem seizures in hydranencephaly. *Neurology* **24**, 1152–1157.

Fernandes, E.T., Custer, M.D., Burton, E.M., Boulden, T.F., Wrenn, E.L. Jr., Whittle, A.P. & Edwards, O.P. (1991): Neuroenteric cyst: surgery and diagnostic imaging. *J. Pediatr. Surg.* **26**, 108–110.

Ferrer, I. & Navarro, C. (1978): Multicystic encephalomalacia of infancy: clinico-pathological report of 7 cases. *J. Neurol. Sci.* **38**, 179–189.

Ferrer, I., Fabregues, I. & Palacios, G. (1982): An autoradiographic study of methyl-azoxy-methanol acetate-induced cortical malformation. *Acta Neuropathol. (Berl.)* **57**, 313–315.

Ferrer, I. (1984): A Golgi analysis of unlayered polymicrogyria. *Acta Neuropathol. (Berl.)* **65**, 69–76.

Ferrer, I., Xumetra, A. & Santamaria, J. (1984): Cerebral malformation induced by prenatal X-irradiation: an autoradiographic and Golgi study. *J. Anat.* **138**, 81–93.

Ferrer, I., Cusi, M.V., Liarte, A. & Campistol, J. (1986): A Golgi study of polymicrogyric cortex in Aicardi syndrome. *Brain Dev.* **8**, 518–525.

Ferrer, I. & Galofre, E. (1987): Dendritic spine anomalies in fetal alcohol syndrome. *Neuropediatrics* **18**, 161–163.

Ferrer, I. & Gullotta, F. (1990): Down's syndrome and Alzheimer's disease: dendritic spine counts in the hippocampus. *Acta Neuropathol. (Berl.)* **79**, 680–685.

Ferrer, I. & Catala, I (1991): Unlayered polymicrogyria: structural and developmental aspects. *Anat. Embryol. (Berl.)* **184**, 517–528.

Fields, W.H. Jr., Metzner, L., Garol, J.D. & Kokich, V.G. (1978): The craniofacial skeleton in anencephalic human fetuses. I. Cranial floor. *Teratology* **17**, 57–65.

Flanigan, R.C., Russell, D.P. & Walsh, J.W. (1989): Urologic aspects of tethered cord. *Urology* **33**, 80–82.

Fletchner, H.M. (1900): A case of megalencephaly. *Trans. Pathol. Soc. London* **51**, 230–232.

Fransen, E., Schrander-Stumpel, C., Vits, L., Coucke, P., Van Camp, G. & Willems, P.J. (1994): X-linked hydrocephalus and MASA syndrome present in one family are due to a single missense mutation in exon 28 of the L1CAM gene. *Hum. Mol. Genet.* **3**, 2255–2256.

French, N.B. (1983): The embryology of the spinal dysraphism. *Clin. Neurosurg.* **30**, 295–340.

Francois, J. (1972): A general introduction. In: *The phakomatoses*, Handbook of clinical neurology, eds. PJ. Vinken & G.W. Bruyn, vol. 14, pp. 1–18. Amsterdam: North-Holland Publishing Co.

Friede, R.L. (1962): A quantitative study of myelination in hydrocephalus (factors controlling glial proliferation in myelination). *J. Neuropathol. Exp. Neurol.* **21**, 645–648.

Friede, R.L. & Roessmann, U. (1976): Chronic tonsillar herniation: an attempt at classifying chronic herniation at the foramen magnum. *Acta Neuropathol. (Berl.)* **34**, 219–235.

Friede, R.L. & Yasargil, M.G. (1977): Supratentorial intracerebral epithelial (ependymal) cysts: review, case reports, and fine structure. *J. Neurol. Neurosurg. Psychiatr.* **40**, 127–137.

Friede, R.L. & Boltshauser, E. (1978): Uncommon syndromes of cerebellar vermis aplasia. I. Joubert syndrome. *Dev. Med. Child. Neurol.* **20**, 758–763.

Friede, R.L. & Briner, J. (1978): Midline hyperplasia with malformation of the fornical system. *Neurology* **28**, 1302–1305.

Friede, R.L. & Mikolasek, J. (1978): Postencephalitic porencephaly, hydranencephaly or polymicrogyria. A review. *Acta Neuropathol. (Berl.)* **43**, 161–168.

Frieden, I.J. (1986): Aplasia cutis congenita: a clinical review and proposal for classification. *J. Am. Acad. Dermatol.* **14**, 646–660.

Friede, R.L. (1989): *Developmental neuropathology*, 2nd rev. and expanded ed., Berlin: Springer Verlag.

Frye, F.L., Mc Farland, L.Z. & Enright, J.B. (1964): Sacrococcygeal agenesis in Swiss mice. *Cornell Vet.* **54**, 487–495.

Fu, Y.H., Kuhl, D.P.A., Pizzuti, A., Pieretti, M., Sutcliffe, J.S., Richards, S., Verkerk, A. *et al.* (1991): Variation of the CGG repeat at the fragile X site results in genetic instability: resolution of the Sherman paradox. *Cell* **67**, 1047–1058.

Fulroth, R., Phillips, B. & Durand, D.J. (1989): Perinatal outcome of infants exposed to cocaine and/or heroin in utero. *Am J. Dis. Child.* **143**, 905–910.

Gadisseux, J.F., Rodriguez, J. & Lyon, G. (1984): Pontoneocerebellar hypoplasia B a probable consequence of prenatal destruction of the pontine nuclei and a possible role of phenytoin intoxication. *Clin. Neuropathol.* **3**, 160–167.

Gaily, E.K., Grunstrom, M.L., Hiilesmaa, V.K. & Bardy, A.H. (1990): Head circumference in children of epileptic mothers: contributions of drug exposure and genetic background. *Epilepsy Res.* **5**, 217–222.

Galaburda, A.M., Sherman, G.F., Rosen, G.D., Aboitz, F. & Geschwind, N. (1985): Developmental dyslexia: four consecutive patients with cortical anomalies. *Ann. Neurol.* **18**, 222–233.

Garcia, J.H. & Anderson, M.L. (1991): Circulatory disorders and their effects on the brain. In: *Textbook of neuropathology*, eds. R.L. Davis & D.M. Robertson, 2nd ed., pp. 621–718. Baltimore: Williams & Wilkins.

Gardner, W.J. (1973): The dysraphic states from syringomyelia to anencephaly. Amsterdam: Excerpta medica.

Giacomini, C. (1885): Contributo allo studio dello microcefalia. *Arch. Psychiatr. (Torino)*, **6**, 63–81.

Gilbert, J.N., Jones, K.L., Rorke, L.B. Chernoff, G.F. & James, H.E. (1986): Central nervous system anomalies associated with meningomyelocele, hydrocephalus and the Arnold-Chiari malformation: reappraisal of theories regarding the pathogenesis of posterior neural tube closure defects. *Neurosurgery* **18**, 559–564.

Gilles, F.H. & Davidson, R.I. (1971): Communicating hydrocephalus associated with deficient dysplastic parasagittal arachnoidal granulations. *J. Neurosurg.* **35**, 421–426.

Gilles, F.H. & Gilles, E.E. (1986): Hydrocephalus in the neonate, infant and child. In: *Disorders of the developing nervous system: diagnosis and treatment*, eds. H.J. Hoffman & F. Epstein, pp. 541–572. Boston: Blackwell Scientific Publications.

Gilles, F.H. (1991): Perinatal neuropathology. In: *Textbook of neuropathology*, 2nd ed., eds. R.L. Davis & D.M. Robertson, pp. 624–633. Baltimore: Williams & Wilkins.

Golden, J.A. & Hyman, B.T. (1994): Development of the superior temporal neocortex is anomalous in trisomy 21. *J. Neuropathol. Exp. Neurol.* **53**, 513–520.

Gomez, M.R. (1988): Tuberous sclerosis, 2nd. edn. New York: Raven Press.

Gorlin, R.J., Cervenka, J. & Pruzansky, S. (1971): Facial clefting and its syndromes. *Birth Defects* **7 (3)**, 3–49.

Grcevic, N. & Robert, F. (1961): Verrucose dysplasia of the cerebral cortex. *J. Neuropathol. Exp. Neurol.* **20**, 399–411.

Gregory, P.E., Gutmann, D.H., Mitchell, A., Park, S., Baguski, M., Jacks, T., Wood, D.L., Jove, R. & Collins, F.S. (1993): Neurofibromatosis type 1 gene product (neurofibromin) associates with microtubules. *Somat. Cell. Mol. Genet.* **19**, 265–274.

Gross, H. & Hoff, H. (1959a): Sur les dysraphics cranioencephaliques. In: *Malformations congenitales du cerveau*, eds. G. Heuyer, M. Feld & J. Gruner, pp. 287–296. Paris: Masson.

Gross, H. & Hoff, H. (1959b): Sur les malformations ventriculaires dependantes des dysgenesies commissurales. In: *Malformations congenitales du cerveau*, eds. G. Heuyer, M. Feld & J. Gruner, pp. 329–351. Paris: Masson.

Gross, G.W. & Goldberg, B.B. (1995): Neurosonography of the fetal neonatal and infant brain and spine. In: *Pediatric neuropathology*, ed. Serge Duckett, pp. 830–881. Baltimore: Williams & Wilkins.

Gruhn, J.G., Gorlin, R.J. & Langer, L.O. (1978): Dyssegmental dwarfism. A lethal anisospondylic camptomicromelic dwarfism. *Am J. Dis. Child.* **132**, 382–386.

Gullotta, F. & Rehder, H. (1974): Chromosomal anomalies and central nervous system. *Beitr. Pathol.* **152**, 74–80.

Gullotta, F., Rehder, H. & Gropp, A. (1981): Descriptive neuropathology of chromosomal disorders in man. *Hum. Genet.* **57**, 337–344.

Guthkelch, A.N. (1970): Occipital cranium bifidum. *Arch. Dis. Child.* **45**, 104–109.

Guttmann, D.H. & Collins, F.S. (1992): Recent progress toward understanding the molecular biology of von Recklinghausen neurofibromatosis. *Ann. Neurol.* **31**, 555–561.

Haberland, C. (1977) : The phakomatoses. 'Congenital malformations of the brain and skull, Part II.' In: *Handbook of clinical neurology*, eds. P.J .Vinken & G.W. Bruyn, vol. 31, pp. 1–34. Amsterdam: North-Holland Publishing Co.

Hagerman, R.J., Amiri, K. & Cronister, A. (1991): Fragile X checklist. *Am. J. Med. Genet.* **38,** 283–287.

Hair, L.S., Symmans, F., Powers, J.M. & Carmel, P. (1992): Immunohistochemistry and proliferative activity in Lhermitte–Duclos disease. *Acta Neuropathol. (Berl.)* **84,** 570–573.

Halimi, P., Sigal, R., Doyon, D. *et al.* (1989): Diagnostique des affections du la moelle et de rachis. *Rev. Prat.* **39,** 751–757.

Hallervorden, J. (1949): Uber eine Kohlenoxydvergiftung im Fetalleben mit Entwicklungsstorung der Hirnrinde. *Allg. Z. Psychiatr.* **124,** 289–298.

Hallervorden, J. & Meyer, J.E. (1956): Cerebrale Kinderlahmung. In: *Handbuch der speziellen pathologischen Anatomie und Histologie*, Bd. 13/+4, eds. F. Henke, O. Lubarsch & R. Rössle, pp. 194–282. Berlin: Springer Verlag

Hallervorden, J. (1959): Uber die Hamartome (Ganglioneurome) des Gehirns. *Deutsch. Z. Nervenheilk.* **179,** 531–563.

Harding, B.N., Dunger, D.B., Grant, D.B. & Erdehazi, M. (1988): Familial olivoponto-cerebellar atrophy with neonatal onset: a recessively inherited syndrome with systemic and biochemical abnormalities. *J. Neurol. Neurosurg. Psychiatr.* **51,** 385–390.

Harding, B.N. (1992): Malformations of the nervous system. In: *Greenfield's neuropathology*, 5th edn., eds. J.H. Adams & L.W. Ducken, pp. 521–638. New York: Oxford University Press.

Harding, B. & Copp, A.J. (1997): Malformations. In: *Greenfield's neuropathology*, 6th edn., eds. D.I. Graham & P.L. Lantos, pp. 397–533. London: Arnold/Oxford University Press NY.

Harris, C.P., Townsend, J.J. & Carey, J.C. (1993): Acalvaria: a unique congenital anomaly. *Am. J. Med. Genet.* **46,** 694–699.

Hart, M.N., Malamud, N. & Ellis, W.G. (1972): The Dandy–Walker syndrome. A clinico-pathological study of 28 cases. *Neurology* **22,** 771–782,

Haslam, R.H.A. (1987): Microcephaly. 'Malformations.' In: *Handbook of clinical neurology*, vol. 50, eds. P.J. Vinken, G.W. Bruyn & H.L. Klawans, pp. 267–284. Amsterdam: Elsevier Science Publishers.

Haworth, J.C., Medovy, H., Lewis, A.J. (1961): Cebocephaly with endocrine dysgenesis. Report of 3 cases. *J. Pediatr.* **59,** 726–733.

Heggie, P., Grossniklaus, H.E., Roesmann, U., Chou, S.M. & Cruse, R.P. (1987): Cerebro-ocular dysplasia – muscular dystrophy syndrome. Report of two cases. *Arch. Ophthalmol.* **105,** 520–524.

Hennekam, R.C., van Rhijn, A. & Hennekam, F.A. (1992): Dominantly inherited microcephaly, short stature and normal intelligence. *Clin. Genet.* **41,** 248–251.

Heyer, R., Ehrich, J., Goebel, H.H., Christen, H.J. & Hanefeld, F. (1986): Congenital muscular dystrophy with cerebral and ocular malformations (cerebro-oculo-muscular syndrome). *Brain Dev.* **8,** 614–619.

Hicks, S.P. (1953): Developmental malformations produced by radiation. A timetable of their development. *Am. J. Roentgenol.* **69,** 272–293.

Hicks, S.P. (1954): Mechanism of radiation anencephaly anophthalmia, and pituitary anomalies: repair in mammalian embryo. *Arch. Pathol.* **57,** 363–378.

Hinton, V.J., Brown, W.T., Wiśniewski, K. & Rudelli, R.D. (1991): Analysis of neocortex in three males with fragile X syndrome. *Am. J. Med. Genet.* **41,** 289–294.

Hirano, A. & Solomon, S. (1960): Arteriovenous aneurysm of the vein of Galen. *AMA Arch. Neurol.* 1960, **3,** 589–593.

Hoffman, H.J. & Tucker, W.S. (1976): Cephalocranial disproportion. A complication of the treatment of hydrocephalus in children. *Child's Brain* **2,** 167–176.

Ho, K.L. & Tiel, R. (1989): Intraspinal bronchogenic cyst: ultrastructural study of the lining epithelium. *Acta Neuropathol. (Berl.)* **78**, 513–520.

Holmes, L.B. (1994): Spina bifida: anticonvulsants and other maternal influences. In: Ciba Found. Symp. 181, pp. 232–238; discussion 239–244.

Hosley, M.A., Abroms, I.F. &, Ragland, R.L. (1992): Schizencephaly: case report of familial incidence. *Pediatr. Neurol.* **8**, 148–150.

Iannetti, P., Schwartz, C.E., Dietz-Band, J., Light, E., Timmerman, J. & Chessa, L. (1993a): Norman-Roberts syndrome: clinical and molecular studies. *Am. J. Med. Genet.* **47**, 95–99.

Iannetti, P., Raucci, U., Basile, L.A., Spalice, A., Di Biasi, C., Trasimoni, G. & Gualdi, G.F. (1993b): Neuronal migration disorders: diffuse cortical dysplasia or the 'double cortex' syndrome. *Acta Pediatr.* **82**, 501–503.

Iashima, A., Kisa, T., Yoshino, K., Takashima, S. & Takeshita, K. (1984): A morphometric CT study of Down's syndrome showing small posterior fossa and calcification of basal ganglia. *Neuroradiology* **26**, 493–498.

Iivanainen, M., Haltia, M. & Lydecken, K. (1977): Atelencephaly. *Dev. Med. Child. Neurol.* **19**, 663–668.

Ikeda, H., Niizuma, H., Suzuki, J., Takabayashi, T. & Ozawa, N. (1987): A case of cebocephaly-holoprosencephaly with an aberrant adenohypophysis. *Child's Nerv. Syst.* **3**, 251–254.

Inagaki, M., Ando, Y., Mito, T., Ieshima, A., Ohtani, K., Takashima, S. & Takeshita, K. (1987): Comparison of brain imaging and neuropathology in cases of trisomy 18 and 13. *Neuroradiology* **29**, 474–479.

Ingraham, F.D. & Swan, H. (1943): Spina bifida and cranium bifidum (encephalocele). A summary of 546 cases. *N. Engl. J. Med.* **228**, 559–563.

Ingraham, F.D. (1944): Spina bifida and cranium bifidum. Papers reprinted from the *New England Journal of Medicine*, with the addition of a comprehensive bibliography. Boston, The Children's Hospital; Cambridge, Harvard University Press.

Izmeth, M.G. & Parameshwar, E. (1989): The Miller–Dieker syndrome: a case report and review of the literature. *J. Ment. Defic. Res.* **33**, 267–270.

Jacob, H. (1936): Faktoren bei der Entstehung der normalen und der entwicklungs-gestorten Hirnrinde. *Z. Neurol. Psychiatr. (Originalien)* **155**, 1–39.

Jacob, H. (1940): Die feinere Oberflachengestaltung der Hirnwindungen, die Hirnwarzenbildung und die Mikropolygyrie. *Z. Neurol. Psychiatr. (Originalien)* **170**, 62–84.

Jacobs, P.A. & Hassold, T.J. (1987): Chromosome abnormalities: origin and etiology in abortions and live births. In: *Human genetics*, Proceedings of the 7th International Congress, eds. F. Vogel & K. Sperling, pp. 233–244. Berlin: Springer-Verlag.

James, C.C.M. & Lassman, L.P. (1981): Spina bifida occulta: orthopaedic, radiological and neurosurgical aspects. New York: Grune & Stratton.

Janzer, R.C. & Friede, R.L. (1982): Dandy–Walker syndrome with atresia of the fourth ventricle and multiple rhombencephalic malformations. *Acta Neuropathol. (Berl.)* **58**, 81–86.

Jay, V., Chan, F.-W. & Becker, L.E. (1990): Dendritic arborization in the human fetus and infant with the trisomy 18 syndrome. *Brain Res. Dev. Brain Res.* **54**, 291–294.

Jellinger, K., Kucsko, L. & Seitelberger, F. (1966): Diffuse meningo-cerebrale Angiodysplasia mit hypoplasiogener Isthmusstenose bei einem eugeborenen. *Beitr. Pathol. Anat.* **133**, 41–72.

Jellinger, K. & Rett, A. (1976): Agyria-pachygyria (lissencephaly syndrome). *Neuropediatric* **7**, 66–91.

Jellinger, K., Gross, H., Kaltenback, E. & Grisold, W. (1981): Holoprosencephaly and agenesis of the corpus callosum: frequency of associated malformations. *Acta Neuropathol. (Berl.)* **55**, 1–10.

Jenkins, E.C., Brown, W.T., Brooks, J., Duncan, C.J., Rudelli, R.D. & Wiśniewski, H.M. (1984): Experience with prenatal fragile X detection. *Am. J. Med. Genet.* **17**, 215–239.

Jenkyn, L.R., Roberts, D.W., Merlis, A.L., Rozycki, A.A. & Nordgren, R.E. (1981): Dandy–Walker malformation in identical twins. *Neurology* **31**, 337–341.

Jeret, J.S., Serur, D., Wiśniewski, K. & Fisch, C. (1986): Frequency of agenesis of the corpus callosum in the developmentally disabled population as determined by computerized tomography. *Pediatr. Neurosci.* **12**, 101–103.

Jeret, J.S., Serur, D., Wiśniewski, K.E. & Lubin, R.A. (1987): Clinicopathological findings associated with agenesis of the corpus callosum. *Brain Dev.* **9**, 255–264.

Jervis, G.A. (1950): Early familial cerebellar degeneration. Report of three cases in one family. *J. Nerv. Ment. Dis.* **111**, 398–407.

Johnson, E.S. & Ludwin, S.K. (1984): Rhabdoneuroglial heterotopia of the pontine leptomeninges in trisomy 13. *Arch. Pathol. Lab. Med.* **108**, 906–908.

Jones, K.L., Smith, D.W., Ulleland, C.N. & Streissguth, P. (1973): Pattern of malformation in offspring of chronic alcoholic mothers. *Lancet* **1**, 1267–1271.

Joubert, M., Eisenring, J.J., Robb, J.P. & Andermann, F. (1969): Familial agenesis of the cerebellar vermis. A syndrome of episodic hypernea, abnormal eye movements, ataxia, and retardation. *Neurology* **19**, 813–825.

Jouet, M. & Kenwrick, S. (1995): Gene analysis of L1 neural cell adhesion molecule in prenatal diagnosis of hydrocephalus. *Lancet* **345**, 161–162.

Karch, S.B. & Urich, H. (1972): Occipital encephalocele: a morphological study. *J. Neurol. Sci.* **15**, 89–112.

Kaufmann, W.E. & Galaburda, A.M. (1989): Cerebrocortical microdysgenesis in neurologically normal subjects: a histopathologic study. *Neurology* **39**, 238–244.

Kazee, A.M., Lapham, L.W., Torres, C.F. & Wang, D.D. (1991): Generalized cortical dysplasia. Clinical and pathologic aspects. *Arch. Neurol.* **48**, 850–853.

Kemper, T.L. (1988): Neuropathology of Down syndrome. In: *The psychobiology of Down Syndrome*, ed. L. Nadel, pp. 269–289. Cambridge, MA: The MIT Press.

Kennedy, C., Grave, G.D., Jehle, J.W. & Sokoloff, L. (1970): Blood flow to white matter during maturation of the brain. *Neurology* **20**, 613–618.

Kida, E., Choi-Miura, N.-H. & Wiśniewski, K.E. (1995): Deposition of apolipoproteins E and J in senile plaques is topographically determined in both Alzheimer's disease and Down's syndrome brain. *Brain Res.* **685**, 211–216.

Kim, T.S., Cho, S. & Dickson, D.W. (1990): Aprosencephaly: review of the literature and report of a case with cerebellar hypoplasia, pigmented epithelial cyst and Rathke's cleft cyst. *Acta Neuropathol. (Berl.)* **79**, 424–431.

Kimura, S., Sasaki, Y., Kobayashi, T., Ohtsuki, N., Tanaka, Y., Hara, M., Miyake, S., Yamada, M., Iwamoto, H. & Misugi, N. (1993): Fukuyama-type congenital muscular dystrophy and the Walker–Warburg syndrome. *Brain Dev.* **15**, 182–191.

King, M.D., Dudgeon, J. & Stephenson, J.B. (1984): Joubert's syndrome with retinal dysplasia: neonatal tachypnoea as the clue to a genetic brain-eye malformation. *Arch. Dis. Child.* **59**, 709–718.

Klingensmith, W.C. & Cioffi-Ragan, D.T. (1986): Schizencephaly: diagnosis and progression in utero. *Radiology* **159**, 617–618.

Kondziolka, D., Humpreys, R.P., Hoffman, H.J., Hendrick, E.B. & Drake, J.M. (1992): Arteriovenous malformations of the brain in children: a forty year experience. *Can. J. Neurol. Sci.* **19**, 40–45.

Kousseff, B.G. (1990): The phakomatoses as a paracrine growth disorders (paracinopathies). *Clin. Genet.* **37**, 97–105.

Kousseff, B.G. (1992): Hypothesis: Jadassohn nevus phakomatosis: a paracrinopathy with variable phenotype. *Am. J. Med. Genet.* **43**, 651–661.

Kozłowski, P.B., Sher, J.H., Nicastri, A.D. & Rudelli, R.D. (1989): Brain morphology in the Galloway syndrome. *Clin. Neuropathol.* **8**, 85–91.

Kozłowski, P.B. (1995): Pediatric human immunodeficiency virus (HIV) infection. In: *Pediatric neuropathology*, ed. S. Duckett, pp. 435–447. Baltimore: William & Wilkins.

Kozłowski, P.B., Brudkowska, J., Kraszpulski, M., Sersen, E.A., Wrzolek, M.A., Anzil, A.P., Rao, C. & Wiśniewski, H.M. (1997): Microencephaly in children congenitally infected with human immunodeficiency virus B a gross anatomical morphometric study. *Acta Neuropathol. (Berl.)* **93**, 136–145.

Krigman, M.R. & Hogan, E.L. (1976): Undernutrition in the developing rat: effect upon myelination. *Brain Res.* **107**, 239–255.

Krijgsman, J.B., Barth, P.G., Stam, F.C., Slooff, J.L. & Jaspar, H.H. (1980): Congenital muscular dystrophy and cerebral dysgenesis in a Dutch family. *Neuropediatrie* **11**, 108–120.

Kruyff, E. & Jeffs, R. (1966): Skull abnormalities associated with the Arnold-Chiari malformation. *Acta Radiol. (Diagn.) (Stockh.)* **5**, 9–24.

Kuban, K.C.K. & Gilles, F.H. (1985): Human telencephalic angiogenesis. *Ann. Neurol.* **17**, 539–548.

Kuchna, I. (1994): Quantitative studies of human newborns' hippocampal pyramidal cells after perinatal hypoxia. *Folia Neuropathol.* **32**, 9–16.

Kuharik, M.A., Edwards, M.K. & Grossman, C.B. (1985–86): Magnetic resonance evaluation of pediatric spinal dysraphism. *Pediatr. Neurosci.* **12**, 213–218.

Kundrat, H. (1882): Arhinencephalie als typische Art von Missbildung. Graz, Leuschner and Lubensky, 1882.

Kuzniecky, R.I. (1994): Magnetic resonance imaging in developmental disorders of the cerebral cortex. *Epilepsia* **35**, (Suppl 6), S44BS56.

Kwiatkowski, D.J., Aklog, L., Ledbetter, D.H. & Morton, C.C. (1990): Identification of the functional profilin gene, its localization to chromosome subband 17p 13.3 and demonstration of its deletion in some patients with Miller–Dieker syndrome. *Am. J. Hum. Genet.* **46**, 559–567.

Larisseau, A., Vanasse, M., Brochu, P. & Jasmin, G. (1984): The Andermann syndrome: agenesis of the corpus callosum associated with mental retardation and progressive sensorimotor neuropathy. *Can. J. Neurol. Sci.* **11**, 257–261.

Lach, B., Russell, N., Atack, D. & Benoit, B. (1989): Intraparenchymal epithelial (enterogenous) cyst of the medulla oblongata. *Can. J. Neurol. Sci.* **16**, 206–210.

Lagger, R.L. (1979): Failure of pyramidal tract decussation in the DandyBWalker syndrome. Report of two cases. *J. Neurosurg.* **50**, 382–387.

Lammer, E.J., Sever, L.E. & Oakley, G.P.Jr. (1987): Teratogen update: valproic acid. *Teratology* **35**, 465–473.

Langman, J. & Shimada, M. (1971): Cerebral cortex of the mouse after prenatal chemical insult. *Am J. Anat.* **132**, 355–374.

Lapras, C., Papet, J.D., Huppert, J. et al. (1985): Tethered conus syndrome or fixed spinal cord syndrome Lumbosacral lipomas. *Rev. Neurol. (Paris)* **141**, 207–215.

Larroche, J.C. (1977): Developmental pathology of the neonate. Amsterdam, Excerpta medica.

Larroche, J.C. (1981): Cerebellum hypoplasia. In: *Handbook of Clinical Neurology*, vol. 42, eds P.J. Vinken & G.W. Bruyn, pp. 18–20. Amsterdam: North Holland.

Larroche, J.C., Bethmann, O., Baudoin, M. & Couchard, M. (1986): Brain damage in the premature infant. Early lesions and new aspects of sequelae. *Ital. J. Neurol. Sci.* (suppl.) **5**, 43–52.

Laure-Kamionowska, M. (1980): [Effect of gestosis on fetal brain.] Published in Polish. *Neuropatol. Pol.* **18**, 239–257.

Laure-Kamionowska, M., Dąmbska, M., Janczewska, E. et al. (1980): [The development of fetuses and their brains from diabetic mothers.] Published in Polish. *Problemy Cukrzycy w Poloznictwie I Neonatologii*, Pożnan, 1980.

Laure-Kamionowska, M. & Majdecki, T. (1982): [Changes in the fetal nervous system as a result of pregnancy complications.] Published in Polish. *Neuropatol. Pol.* **20**, 475–481.

Laure-Kamionowska, M. & Dąmbska, M. (1992): Damage of maturing brain in the course of toxoplasmic encephalitis. *Neuropatol. Pol.* **30**, 307–314.

Laverda, A.M., Saia, O.S., Drigo, P., Danieli, E., Clementi, M. & Tenconi, R. (1984): Chorioretinal coloboma and Joubert syndrome: a nonrandom association. *J. Pediatr.* **105**, 282–284.

Leach, R.W. et al. (1975): Normal and abnormal development of the human nervous system. Hagerstown, MD: Harper & Row.

Leech, R.W. & Shuman, R.M. (1986): Holoprosencephaly and related midline cerebral anomalies: a review. *J. Child Neurol.* **1**, 3–8.

Leech, R.W., Christoferson, L.A. & Gilbertson, R.L. (1977): Dysplastic gangliocytoma (Lhermitte–Duclos disease) of the cerebellum. Case report. *J. Neurosurg.* **47**, 609–612.

Lejeune, J., Gauthier, M. & Turpin, R. (1959): Etude des chromosomes somatiques de neuf enfants monogoliens. *CR Acad. Sci.* **248**, 1721–1722.

Lemire, R.J., Beckwith, J.B. & Shepard, T.H. (1972): Iniencephaly and anencephaly with spinal retroflexion. A comparative study of eight human specimens. *Teratology* **6**, 27–36.

Lemire, R.J., Beckwith, J.B. & Warkany J (1978): Anencephaly. New York: Raven Press.

Lemire, R.J. (1987): Anencephaly. 'Malformations.' In: *Handbook of clinical neurology*, vol. 50, eds. P.J. Vinken, G.W. Bruyn & H.L. Klawans, pp. 71–95. Amsterdam: Elsevier Science Publishers.

Lemire, R.J., Loeser, J.D., Leonard, C.M., Voeller, K.K.S., Lombardino, L.J., Morris, M.K., Hynd, G.W., Alexander, A.W., Anderson, H.G., Garofalakis, M., Honeyman, J.C., Mao, J. et al. (1993): Anomalous cerebral structure in dyslexia revealed with magnetic resonance imaging. *Arch. Neurol.* **50**, 461–469.

Levine, D.N., Fischer, M.A. & Caviness, V.C. Jr, (1974): Porencephaly with microgyria: a pathologic study. *Acta Neuropathol. (Berl.)* **29**, 99–113.

Levy, H.L., Lobbregt, D., Sansaricq, C. & Snyderman, S.E. (1992): Comparison of phenylketonuric and nonphenylketonuric sibs from untreated pregnancies in a mother with phenylketonuria. *Am. J. Med. Genet.* **44**, 439–442.

Lhermitte, J. & Duclos, P. (1920): Sur une ganglioneurome diffus du cortex du cervelet. *Bull. Assoc. Fr. Cancer* **9**, 99–107.

Lindhout, D. & Barth, P.G. (1985): Chorioretinal coloboma and Joubert syndrome. *J. Pediatr.* **107**, 158–159 (letter).

Loeser, J.D. & Alvord, E.C. Jr. (1968): Clinicopathological correlations in agenesis of the corpus callosum. *Neurology* **18**, 745–756.

Lonton, A.O. (1984): In infantile hydrocephalus how much brain mantle is needed for normal development? In: *Dilemmas in the management of the neurological patient*, eds. C. Warlow & J. Garfield, pp. 260–269. New York: Churchill Livingstone.

Lorber, J. (1967): The prognosis of occipital encephalocele. *Dev. Med. Child. Neurol.* (suppl.) **13**, 75–86.

Lott, I.T., Williams, R.S., Schnur, J.A. & Hier, D.B. (1979): Familial amentia, unusual ventricular calcifications, and increased cerebrospinal fluid protein. *Neurology* **29**, 1571–1577.

Lou, H.C. (1988): The 'lost autoregulation hypothesis' and brain lesions in the newborn B an update. *Brain Dev.* **10**, 143–146.

Lurie, I.W., Nedzed, M.K., Lazjuk, G.I., Kirillova, I.A., Cherstvoy, E.D., Ostrovskaja, T.I. & Shved, I.A. (1980): The XK-aprosencephaly syndrome. *Am. J. Med. Genet.* **7**, 231–234.

Lyon, G., Raymond, G., Mogami, K., Gadisseux, J.F. & Della Giustina, E. (1993): Disorder of cerebellar foliation in Walker's lissencephaly and neu-laxova syndrome. *J. Neuropathol. Exp. Neurol.* **52**, 633–639.

Macchi, G. & Bentivoglio, M. (1987): Agenesis or hypoplasia of cerebellar structures. 'Malformations.' In: *Handbook of clinical neurology*, vol. 50, eds. P.J. Vinken, G.W. Bruyn, H.L. Klavans, pp. 175–196. Amsterdam: Elsevier Science Publishers.

MacFarlane, A. & Maloney, A.F.J. (1957): The appearance of aqueduct and its relationship to hydrocephalus in the Arnold-Chiari malformation. *Brain* **80**, 479–491.

Mackiewicz, S. (1935): Uber ein Fall von halbseitiger Aplasia des Kleinhirns. *Schweiz Arch. Neurol. Psychiatr.* 36, 81–111.

Madonick, M.J. & Ruskin, A.P. (1962): Recurrent oculomotor paresis. Paresis associated with a vascular anomaly, carotid-basilar anastomosis. *Arch. Neurol.* **6**, 353–357.

Main, D.M. & Mennuti, M.T. (1986): Neural tube defects: issues in prenatal diagnosis and counseling. *Obstet. Gynecol.* **67**, 1–16.

Mann, D.M. & Esiri, M.M. (1989): The pattern of acquisition of plaques and tangles in the brains of patients under 50 years of age with Down's syndrome. *J. Neurol. Sci.* **89**, 169–179.

Manson, J., Speed, I., Abbott. K. & Crompton, J. (1988): Congenital blindness, porencephaly, and neonatal thrombocytopenia: a report of four cases. *J. Child Neurol.* **3**, 120–124.

Manz, H.J., Phillips, T.M., Rowden, G. & McCullough, D.C. (1979): Unilateral megalencephaly, cerebral cortical dysplasia, neuronal hypertrophy, and heterotopia: cytomorphometric, fluorometric cytochemical, and biochemical analyses. *Acta Neuropathol. (Berl.)* **45**, 97–103.

Marchuk, D.A., Saulino, A.M., Tavakkol Swaroop, M., Wallace, M.R., Anderson, L.B., Mitchell, A.L., Gutmann, D.H., Boguski, M. & Collins, F.S. (1991): cDNA cloning of the type 1 neurofibromatosis gene: complete sequence of the NF1 gene product. *Genomics* **11**, 931–940.

Marin-Padilla, M. (1975): Abnormal neuronal differentiation (functional maturation) in mental retardation. *Birth Defects OAS* **11**, (7), 133–153.

Marin-Padilla, M. & Marin-Padilla, T.M. (1981): Morphogenesis of experimentally induced Arnold-Chiari malformation. *J. Neurol. Sci.* **50**, 29–55.

Marques Dias, M.J., Harmant-van Rijckevorsel, G., Landrieu, P. & Lyon, G. (1984): Prenatal cytomegalovirus disease and cerebral microgyria: evidence for perfusion failure, not disturbance of histogenesis, as the major cause of fetal cytomegalovirus encephalopathy. *Neuropediatrics* **15**, 18–24.

Masliah, E., Achim, C.L., Ge, N., DeTeresa, R. & Wiley, C.A. (1994): Cellular neuropathology in HIV encephalitis. In: *HIV, AIDS, and the Brain,* vol. 72, eds. R.W. Price & S.W. Perry, pp. 119–131. New York: Raven Press. Research publications (Association for Research in Nervous and Mental Disease).

Matson, D.D. & Ingraham, F.D. (1951): Intracranial complication of congenital dermal sinuses. *Pediatrics* **8**, 463–474.

Matson, D.D. (1969): *Neurosurgery of infancy and childhood,* 2nd ed. Springfield, Ill: Thomas.

Matsubara, O., Tanaka, M., Ida, T. & Okeda, R. (1983): Hemimegalencephaly with hemihypertrophy (Klippel–Trenaunay–Weber syndrome). *Virchows. Archiv. A. Pathol. Anat. Histopathol.* **400**, 155–162.

McBride, M.C. & Kemper, T.L. (1982): Pathogenesis of four-layered microgyric cortex in man. *Acta Neuropathol. (Berl.)* **57**, 93–98.

McComb, J.G. & Davis, R.L. (1990): Choroid plexus cerebrospinal fluid hydrocephalus cerebral edema and herniation phenomenon. In: *Textbook of neuropathology*, eds. R.L. Davis & M.D. Robertson, pp. 175–206. Baltimore: Williams & Williams,

McCormick, P.C., Michelsen, W.J., Post, K.D., Carmel, P.W. & Stein, B.M. (1988): Cavernous malformations of the spinal cord. *Neurosurgery* **23**, 459–463.

McLaurin, R.L. (1987): Encephalocele and cranium bifidum. 'Malformations.' In: *Handbook of clinical neurology*, vol. 50, eds. P.J. Vinken, G.W. Bruyn & H.L. Klawans, pp. 97–111. Amsterdam: Elsevier Science Publishers.

McLendon, R.E., Crain, B.J., Oakes, W.J. & Burger, P.C. (1985): Cerebral polygyria in the Chiari Type II (Arnold-Chiari) malformation. *Clin. Neuropathol.* **4**, 200–205.

Menkes, J.H., Philippart, M. & Clark, D.B. (1964): Hereditary partial agenesis of the corpus callosum: biochemical and pathological studies. *Arch. Neurol.* **11**, 198–208.

Michaud, J., Mizhari, E.M. & Urich, H. (1982): Agenesis of the vermis with fusion of the cerebellar hemispheres, septo-optic dysplasia and associated anomalies. Report of a case. *Acta Neuropathol. (Berl.)* **56**, 161–166.

Miller, J.Q. (1963): Lissencephaly in 2 siblings. *Neurology* **13**, 841–850.

Miller, R.W. (1990): Effects of prenatal exposure to ionizing radiation. *Health Phys.* **59**, 57–61.

Mischel, P.S., Nguyen, L.P. & Vinters, H.V. (1992): Cerebral cortical dysplasia, associated with pediatric epilepsy. Review of neuropathologic features and proposal for a grading system. *J. Neuropathol. Exp. Neurol.* **54**, 137–153.

Modesti, L.M., Glasauer, F.E. & Terplan, K.L. (1977): Sphenoethmoidal encephalocele. *Child's Brain* **3**, 140–153.

Moebius, J.P. (1888): Ueber angeborene doppelseitige Abducens-Facialis-Lahmung. *Muncher. Med. Wochenschr.* **35**, 91–94, 108–111.

Moessinger, A.C. (1983): Fetal akinesia deformation sequence: an animal model. *Pediatrics* **72**, 857–863.

Mohr, P.D., Strang, F.A., Sambrook, M.A. & Boddie, H.G. (1977): The clinical and surgical feature in 40 patients with primary cerebellar ectopia (adult Chiari malformation). *Q. J. .Med.* **46**, 85–96.

Morel, F. & Wildi, E. (1952): Dysgenesis nodulaire disseminee de l'ecorce frontale. *Rev. Neurol.* **87**, 251–270.

Moreland, D.B., Glasauer, F.E., Egnatchik, J.G., Heffner, R.R. & Alker, G.J. Jr. (1988): Focal cortical dysplasia. Case report. *J. Neurosurg.* **68**, 487–490.

Müller, F. & O'Rahilly, R. (1984): Cerebral dysraphia (future anencephaly) in a human twin embryo at stage 13. *Teratology* **30**, 167–177.

Müller, F. & O'Rahilly, R. (1989): Mediobasal prosencephalic defects, including holoprosencephaly and cyclopia, in relation to the development of the human forebrain. *Am. J. Anat.* **185**, 391–414.

Munchoff, C. & Noetzel, H. (1965): Uber eine nahezu totale Agyrie bei einem 6 Jahre alt gewordenen Knaben. *Acta Neuropathol. (Berl.)* **4**, 469–475.

Myrianthopoulos, N.C. (1981): 'Craniosynostosis. Neurogenetic directory, Part 1.' In: *Handbook of clinical neurology*, vol. 42, eds. P.J. Vinken & G.W. Bruyn, pp. 20–21. Amsterdam: North Holland Publishing Co.

Myrianthopoulos, N.C. & Melnik, M. (1987): Studies in neural tube defects. I. Epidemiologic and etiologic aspects. *Am. J. Med. Genet.* **26**, 783–796.

Naidich, T.P., Pudlowski, R.M., Naidich, J.B., Garnish, M. & Rodriguez, F.J. (1980a): Computed tomographic signs of the Chiari II malformation. Part I. Skull and dural partitions. *Radiology* **134**, 65–71.

Naidich, T.P., Pudlowski,R.M. & Naidich, J.B. (1980b): Computed tomographic signs of the Chiari II malformation. Part II. Midbrain and cerebellum. *Radiology* **134**, 391–398.

Naidich, T.P., Pudlowski, R.M. & Naidich, J.B.(1980c): Computed tomographic signs of the Chiari II malformation. Part III. Ventricles and cisterns. *Radiology* **134**, 657–663.

Naidich, T.P., McLone, D.G. & Fulling, K.H. (1983): The Chiari II malformation: Part IV. The hindbrain deformity. *Neuroradiology* **25**, 179–197.

Naidich, T.P., McLone, D.G., Bauer, B.S. *et al.* (1983): Midline craniofacial dysraphism. Midline cleft upper lip basal encephalocele, callosal agenesis and optic nerve dysplasia. *Concepts Pediatr. Neurosurg.* **4**, 186–207.

Nakamura, T. (1984): [Diagnosis and treatment of tethered spinal cord syndrome C based on experience of 77 cases.] Published in Japanese. *Nippon Seikeigeka Gakkai Zasshi.* **58**, 1237–1251.

Nakamura, Y., Hashimoto, T., Sasaguri, Y., Yamana, K., Tanaka, S., Morodomi, T., Murakami, T., Maehara, F., Nakashima, T., Fukuda, S. *et al.* (1986a): Brain anomalies found in 18 trisomy: CT scanning, morphologic and morphometric study. *Clin. Neuropathol.* **5**, 47–52.

Nakamura, Y., Fujiyoshi, Y., Fukuda, S., Matsunaga, T., Hashimoto, T., Manabe, A. & Nakashima, T. (1986b): Cystic brain lesions in utero. *Acta Pathol. Jpn.* **36**, 613–620.

Nakano, K.K. (1973): Anencephaly: a review. *Dev. Med. Child. Neurol.* **15**, 383–400.

Nau, H. (1994): Valproic acid-induced neural tube defects. In: *Neural tube defects*, Ciba Found. Symp. 181, pp. 144–151.

Nelen, M.R., Padberg, G.W., Peeters, E.A.J., Lin, A.Y., van den Helm, B., Frants, R.R., Coulon, V., Goldstein, A.M., van Reen, M.M., Easton, D.F., Eales, R.A., Hodgsen, S., Mulvihill, J.J., Murday, V.A., Tucker, M.A., Mariman, E.C., Starink, T.M., Ponder, B.A., Ropers, H.H, Kremer, H., Longy, M. & Eng, C. (1996): Localization of the gene for Cowden disease to chromosome 10q 22–23. *Nat. Genet.* **13**, 114–116.

Neuburger, T. & Edinger, L. (1898): Einseltiges fast totaler Mangel des Cerebellums. Varix oblongata Herztod durch Accessoriumreizung. *Berliner Klin. Wochenschr.* **35**, 69–72, 100–103.

Newman, G.C., Buschi, A.I., Sugg, N.K., Kelly, T.E. & Miller, J.Q. (1982): Dandy-walker syndrome diagnosed in utero by ultrasonography. *Neurology* **32**, 180–184.

Nishimura, H. & Okamoto, N. (1977): Iniencephaly. 'Congenital malformations of the brain and skull, Part I.' In: *Handbook of clinical neurology*, vol. 30, eds. P.J. Vinken & G.W. Bruyn, pp. 257–268. Amsterdam: North-Holland Publishing Company.

Nora, J.J. & Fraser, F.C. (1994): In: *Medical genetics: principles and practice*, 4th edn., eds. J.J. Nora & F.C. Fraser. Philadelphia: Lea and Febiger.

Norman, R.M. (1966): Neuropathological findings in trisomies 13–15 and 17–18 with special reference to cerebellum. *Dev. Med. Child. Neurol.* **8**, 170–177.

Norman, M.G. (1972): Antenatal neuronal loss and gliosis of the reticular formation, thalamus and hypothalamus. A report of three cases. *Neurology* **22**, 910–916.

Norman, M.G. & Becker, L.E. (1974): Cerebral damage in neonates resulting from arteriovenous malformation of the vein of Galen. *J. Neurol. Neurosurg. Psychiatr.* **37**, 252–258.

Norman, M.G., Roberts, M., Sirois, J. & Tremblay, L.J. (1976): Lissencephaly. *Can. J. Neurol. Sci.* **3**, 39–46.

Norman, M.G. & Schoene, W.C. (1977): The ultrastructure of Sturge–Weber disease. *Acta Neuropathol. (Berl.)* **37**, 199–205.

Norman, M.G. (1978): Perinatal brain damage. *Perspect. Pediatr. Pathol.* **4**, 41–92.

Norman, M.G. (1980): Bilateral encephaloclastic lesions in a 26 week gestation fetus: effect on neuroblast migration. *Can. J. Neurol. Sci.* **7**, 191–194.

Norman, M.G., Thurber, L.A. & Woolley, H.E. (1981): Abnormal leptomeninges and vessels causing fetal hydrocephalus: diagnosis of hydrocephalus at 19 weeks gestation by ultrasound. *Acta Neuropathol. (Berl.)* **54**, 283–285.

Norman, M.G. & O'Kusky, J.R. (1986): The growth and development of microvasculature in human cerebral cortex. *J. Neuropathol. Exp. Neurol.* **45**, 222–232.

Norman, M.G. & McGillivray, B. (1988): Fetal neuropathology of proliferative vasculopathy and hydranencephaly-hydrocephaly with multiple limb pterygia. *Pediatr. Neurosci.* **14**, 301–306.

Norman, M.G. & Ludwin, S.K. (1991): Congenital malformations of the nervous system. In: *Textbook of neuropathology*, eds R.L. Davis & D.M. Robertson, pp. 207–280. Baltimore: Williams & Wilkins.

Norman, M.G., Mc Gillivray, B.C., Kalousek, D.K., Hill, A. & Paskitt, K.J. (1995): Congenital Malformations of the Brain: Pathologic, Embryologic, Clinical, Radiologic, and Genetic Aspects. New York: Oxford University Press.

Nyland, H. & Krogness, K.G. (1978): Size of posterior fossa in Chiari type I malformation in adults. *Acta Neurochir. (Wein)* **40**, 233–242.

Oakley, G.P. Jr., Erickson, J.D., James, L.M., Mulinare, J. & Cordero, J.F. (1994): Prevention for folic acid-preventable spina bifida and anencephaly. Ciba Found. Symp. 181, pp. 212–223; discussion 223–231.

Ogunmekan, A.O., Hwang, P.A. & Hoffman, H.J. (1989): Sturge–Weber–Dimitri disease: role in hemispherectomy in prognosis. *Can. J. Neurol. Sci.* **16**, 78–80.

Opitz, J.M. & Sutherland, G.R. (1984): Conference report: International workshop on the fragile X and X-linked mental retardation. *Am. J. Med. Genet.* **17**, 5–94.

Opitz, J.M. & Gilbert-Barness, E.F. (1990): Reflections on the pathogenesis of Down syndrome. *Am. J. Med. Genet. Suppl.* **7**, 38–51.

O'Rahilly, R. & Müller, F. (1989): Interpretation of some median anomalies as illustrated by cyclopia and symmelia. *Teratology* **40**, 409–421.

O'Rahilly, R. & Müller, F. (1994): Neurulation in the normal human embryo. Ciba Found. Symp. 181, pp. 70–82 discussion 82–89.

Osaka, K., Tanimura, T., Hirayama, A. & Matsumoto, S. (1978): Myelomeningocele before birth. *J. Neurosurg.* **49**, 711–724.

Ostertag, B. (1956): Uber die grundlagen der Formbildung und der Fehlentwicklung im Zentralnervensystems. *Ztbld. ges. Neurol. Psychiat.* **135**, 257–259.

Ostertag, B. (1957): Missbildungen. Handbuch der speziella pathologischen Anatomic und Histologic, vol. XII/4, eds. F. Henke, O. Lubarsch & R. Rössle, pp. 282–601. Berlin: Springer Verlag.

Ostlere, S.J., Irving, H.C. & Lilford, R.J. (1990): Fetal choroid plexus cysts: a report of 100 cases. *Radiology* **175**, 753–755.

Ostrovskaya, T.I. & Lazjuk, G.I. (1988): Cerebral abnormalities in the Neu–Laxova syndrome. *Am. J. Med. Genet.* **30**, 747–756.

Paetau, A., Salonen, R. & Haltia, M. (1985): Brain pathology in the Meckel syndrome: a study of 59 cases. *Clin. Neuropathol.* **4**, 56–62.

Padberg, G.W., Schot, J.D., Vielvoye, G.J., Bots, G.T. & de Beer, F.C. (1991): Lhermitte–Duclos disease and Cowden disease: a single phakomatosis. *Ann. Neurol.* 1991, **29**, 517–523.

Padget, D.H. (1972): Development of so-called dysraphism; with embryologic evidence of clinical Arnold-Chiari and Dandy–Walker malformations. *Johns Hopkins Med. J.* **130**, 127–165.

Palmini, A., Andermann, F., Olivier, A., Tampieri, D., Robitaille, Y., Andermann, E. & Wright, G. (1991): Focal neuronal migration disorders and intractable partial epilepsy: a study of 30 patients. *Ann. Neurol.* **30**, 741–749.

Paneth, N., Rudelli, R., Kazam, E. & Monte, W. (1994): Brain damage in the preterm infant. In: *Clin. Dev. Med.*, no. 131. London: Mac Keith Press. Distributed by Cambridge University Press, Cambridge, England.

Pang, D., Dias, M.S. & Ahab-Barmada, M. (1992): Split cord malformation. Part I: A unified theory of embryogenesis for double spinal cord malformations. *Neurosurgery* **31**, 451–480.

Park, I.S., Cail, W.S., Delashaw, J.B. & Kattwinkel, J. (1986): Spinal cord arteriovenous malformation in a neonate. Case report. *J. Neurosurg.* **64**, 322–324.

Parish, W.R. (1989): Intrauterine herpes simplex virus infections: Hydranencephaly and a nonvesicular rash in an infant. *Int. J. Dermatol.* **28**, 397–401.

Passarge, E. & Lenz, W. (1966): Syndrome of caudal regression in infants of diabetic mothers: observations of further cases. *Pediatrics* **37**, 672–675.

Paul, K.S., Lye, R.H., Strang, F.A. & Dutton, J. (1983): Arnold-Chiari malformation. Review of 71 cases. *J. Neurosurg.* **58**, 183–187.

Pavone, L., Gullotta, F., Incorpora, G., Grasso, S. & Dobyns, W.B. (1990): Isolated lissencephaly: report of four patients from two unrelated families. *J. Child Neurol.* **5**, 52–59.

Pavone, L., Curatolo, P., Rizzo, R., Micali, G., Incorpora, G., Garg, B.P., Dunn, D.W. & Dobyns, W.B. (1991): Epidermal nevus syndrome: a neurologic variant with hemimegalencephaly gyral malformation, mental retardation, seizures, and facial hemihypertrophy. *Neurology* **41**, 266–271.

Peach, B. (1965): The Arnold-Chiari malformation. Morphogenesis. *Arch. Neurol.* **12**, 527–535.

Persutte, W.H., Kurczynski, T.W., Chandhuri, K., Lenke, R.R., Woldenberg, L. & Brinker, R.A. (1990): Prenatal diagnosis of autosomal dominant microcephaly and postnatal evaluation with magnetic resonans imaging. *Prenat. Diagn.* **10**, 631–642.

Pfeiffer, J., Majewski, F., Fischbach, H., Bierich, J.R. & Volk, B. (1979): Alcohol embryo- and fetopathy. Neuropathology of 3 children and 3 fetuses. *J. Neurol. Sci.* **41**, 125–137.

Pfeiffer, G. & Friede, R.L. (1984): Unilateral hydrocephalus from early developmental occlusion of one foramen of Monro. *Acta Neuropathol. (Berl.)* **64**, 75–77.

Pollock, J.A., Newton, T.H. & Hoyt, W.F. (1968): Transsphenoidal and transethnoidal encephaloceles. A review of clinical and roentgen features in 8 cases. *Radiology* **90**, 442–453.

Prayson, R.A. & Estes, M.L. (1992): Dysembryoplastic neuroepithelial tumor. *Am. J. Clin. Pathol.* **97**, 398–401.

Prayson, R.A., Estes, M.L. & Morris, H.H. (1993): Coexistence of neoplasia and cortical dysplasia in patients presenting with seizures. *Epilepsia* **34**, 609–615.

Prevot, J., Gueriot, S., Mataizeau, J.P. & Leveau, P. (1984): [Duplication of the complete lumbosacral spine. A propos of 1 case.] Published in French. *Chir. Pediatr.* **25**, 87–89.

Probst, M. (1901): Ueber den Bau des vollstandig balkenlasen Grosshirns sowie uber mikrogyrie und Heterotopie der grauen Substanz. *Arch. Psychiatr. Nervenkrankheit.* **34**, 709–786.

Purpura, D.P. (1975): Dendritic differentiation in human cerebral cortex: normal and aberrant developmental patterns. *Adv. Neurol.* **12**, 91–134.

Qazi, Q.H. & Reed, T.E. (1975): A possible major contribution to mental retardation in the general population by the gene for microcephaly. *Clin. Genet.* **7**, 85–90.

Raghavan, N., Barkovich, A.J., Edwards, M. & Norman, D. (1989): MR imaging in the tethered spinal cord syndrome. *AJR Am. J. Roentgenol.* **152**, 843–852.

Rakic, P. (1988): Defects of neuronal migration and the pathogenesis of cortical malformations. *Prog. Brain Res.* **73**, 15–37.

Raymond, A.A., Fisch, D.R., Sisodiya, S.M., Alsanjari, N., Stevens, J.M. & Shorvon, S.D. (1995): Abnormalities gyration, heterotopia, tuberous sclerosis, focal cortical dysplasia, microdysgenesis dysembryoplastic neuroepithelial tumour and dysgenesis of the archicortex in epilepsy. Clinical, EEG, and neuroimaging features in 100 adult patients. *Brain* **118**, 629–660.

Raz, N., Torres, I.J., Briggs, S.D., Spencer, W.D., Thornton, A.E., Loken, W.J., Gunning, F.M., McQuinn, J.D., Oriesen, N.R. & Acker, J.D. (1995): Selective neuroanatomic abnormalities in Down's syndrome and their cognitive correlations: evidence from MRI morphometry. *Neurology* **45**, 356–366.

Rengachary, S.S. & Watanabe, I. (1981): Ultrastructure and pathogenesis of intracranial arachnoid cysts. *J. Neuropathol. Exp. Neurol.* **40**, 61–83.

Reil, J.C. (1812): Mangel des mittleven und freyentheils des Balkens im Menschengchirn. *Arch. Physiol.* **11**, 341–344.

Reznik, M. & Pierard, G.E. (1995): Neurophakomatoses and allied disorders. In: *Pediatric neuropathology*, ed. W. Duckett, pp. 734–755. Baltimore: Williams & Wilkins.

Reznikoff-Etievant, M.F. (1988): Management of alloimmune neonatal and antenatal thrombocytopenia. *Vox Sang* **55**, 193–201.

Ricci, S., Cusmai, R., Fariello, G., Fusco, L. & Vigevano, F. (1992): Double cortex. A neuronal migration anomaly as a possible cause of Lennox-Gastaut syndrome. *Arch. Neurol.* **49**, 61–64.

Richman, D.P., Stewart, R.M. & Caviness, V.S., Jr. (1974): Cerebral microgyria in a 27-week fetus: an architectonic and topographic analysis. *J. Neuropathol. Exp. Neurol.* **33**, 374–384.

Roach, E.S., Smith, M., Huttenlocher, P., Bhat, M., Alcorn, D. & Hawley, L. (1992): Diagnostic criteria: tuberous sclerosis complex. Report of the Diagnostic Criteria Committee of the National Tuberous Sclerosis Association. *J. Child Neurol.* **7**, 221–224.

Robain, O. & Lyon, G. (1972): Les microcephalies familiales par malformation cerebrale. Etude anatomo-clinique. *Acta Neuropathol. (Berl.)* **20**, 96–109.

Robain, O. & Pansot, G. (1978): Effects of undernutrition on glial maturation. *Brain Res.* **149**, 379–397.

Robain, O. & Deonna, T. (1983): Pachygyria and congenital nephrosis disorder of migration and neuronal orientation. *Acta Neuropathol. (Berl.)* **60**, 137–141.

Robinson, R.O. (1991): Familial schizencephaly. *Dev. Med. Child. Neurol.* **33**, 1010–1020.

Rodriguez, J.I., Garcia, M., Morales, C., Morillo, A. & Delicado, A.(1990): Trisomy 13 syndrome and neural tube defects. *Am. J. Med. Genet.* **36**, 513–516.

Roessmann, U. & Wongmongkolrit, T. (1984): Dysplastic gangliocytoma of cerebellum in a newborn. Case report. *J. Neurosurg.* **60**, 845–847.

Roessmann, U., Velasco, M.E., Small, E.J. & Hori, A. (1987): Neuropathology of 'septo-optic dysplasia' (de Morsier syndrome) with immunohistochemical studies of the hypothalamus and pituitary gland. *J. Neuropathol. Exp. Neurol.* **46**, 597–608.

Rorke, L.B. & Spiro, A.J. (1967): Cerebral lesions in congenital rubella syndrome. *J. Pediatr.* **70**, 243–255.

Rorke, L.B. (1992a): Anatomical features of the developing brain implicated in pathogenesis of hypoxic-ischemic injury. *Brain Pathol.* **2**, 211–221.

Rorke, L.B. (1992b): Perinatal brain damage. In: *Greenfield's neuropathology*, 5th edn., eds. J.H. Adams & L.W. Duchen, pp. 639–708. New York: Oxford University Press.

Rorke, L.B. (1994): A perspective: the role of disordered genetic control of neurogenesis in the pathogenesis of migration disorders. *J. Neuropathol. Exp. Neurol.* **53**, 105–117.

Rosa, F.W. (1991): Spina bifida in infants of women treated with carbamizepine during pregnancy. *N. Engl. J. Med.* **324**, 674–677.

Ross, J.J. & Frias, J.L. (1977): Microcephaly. 'Congenital malformations of the brain and skull, Part I.' In: *Handbook of clinical neurology*, vol. 30, eds. P.J. Vinken & G.W. Bruyn, pp. 507–524. Amsterdam: North Holland Publishing Co.

Ross, M.H., Galaburda, A.M. & Kemper, T.L. (1984): Down's syndrome: is there a decreased population of neurons? *Neurology* **34**, 909–916.

Rouleau, G.A., Wertelecki, W., Haines, J.L., Hobbs, W.J., Trofatter, J.A., Seizinger, B.R., Martuza, R.L.,Superneau, D.W., Conneally, P.M. & Gussella, J.F. (1987): Genetic linkage of bilateral acustic neurofibromatosis to a DNA marker on chromosome 22. *Nature* **329**, 246–248.

Rowlatt, U. & Pruzansky, S. (1980): Premaxillary agenesis, ocular hypotelorism, holoprosencephaly, and extracranial anomalies in an infant with a normal karyogram. *Cleft Palate J.* **17**, 197–204.

Rubinstein, H.S. & Freeman, W. (1940): Cerebellar agenesis. *J. Nerv. Ment. Dis.* **92**, 489–502.

Rubinstein, L.J. (1986): The malformative central nervous system lesions in the central and peripheral forms of neurofibromatosis. A neuropathological study of 22 cases. *Ann. N. Y. Acad. Sci.* **486**, 14–19.

Rudelli, R.D., Brown, W.T., Wiśniewski, K., Jenkins, E.C., Laure-Kamionowska, M., Connell, F. & Wiśniewski, H.M. (1985): Adult fragile X syndrome. Clinico-neuropathologic findings. *Acta Neuropathol. (Berl.)* **67**, 289–295.

Russell, D.S. & Donald, C. (1935): The mechanism of internal hydrocephalus in spina bifida. *Brain* **58**, 203–215.

Russell, D.S. (1949): Observations on the pathology of hydrocephalus. London: Med Res Council Spec Report Series No. 265, HMSO.

Russell, D.S. (1968) Observation on the pathology of hydrocephalus. Med. Res. Council Spec. Report Series No. 265, Her Majesty's Stationary Office, London 4th Impression.

Russell, D.S. & Rubinstein, L.J. (1989): The pathology of tumours of the central nervous system, 5th edn., pp. 766–808. London: Ed. Edward Arnold.

Salonen, R., Herva, R. & Novio, R. (1981): The hydrolethalus syndrome: delineation of a 'new' lethal malformation syndrome based on 28 patients. *Clin. Genet.* **19**, 321–330.

Sampson, J.R., Janssen, L.A. & Sandkuijl, L.A. (1992): Linkage investigation of three putative tuberous sclerosis determining loci on chromosomes 9q, 11q, and 12q. The Tuberous Sclerosis Collaborative Group. *J. Med. Genet.* **29**, 861–866.

Santavuori, P., Somer, H., Sainio, K., Rapola, J., Kruus, S., Nikitin, T., Ketonen, L. & Leisti, J. (1989): Muscle-eye-brain disease (MEB). *Brain Dev.* **11**, 147–153.

Sarma, M.K. & Rao, K.S. (1974): Biochemical composition of different regions in brains of small-for-date infants. *J. Neurochem.* **22**, 671–677.

Sarnat, H.B. (1922): Cerebral dysgenesis: embryology and clinical expression. New York: Oxford University Press.

Sarnat, H.B., Case, M.E. & Graviss, R. (1976): Sacral agenesis. Neurologic and neuropathologic features. *Neurology* **26**, 1124–1129.

Sarnat, H.B. & Alcala, H. (1980): Human cerebellar hypoplasia: a syndrome of diverse causes. *Arch. Neurol.* **37**, 300–305.

Sarwar, M., Virapongsa, C. & Bhimani, S. (1984): Primary tethered cord syndrome: a new hypothesis of its origin. *AJNR Am. J. Neuroradiol.* **5**, 235–242.

Schachenmayr, W. & Friede, R.L. (1979): Fine structure of arachnoid cysts. *J. Neuropathol. Exp. Neurol.* **38**, 434–446.

Schachenmayr, W. & Friede, R.L. (1982): Rhombencephalosynapsis: a Viennese malformation? *Dev. Med. Child. Neurol.* **24**, 178–182.

Schady, W., Metcalfe, R.A. & Butler, P. (1987): The incidence of craniocervical bone anomalies in the adult Chiari malformation. *J. Neurol. Sci.* **82**, 193–203.

Scherer, E. (1935a): Uber pialen Lipome des Gehirns. Beitrag eines Fales von ausgedehnter meningeoler Lipomatose eines Grasshirnhemisphere bei Microgyric. *Z. Neurol. Psychiatr.* **154**, 45–61.

Scherer, E. (1935b): Uber Cystenbildung der weichen Hirnhaute in Liquorraum der Sylvischen Furche mit hochgradiger Deformierung des Gehirns. *Arch. Psychiatr. Nervenkr.* **152**, 787–799.

Scherrer, C.C., Hammer, F., Schinzel, A. & Briner, J. (1992): Brain stem and cervical cord dysraphic lesions in iniencephaly. *Pediatr. Pathol.* **12**, 469–476.

Schinzel, A. (1988): Microdeletion syndromes, balanced translocations and gene mapping. *J. Med. Genet.* **25**, 454–462.

Schinzel, A. & Kaufmann, U. (1986): The acrocallosal syndrome in sisters. *Clin. Genet.* **30**, 399–405.

Schmidt-Sidor, B., Wiśniewski, K.E., Shepard, T.H. & Sersen, E.A. (1990): Brain growth in Down syndrome subjects 15 to 22 weeks of gestational age and birth to 60 months. *Clin. Neuropathol.* **9**, 181–190.

Scott, B.S., Petit, T.L., Becker, L.E. & Edwards, B.A. (1982): Abnormal electric membrane properties of Down's syndrome DRG neurons in cell culture. *Brain Res.* **2**, 257–270.

Scott, B.S., Becker, L.E. & Petit, T.L. (1983): Neurobiology of Down's syndrome. *Prog. Neurobiol.* **21**, 199–237.

Segall, H.D., Pitts, F.W., Rumbaugh, C.L., Bergeron, R.T., Teal, J.S. & Gwinn, J.L. (1974): Foramen of Monro obstruction in children. Intra-axial lesions. *Radiology* **110**, 125–134.

Seizinger, B.R., Rouleau, G.A., Ozelius, L.J., Lane, A.H., Farmer, G.E., Lamiell, J.M., Haines, J., Yuen, J.W., Collins, D., Majoor-Krakauer, D. *et al.* (1988): Von Hippel–Lindau disease maps to the region of chromosome 3 associated with renal cell carcinoma. *Nature* **332**, 268–269.

Serur, D., Jeret, J.S. & Wiśniewski, K. (1988): Agenesis of the corpus callosum: clinical, neuroradiological and cytogenetic studies. *Neuropediatrics* **19**, 87–91.

Shapiro, W.R., Williams, G.H. & Plum, F. (1969): Spontaneous recurrent hypothermia accompanying agenesis of the corpus callosum. *Brain* **92**, 423–436.

Shaw, C.M. & Alvord, E.C. Jr. (1995): Hydrocephalus. In: *Pediatric neuropathology*, ed. W. Duckett, pp. 149–211. Baltimore: Williams & Wilkins.

Shepard, T.H. (1986): Teratogenesis: general principles. In: *Drug and chemical action in pregnancy: pharmacologic and toxicologic principles*, eds. S. Fabro & A.R .Scialli, pp. 237–250. New York: M. Dekker.

Shepard, T.H. (1992): *Catalog of Teratogenic Agents*, 7th ed. Baltimore: Johns Hopkins University Press.

Sidman, R.L. & Rakic, P. (1982): Development of the human central nervous system. In: *Histology and histopathology of the nervous system*, vol. 1, eds. W. Haymaker & R.D. Adams, pp. 3–145. Illinois: Thomas, Springfield.

Siebert, J.R., Warkany, J. & Lemire, R.J. (1986): Atelencephalic microcephaly in a 21-week human fetus. *Teratology* **34**, 9–19.

Siebert, J.R., Kokich, V.G., Warkany, J. & Lemire, R.J. (1987): Atelencephalic microcephaly: craniofacial anatomy and morphologic comparisons with holoprosencephaly and anencephaly. *Teratology* **36**, 279–285.

Siebert, J.R., Cohen, M.M. Jr., Sulik, K.K. *et al.* (1990): Holoprosencephaly: an overview and atlas of cases. pp. 135–139 and 365–366. New York: Wiley-Liss.

Smith, M.T. & Huntington, H.W. (1977): Inverse cerebellum and occipital encephalocele. A dorsal fusion defect uniting the Arnold-Chiari and DandyBWalker spectrum. *Neurology* **27**, 246–251.

Smith, M.T. & Huntington, H.W. (1981): Morphogenesis of experimental anencephaly. *J. Neuropathol. Exp. Neurol.* **40**, 20–31.

Spatz, M. & Laqueur, G.L. (1968): Transplacental chemical induction of microencephaly in two strains of rats. *I Proc. Soc. Exp. Biol. Med.* **129**, 705–710.

Spillane, J.D., Pallis, C. & Jones, A.M. (1957): Developmental abnormalities in the region of the foramen magnum. *Brain* **80**, 11–48.

Squier, M.V. (1993): Development of cortical dysplasia of type II lissencephaly. *Neuropatol. Appl. Neurobiol.* **19**, 209–213.

Steinbok, B. & Cochrane, D.D. (1991): The nature of congenital posterior cervical or cervicothoracic midline cutaneous mass lesions. *J. Neurosurg.* **75**, 206–212. [Published erratum appears in *J. Neurosurg.* **75**, 1003].

Sternberg, C. (1912): Ueber vollstandigen Defekt des Kleinhirnes. *Verhundlungen. Dtsch. Pathol. Ges.* **15**, 353–359.

Stewart, R.M. Richman, D.P. & Caviness, V.C. Jr. (1975): Lissencephaly and Pachygyria: an architectonic and topographical analysis. *Acta Neuropathol. (Berl.)* **31**, 1–12.

Suchet, I.B. (1994): Schizencephaly: antenatal and postnatal assessment with colour-flow Doppler imaging. *Can. Assoc. Radiol. J.* **45**, 193–200.

Suetsugu, M. & Mehraein, P. (1980): Spine distribution along the apical dendrites of the pyramidal neurons in Down's syndrome. A quantitative Golgi Study. *Acta Neuropathol. (Berl.)* **50**, 207–210.

Sugimoto, T., Yasuhara, A., Nishida, N., Murakami, K., Woo, M. & Kobayaski, J. (1993): MRI of the head in the evaluation of microcephaly. *Neuropediatrics* **24**, 4–7.

Sulik, K.K. & Johnston, M.C. (1982): Embryonic origin of holoprosencephaly: interrelationship of the developing brain and face. *Scan. Electron. Microsc.* **pt 1**, 309–322.

Sutherland, G.R., Gedeon, A., Kornman, L., Donnelly, A., Byard, R.W., Mulley, J.C., Kremer, E., Lynch, M., Pritchard, M., Yu, S. *et al.* (1991): Prenatal diagnosis of fragile X syndrome by direct detection of the unstable DNA sequence. *N. Engl. J. Med.* **325**, 1720–1722.

Suwanwela, C. & Suwanwela, N. (1972): A morphological classification of sincipital encephalomeningoceles. *J. Neurosurg.* **36**, 201–211.

Taggart, J.K. & Walker, A.E. (1942): Congenital atresia of the foramina of Luschka and Magendie. *Arch. Neurol. Psychiatr.* **48**, 583–612.

Tajima, M., Yamada, H. & Kageyama, N. (1977): Craniolacunia in newborn with myelomeningocele. *Child's Brain* **3**, 297–303.

Takada, K., Nakamura, H. & Tanaka, J. (1984): Cortical dysplasia in congenital muscular dystrophy with central nervous system involvement (Fukuyama type). *J. Neuropathol. Exp. Neurol.* **43**, 395–407.

Takashima, S. & Becker, L.E. (1980): Neuropathology of cerebral arteriovenous malformations in children. *J. Neurol. Neurosurg. Psychiatr.* **43**, 380–385.

Takashima, S., Chan, F., Becker, L.E. & Armstrong, D.L. (1980): Morphology of the developing visual cortex of the human infant: a quantitative and qualitative Golgi study. *J. Neuropathol. Exp. Neurol.* **39**, 487–501.

Takashima, S. & Becker, L.E. (1985): Basal ganglia calcification in Down syndrome. *J. Neurol. Neurosurg. Psychiatr.* **48**, 61–64.

Takashima, S., Becker, L.E., Chan, F. *et al.* (1987): A Golgi study of the cerebral cortex in Fukuyama-type congenital muscular dystrophy, Walker-type 'lissencephaly,' and classical lissencephaly. *Brain Dev.* **9**, 621–626.

Takeuchi, I.K. & Takeuchi, Y.K. (1985): 5-Azacytidine-induced exencephaly in mice. *J. Anat.* **140**, 403–412.

Takada, K., Becker, L.E. & Chan, F. (1988): Aberrant dendritic development in the human agyric cortex: a quantitative and qualitative Golgi study of two cases. *Clin. Neuropathol.* **7**, 111–119.

Tal, Y., Freigang, B., Dunn, H.G., Durity, F.A. & Moyes, P.D. (19800: Dandy–Walker syndrome: analysis of 21 cases. *Dev. Med. Child. Neurol.* **22**, 189–201.

Tamaki, N., Shirataki, K., Kojima, N., Shouse, Y. & Matsumoto, S. (1988): Tethered cord syndrome of delayed onset following repair of myelomeningocele. *J. Neurosurg.* **69**, 393–398.

Tanaka, T., Takamura, H., Takashima, S., Kodama, T. & Hasegawa, H. (1985): A rare case of Aicardi syndrome with severe brain malformation and hepatoblastoma. *Brain Dev.* **7**, 507–512.

Taylor, D.C., Falconer, M.A., Bruton, C.J. & Corsellis, J.A. (1971): Focal dysplasia of the cerebral cortex in epilepsy. *J. Neurol. Neurosurg. Psychiatr.* **34**, 369–387.

Terplan, K.L., Sandberg, A.A. & Aceto, T. Jr. (1966): Structural anomalies in the cerebellum in association with trisomy. *JAMA* **197**, 557–568.

Toda, T., Segawa, M., Nomura, Y., Nonaka, I., Musuda, K., Ishihara, T., Sakai, M., Tomita, I., Origuchi, Y. & Suzuki, M. (1993): Localization of a gene for Fukuyama–type congenital muscular dystrophy to chromosome 9q 31–33. *Nat. Genet.* **5**, 283–286. [published erratum appears in *Nat. Genet.* (1994) **7**, 113.]

Toda, T., Yoshioka, M., Nakahori, Y., Kanazawa, I., Nakamura, Y. & Nakagome, Y. (1995): Genetic identity of Fukuyama-type congenital muscular dystrophy and Walker–Warburg syndrome. *Ann. Neurol.* **37**, 99–101.

Towfighi, J., Marks, K., Palmer, E. & Vannucci, R. (1979): Mobins syndrome. Neuropathologic observations. *Acta Neuropathol. (Berl.)* **48**, 11–17.

Towfighi, J. & Hausman, C. (1991): Spinal cord abnormalities in caudal regression syndrome. *Acta Neuropathol.* **81**, 458–466.

Trofatter, J.A., MacCollin, M.M., Rutter, J.L., Murrell, J.R., Duyao, M.P., Parry, D.M., Eldridge, R., Kley, N., Menon, A.G., Pulaski, K. *et al.* (1993): A novel moesin-, ezrin-, radixin-like gene is a candidate for the neurofibromatosis 2 tumor suppressor. *Cell* **72**, 791–800. [published erratum appears in *Cell* **75**, 826.]

Trounce, J.Q., Rutter, N. & Mellor, D.H. (1991): Hemimegalencephaly: diagnosis and treatment. *Dev. Med. Child. Neurol.* **33**, 261–266.

Truhan, A.P. & Filipek, P.A. (1993): Magnetic resonance imaging. Its role in neuroradiologic evaluation of neurofibromatosis, tuberous sclerosis, and Sturge–Weber syndrome. *Arch. Dermatol.* **129**, 219–226.

Trumble, E.R., Myseros, J.S., Smoker, W.R.K., Ward, J.D. & Mickell, J.J. (1994): Atlantooccipital subluxation in a neonate with Down's syndrome. Case report and review of the literature. *Pediatr. Neurosurg.* **21**, 55–58.

Turner, G. & Jacobs, P. (1983): Marker (X)-linked mental retardation. *Adv. Hum. Genet.* **13**, 83–112.

Twining, P., Zuccollo, J., Clewes, J. & Swallow, J. (1991): Fetal choroid plexus cysts: a prospective study and review of the literature. *Br. J. Radiol.* **64**, 98–102.

Unterharnscheidt, F., Jachnik, D. & Gott, H. (1968): Der Balkenmangel. Bericht uber Klink, Pathomorphologie und pathophysiologie der bisher mitgeteilten sowie won 33 eigenen Fallen von Balkenmangel und ihre differential diagnostische Abgrenzung. *Monogr. Gesamtgeb. Neurol. Psychiatr.* **128**, 1–232.

Urich, H. (1976): Malformations of the nervous system, perinatal damage and related conditions in early life. In: *Greenfield's neuropathology*, 3rd edn., eds. W. Blackwood & Jan Corsellis, pp. 362–469. London: Edward Arnold.

Van Allen, M.I. & Myhre, S. (1985): Ectopia cordis thoracalis with craniofacial defects resulting from early amnion rupture. *Teratology* **32**, 19–24.

van Bogaert, L. (1949): Les dysplasies a tendence blastomatense. In: *Traite de médicine*, vol. 16, pub. sous la direction de A. Lemierre [*et al.*], pp. 77–116. Masson: Paris.

van Bogaert, L. & Radermecker, M.A. (1955): Une dysgenesie cerebelleuse chez un enfant du radium. *Rev. Neurol.* **93**, 65–82.

van Bogaert, L. (1961): Neuropathologie generale des phacomatoses et de quelque dystrophie neuro-cutannees moins bien connnes chez l'enfant. *18 Congres de l'Association des Pediatres de Languefrancaise*, Geneve, vol. 2. pp. 349–386. Bale-New York: S Karger.

van Tuinen, P., Dobyns, W.B., Rich, D.C., Robinson, J.J. & Ledbetter, D.H. (1988): Frequent submicroscopic delections are detected DNA probes in Miller–Dieker syndrome but not in isolated lissencephaly syndrome. *Am. J. Hum. Genet.* **43**, A98. (Abstract)

Variend, S. & Emery, J.L. (1974): The pathology of the central lobes of the cerebellum in children with myelomeningocele. *Dev. Med. Child. Neurol.* **16** (suppl. 32), 99–106.

Verkerk, A.J.M.H., Pieretti, M., Sutcliffe, J.S., Fu, Y.H., Kuhl, D.P.A., Pizzuti, A., Reiner, O. *et al.* (1991): identification of a gene (FMR–1) containing a CGG repeat coincident with a breakpoint cluster region exhibiting length variation in fragile X syndrome. *Cell* **65**, 905–914.

Vigevano, F., Bertini, E., Boldrini, R., Bosman, C., Claps, D., di Capua, M., di Rocco, C. & Rossi, G.F. (1989): Hemimegalencephaly and intractable epilepsy: benefits of hemispherectomy. *Epilepsia* **30**, 833–843.

Vincent, C., Kalatzis, V., Compain, S., Levilliers, J., Slim, R., Graia, F., Pereira, M.L., Nivelon, A., Croquette, M.F., Lacombe, D. *et al.* (1994): A proposed new contiguous gene syndrome on 8q consists of branchio-oto-renal (BOR) syndrome, Duane syndrome, a dominant form of hydrocephalus and trapeze aplasia; implications for the mapping of the BOR gene. *Hum. Mol. Genet.* **3**, 1859–1866.

Vinters, H.V. (1995): Vascular diseases. In: *Pediatric neuropathology*, ed. S. Duckett, pp. 302–333. Baltimore: Williams and Wilkins.

Vogt, H. & Astwaraturow, M. (1912): Ueber angeborene Kleinhirnerkrankungen mit Beitragen zur Entwicklungs geschichte des Kleinhirns. *Arch. Psychiatr. Nervenkrankheit.* **49**, 175–203.

Volpe, J.J. & Adams, R.D. (1972): Cerebro-hepato-renal syndrome of Zellweger: an inherited disorder of neuronal migration. *Acta Neuropathol. (Berl.)* **20**, 175–198.

von Recklinghausen, F. (1886): Untersuchungen uber die spina bifida. II. Uber die art und die Entstchung der Spina Bifida ihre Beziehung zur Ruckenmarks und Dermsplatte. *Virchows. Arch. fur Pathol. u Anat.* **105**, 296–330.

Wald, N.J. (1994): Folic acid and neural tube defects: the current evidence and implications for prevention. Ciba Found. Symp. 181, pp. 192–208.

Walker, A.E. (1942): Lissencephaly. *Arch. Neurol. Psychiatry* **48**, 13–29.

Wallace, M.R., Marchuk, D.A., Andersen, L.B., Letcher, R., Odeh, H.M., Saulino, A.M., Fountain, J.W., Brereton, A., Nicholson, J., Mitchell, A.L. *et al.* (1990): Type 1 neurofibromatosis gene: identification of a large transcript disrupted in three NF1 patients. [published erratum appears in *Science* 1990, **250**, 1749.] *Science* **249**, 181–186.

Warburg, M. (1987): Ocular malformations and lissencephaly. *Eur. J. .Pediatr.* **146**, 450–452.

Warkany, J. (1971): Congenital malformations, pp. 176–190. Chicago: Year Book Medical Publishers.

Warkany, J. (1977): Morphogenesis of spina bifida. In: *Myelomeningocele*, ed. R.L. McLaurin, pp. 31–39. New York: Grune & Stratton.

Warkany, J. & Dignan, P.S.J. (1973): Congenital malformations: microcephaly. *Mental Retard Dev. Disabil.* **5**, 113–135.

Warkany, J. & Bofinger, M. (1975): Le role de coumadine dans les malformations congenitales. *Med. Hyg.* **33**, 1454–1457.

Warkany, J. & Lemire, R.J. (1984): Arteriovenous malformations of the brain: a teratologic challenge. *Teratology* **29**, 333–353.

Waterson, J.R., DiPietro, M.A. & Barr, M. (1985): Apert syndrome with frontonasal encephalocele. *Am. J. Med. Genet.* **21**, 777–783.

Weller, R.O. & Shulman, K. (1972): Infantile hydrocephalus: clinical, histological, and ultrastructural study of brain damage. *J. Neurosurg.* **36**, 255–265.

Whiting, D.M., Chou, S.M., Lanzieri, C.F., Kalfas, I.H. & Hardy, R.W. (1991): Cervical neurenteric cyst associated with Klippel–Feil syndrome: a case report and review of the literature. *Clin. Neuropathol.* **10**, 285–290.

Wiese, G.M., Kempe, L.G. & Hammon, W.M. (1972): Transsphenoidal meningohydroencephalocele. Case report. *J. Neurosurg.* **37**, 475–478.

Wiggins, R.C. (1982): Myelin development and nutritional insufficiency. *Brain Res. Rev.* **4**, 151–175.

Willis, R.A. (1958): The borderland of embryology and pathology. London: Butterworth.

Williams, R.S., Ferrante, R.J. & Caviness, V.S. Jr. (1976): The cellular pathology of microgyria. A Golgi analysis. *Acta Neuropathol. (Berl.)* **36**, 269–283.

Williams, B. & Fahy, G. (1983): A critical appraisal of 'terminal ventriculostomy' for the treatment of syringomyelia. *J. Neurosurg.* **58**, 188–197.

Williams, R.S., Swisher, C.N., Jennings, M., Ambler, M. & Caviness, V.S. Jr. (1984): Cerebro-ocular dysgenesis (WalkerBWarburg syndrome): neuropathologic and etiologic analysis. *Neurology* **34**, 1531–1541.

Wilson, P.W., Easley, R.B., Bolander, F.F. & Hammond, C.B. (1978): Evidence for a hypothalamic defect in septo-optic dysplasia. *Arch. Intern. Med.* **138**, 1276–1277.

Wiśniewski, K.E., French, J.H., Rosen, J.F., Kozłowski, P.B., Tenner, M. & Wiśniewski, H.M. (1982): Basal ganglia calcification (BGC) in Down's syndrome (DS) B Another manifestation of premature aging. *Ann. N.Y. Acad. Sci.* **396**, 179–189.

Wiśniewski, K., Dąmbska, M., Sher, J.H. & Qazi, Q. (1983): A clinical neuropathological study of the fetal alcohol syndrome. *Neuropediatrics* **14**, 197–201.

Wiśniewski, K.E., Laure-Kamionowska, M. & Wiśniewski, H.M. (1984): Evidence of arrest of neurogenesis and synaptogenesis in brains of patients with Down's syndrome. *N. Engl. J. Med.* **311**, 1187–1188. [letter]

Wiśniewski, K.E., Dalton, A.J., McLachlan, C., Wen, G.Y. & Wiśniewski, H.M. (1985a): Alzheimer disease in Down syndrome: clinico-pathological studies. *Neurology* **35**, 957–961.

Wiśniewski, K.E., Wiśniewski, H.M. & Wen, G.Y. (1985b): Occurrence of neuropathological changes and dementia of Alzheimer's disease in Down's syndrome. *Ann. Neurol.* **17**, 278–282.

Wiśniewski, K.E., French, J.H., Fernando, S., Brown, W.T., Jenkins, E.C., Friedman, E., Hill, A.L. & Miezejeski, C.M. (1985c): Fragile X syndrome: associated neurological abnormalities and developmental disabilities. *Ann. Neurol.* **18**, 665–669.

Wiśniewski, K.E., Laure-Kamionowska, M., Connell, F. & Wen, G.Y. (1986): The neuronal density and synaptogenesis in the postnatal stage of brain maturation in Down syndrome. In: *The neurobiology of Down Syndrome*, ed. C.J. Epstein, pp. 29–44. New York: Raven Press.

Wiśniewski, K.E. & Schmidt-Sidor, B. (1989): Postnatal delay of myelin formation in brains from Down syndrome infants and children. *Clin. Neuropathol.* **8**, 55–62.

Wiśniewski, K.E. (1990): Down syndrome children often have brain with maturation delay, retardation of growth, and cortical dysgenesis. *Am. J. Med. Genet. Suppl.* **7**, 274–281.

Wiśniewski, K.E. & Dąmbska, M. (1992): Development and aging in Down's syndrome. In: *Neurodevelopment, aging, and cognition*, eds. I. Kostovic, S. Knezevic, H.M. Wiśniewski & G.J. Spilich, pp. 141–156. Boston: Birkhauser.

Wiśniewski, K.E. & Jeret, J.S. (1994): Callosal agenesis: review of clinical, pathological and cytogenetic features. In: *Callosal agenesis*, eds. M. Lassonde & M.A. Jeeves, pp. 1–6. New York: Plenum Press.

Wiśniewski, K.E. & Kida, E. (1994): Abnormal neurogenesis and synaptogenesis in Down syndrome brain. OASI International for Research on Mental Retardation & Brain Aging, Troina, Italy. *Dev. Brain. Dysfunct.* **7**, 289–301.

Wiśniewski, H.M., Węgiel, J. & Popovitch, E.R. (1994): Age associated development of diffuse and thioflavin-S-positive plaques in Down syndrome. *Dev. Brain Dysfunct.* **7**, 330–339.

Wiśniewski, T., Golabek, A.A., Kida, E., Wiśniewski, K.E. & Frangione, B. (1995): Conformational mimicry in Alzheimer's disease. Role of apolipoproteins in amyloidogenesis. *Am. J. Pathol.* **147**, 238–244.

Wiśniewski, K.E. & Kida, E. (1995): Prenatal and early postnatal abnormalities of Down syndrome brain development and maturation. *Ann. Neurol.* **38**, 536. (Abstract)

Wood, J.W., Johnson, K.G. & Omari, Y. (1967): In utero exposure to the Hiroshima atomic bomb. An evaluation of head size and mental retardation: twenty years later. *Pediatrics* **39**, 385–392.

Wood, R.L. & Smith, M.T. (1984): Generation of anencephaly. 1. Aberrant neurulation and 2. conversion of exencephaly to anencephaly. *J. Neuropathol. Exp. Neurol.* **43**, 620–633.

Woody, R.C., Perrot, L.J. & Beck, S.A. (1992): Neurofibromatosis cerebral vasculopathy in an infant: clinical, neuroradiographic, and neuropathologic studies. *Pediatr. Pathol.* **12**, 613–619.

Yakovlev, P.I. (1959): Pathoarchitectonic studies of the cerebral malformations. III. Arhinencephalies (holotelencephalies). *J. Neuropathol. Exp. Neurol.* **18**, 22–55.

Yakovlev, P.I. & Wadsworth, R.C. (1946a): Schizencephalies. A study of the congenital clefts in the cerebral mantle. I. Clefts with fused lips. *J. Neuropathol. Exp. Neurol.* **5**, 116–130.

Yakovlev, P.I. & Wadsworth, R.C. (1946b): Schizencephalies. A study of the congenital clefts in the cerebral mantle. II. Clefts with hydrocephalus and clefts separated. *J. Neuropathol. Exp. Neurol.* **5**, 169–206.

Yakovlev, P.J. & Rakic, P. (1966): Patterns of decussation of bulbar pyramids and distribution of pyramidal tracts on two sides of the spinal cord. *Trans. Am. Neurol. Assoc.* **91**, 366–367.

Yamazaki, J.N. (1966): A review of the literature on the radiation dosage required to cause manifest central nervous system disturbances from in utero and postnatal exposure. *Pediatrics* **37** (suppl 37), 877–903.

Zaremba, J., Wislawski, J., Bidzinski, J., Kansy, J. & Sidor, B. (1978): Jadassohn's nevus phakomatosis: I. A report of two cases. *J. Ment. Defic. Res.* **22**, 91–102.

Zhong, N., Yang, W., Dobkin, C. & Brown, W.T. (1995): Fragile X gene instability: Anchoring AGGs and linked microsatellites. *Am. J. Hum. Genet.* **57**, 351–361.

Zülch, K.J. (1958): Die Hirngeschwülste in biologischer und morphologischer Darstellung, 3rd ed. Leipzig: Barth.

Index

A

abnormal central nervous system (CNS) development
  etiology factors of 89–92
  genetic causes 89–90
  exogenous factors 90
acrocallosal syndrome 116
agyria/lissencephaly type I 119
  cerebro-cerebellar syndrome 122
  four layered 119
  uni layered 120
  Miller–Dieker syndrome 121
  Norman–Roberts syndrome 121
Aicardi syndrome 116, 126, 131
Ammon's horn development 43
amygdaloid complex, development 39
Anderman syndrome 116
anencephaly 103
angiogenesis 22
angiomatosis cerebrofacialis (Sturge–Weber disease) 97
anomalies
  brain stem 142–143
  dysraphic and related spinal cord 108–111
  focal cortical development 129–131
  meningeal 148
  skull bone 147–148
  spinal cord 108–111, 142–143
  vascular 146–147
  see also cerebellum; cortical malformations; developoment; malformations
anterior perforate substance 42
Apert syndrome 116
aplasia of the cerebellar vermis 133
apoptosis 9
  see cell death
aprosencephaly/atelencephaly 117–118
aqueduct formation 32
arachnoid cysts 148
archicortex 43, 46
  hippocampal complex 43
area cerebro vasculosa 104
arhinencephaly 113–115
arthrogryposis neurogenic form 143
astrocyte 11–13
  generation 3
axon growth 8

B

blood–brain barrier 66–68
Bourneville disease (tuberous sclerosis) 94–95
brain stem 29–32
  development 29–31

dysplasia	142	fragile X syndrome	152
Moebius syndrome	142	claustrum	57
brain warts	130	cortex cerebral	39

C

carnegie stages	23, 24
caudal eminence	26
cavum septi interpositi	59
cavum septi pellucidi	59
cell death programmed	9
central nervous system maturation delay	157–158
cerebellar	
agenesis, aplasia	132, 133
cortex malformations	136–139
cortical dysplasia	137
hypoplasia	135
cortical diffuse hypertrophy (Lhermitte–Duclos)	138
malformations	132–136
cerebellum: primitive and secondary	
development abnormalities	132–139
Joubert syndrome	135
rhombencephalosynapsis	135–136
tectocerebellar dysraphia	135
see also cerebellar apalasia and hypoplasia	
cerebrohepatorenal syndrome of Zellweger	131
cerebrospinal fluid	58–60
Chiari (Arnold–Chiari) malformation	106–108
spinal cord anomalies	107
type I	106
type II	107
types III and IV	106
choroid plexus	58–60
chromosomal aberration	89, 149
abnormal number	89
abnormal structure	89, 90
trisomy 13 (Patau syndrome)	149
trisomy 18 (Edward's syndrome)	150
trisomy 21 (Down syndrome)	150–152

development (*see*: migration – 47)	39–57
superficial accesory layer	52
regional development	53
gyri development	55, 56
see also: cortical dysplasia, malformation, hemimegalencephaly, lissencephaly I, II, pachygyria	
commissural system, developmental anomalies of	115–117
communicating	144–146
corpus callosum	64
agenesis	115
development	46, 59
with dysgenetic syndromes	116
see forebrain commissures	
cortical developmental, anomalies	129–131
early-occurring dysplasia	118
and phakomatoses	119
laminar and focal anomalies	129–131
particular or complex cortical anomalies	131–132
polymicrogyria	123–126
subcortical heterotopia	122–123
cortical malformations and dysplasia	118–132
disorganized cortical structure lissencephaly type II	127–129
cortical stripe maturation	51–56
regional development	53–56
craniolacuniae	148
in Chiari malformation	107
craniosynostosis	148
craniorachischisis	103
cranium bifidum	105
cystic encephalopathy	156

D

Dandy–Walker malformation	132 – 134

delay of the CNS maturation	157	exogenous factors	90–91
dendrytes	8	external glanular layer (Obersteiner)	136
developing brain damage, correlations between time and type	91–92	eyes, development	39
developmental age	70		
developmental anomalies commissural system	115–117	**F**	
		floor plate	17
diastomatomyelia	110	focal cortical developmental anomalies	129–131
diencephalon development	24–28, 36–39	forebrain, see prosencephalon	35 – 60
diencephalic structures	36–39	forebrain commissures	59
epithalamus	38	formation aqueduct	32
hypothalamus	37	fornix, development	46
subthalamus	37–38	fragile X syndrome	152
diplomyelia	110	Fukuyama syndrome congenital muscular dystrophy (FCMI)	129
dorsal thalamus development	38–39		
Down syndrome (trisomy 21)	150–152		
dysplasia see cortical malformations and anomalies	118–132	**G**	
		Galloway–Movat syndrome	132
dsysplastic gangliocytoma of the cerebellum (Lhermitte–Dulcos disease)	98–99	gene mutation	90
		gene factors	89–90, 140
		germinal cells	3
dysraphic cerebral changes	103–106	glial pial barrier	49, 127
related spinal cord anomalies	108–111	glio neuronal heterotopias	127, 130, 131
syndromes, see neural tube defects	101–113	globus pallidus development	57–58
E		**H**	
Edward syndrome (trisomy 18)	150	HARD E syndrome	128
encephalocele	105	hemimegalencephaly	96, 98
occipital	105	heterotopias	121–123
anterior	105	cerebellar	137
midline	106	double cortex	123
in Menckel Gruber syndrome	106	laminar	122
in Joubert syndrome	106	nodular	123
Walker–Warburg syndrome	106	subcortical	122
With fronto nasal dysplasia	106	holoacrania	104
Apert syndrome	106	holoprosencephaly (HPE)	113
environmental factors	140–141	alobar	113
ependymal cells differentiation	17–18	lobar	114
epithalamus development	38	in Meckel–Gruber syndrome	115
etiologic factors	89–92	semilobar	114
exencephaly	104		

hydranencephaly	154	malformations	
hydrocephalus	143–146	brain stem and spinal cord anomalies	142–143
communicating	144	cerebellum: primitive and secondary developmental abnormalities	132–139
non communicating	144	of the CNS	101–148
hydromyelia	109	hydrocephalus	143–146
hypophysis	39	megalencephaly	141–142
hypoplasia of the cerebellum	132–136	meningeal anomalies	148
hypothalamus, development	37	micrencephaly caused by genetic factors	140
I		midline malformations	113–118
inheritance	140	neural tube defects (dysraphic syndromes)	101–113
iniencephaly	104	skull bone anomalies	147–148
insular cortex development	56	vascular anomalies	146–147
isthmus	30	*see also* cortical malformations	118–132
J		Mecker–Gruber syndrome	106
Jadassohn linear nevus	98	meninges development	68
Joubert syndrome	135	meningocele	108
K		meningocystocele	108
Klippel–Feil anomaly	112	meningomyelocele	108
L		Menkes syndrome	116
lamina terminalis	25, 26, 35	meroacrania	104
laminar cortical developmental anomalies	129–131	mesencephalon development	24–28
late developmental anomalies	153–156	metencephalon development	24–28
cystic encephalopathy, variants of	156	micrencephaly	139–141
hydraencephaly	153–156	autosomal inheritance	140
schizencephaly and porencephaly	154–156	chromosomal abnormalities	141
Lhermitte–Duclos disease dysplastic gangliocytoma of cerebellum	98, 138	environmental factors	140
Cowden-disease	99	microglia	18–22
lissencephaly type II disorganized cortical structure	127	origin	19
in Walker–Warburg syndrome	128	midline structures, anomalies	117
in Fukuyama distrophy	129	migration	4
in HARD E syndrome	128	of neuroblasts	47
		Moebius syndrome (congenital facio ofthalmoplegia)	142
		muscle-eye-brain disease of Santavouri	129
		myelination	10, 14–16, 60, 64
		glia	13
M		**N**	
macrophages	20–21	neocortex	39, 47

Index

nerve tissue 1–18
   ependymal cells 17–18
   neuroglia 10–17
   neurons and neuronal development 1–10
Neu–Laxova syndrome 132
neural crest, origine 25
neural groove 24
neural plate 24
neural tube development 25, 102
   defects 101
neurocutaneous melanosis 98
neuroenteric cyst 112
neuroepithelium 3
neurofibromatosis 95–97
   NF 1 = von Recklinghausen disease 96
   NF 2 B – the central form 96
neuroglia 10–17
   astroglia 11–13
   development 10
   oligodendroglia and myelin sheaths formations 13–17
   radial 4, 10, 47
neuromesodermal syndromes, see phakomatoses 93–99
neuron
   generation 3
   migration 4, 47
   neuronal death 9, 52
neuronal induction 23
neuromeres 26
neuropores 25, 26
neurulation
   primary 27
   secondary 27

O

olfactory bulb
   development 42
   aplasia 113
oligodendrocyte 3, 13
   generation 13
oligodendroglia 13–17

P

pachygyria 119 – 120
paleocortex 39, 40
pallium 39–43
   gyrification 56
parasubiculum 46
periamygdaloid cortex 42
periarchicortex 46 – 47
periventricular matrix 47–50
phakomatoses – neuromesodermal syndromes 93 – 99
   hemimegalencephaly 98
   Jadassohn linear nevus 98
   Lhermitte–Dulcos disease (dysplasstic gangliocytoma of the cerebellum) 98–99
   neurocutaneous melanosis 98
   Sturge–Weber disease (angiomatosis cerebrofacialis) 97
   tuberous sclerosis (Bourneville disease) 94–95
   von Hippel–Lindau disease 97
polymicrogyria (PMG) 123–126
   adrenoleukodystrophy 126
   in Aicardi syndrome 126
   four layered 124
   in Meckel syndrome 126
   unilayered 123
porencephaly 154–155
presubiculum 46
proliferative vasculopathy 132
prosencephalon (forebrain) 35–60
   development 35
   lateral eminence 36
   medial eminence 36

R

rhombencephalon 24
rhombencephalosynapsis 135–136
rhombic lip 31–33

S

sacral agenesis 112

schizencephaly	154–155
septo-optic dysplasia (De Morsier syndrome)	117
Shapiro syndrome	116
skull bones	66–70
anomalies	147
craniosynostosis	148
spina bifida	108
combined anterior and posterior	112
spinal cord	28–29, 61
brain stem (except for cerebellar pathways)	61
development	28–29
spinal dysraphism	108
spinal dysraphism occult	102, 112
spinal dermal sinus	112
Sturge–Weber disease	97
subcortical heterotopia	122–123
laminar	122
nodular	123
subpial layer	52
subplate zone	49, 54, 55
subthalamus development	37
superficial layer of Ranke	52
synaps	
elimination	53
synaptogenesis	8–9, 52
syringomyelia	109
in Chiari malformation	107
in NF	96

T

tectocerebellar dysraphia	135
telencephalic structures	39–57
archicortex (hippocampal complex)	43–46
cortical stripe maturation	51–56
insular cortex	56–57
pallium	39–43
periarchicortex	46–47
rotation	44
teratogens	90
tethered cord syndrome	112
thalamus	
dorsal	38–39
ventral	37–38
trisomy 13 (Patau syndrome)	149–150
trisomy 18 (Edwards syndrome)	150
trisomy 21 (Down dyndrome)	150–152
tuberous sclerosis	94–95

V

vascular anomalies	146–147
arteriovenous malformations	146
fetal meningeal vessels	146
neonatal angiomata	148
Sturge–Weber disease	97
teleangiectasia	148
vascularization	64–68
blood brain barrier development	66–68
vasculogenesis	22
ventral thalamus, development	37–38
ventricles, development	30, 57–59
vessels	22
origin	22
vascularization of the CNS	64–66
see also anomalies	
von Hippel–Lindau disease	97
von Recklinghausen disease (peripheral form)	96

W

Walker–Warburg syndrome	106, 128

Z

Zellweger syndrome	131